Calculating Medication Dosages

Formula 1

$$\frac{\text{dose ordered (desired)}}{\text{dose on hand (have)}} \times \text{amount available (quantity)} = \text{amount to give}$$

Formula 2 (ratio and proportion)

$$\frac{\text{dose ordered}}{\text{dose on hand}} = \frac{x}{\text{quantity available}}$$

Formula 3 (dimensional analysis)

Rule 1: Multiplying one side of an equation by a conversion factor will not change the value of the equation.

Rule 2: Set up the problem so that all labels cancel from the numerator and denominator except the label desired in the answer.

Calculating IV Drip Rates

$$\frac{\text{volume (of fluid)}}{\text{time (in minutes)}} \times \text{drop factor} = \text{flow rate}$$

Critical Points in Measuring Vital Signs

Temperature	To convert Fahrenheit to centigrade: (degrees in F − 32) X $\frac{5}{9}$. To convert centigrade to Fahrenheit: (degrees in C X $\frac{9}{5}$) + 32. Ensure no eating or drinking within last 20 minutes for oral temp. to avoid errors. Follow manufacturer directions if electronic measuring devices used. Wear gloves and use lubricating gel if taking a rectal temperature.
Heart rate	Measure apical rate for 1 full minute at apex (5th intercostal space [ICS], mid-clavicular line [MCL]). Measure radial rate for 30 seconds and multiply by 2 if heart rate regular; if irregular, measure for one full minute and take an apical rate as well.
Respiratory rate	Measure respiratory rate for one minute; note pattern also; try to be unobtrusive because rate can change if client is nervous or self-conscious; also take note of any oxygen therapy the client is receiving.
Blood pressure	Measure in both arms initially to determine differences between sides. Measure orthostatic blood pressures in lying, sitting, and standing positions. Have arm resting at heart level and use a proper size cuff (cuff width = $\frac{2}{3}$ length of client's upper arm). Ensure no smoking in last 15-20 minutes to avoid false high readings. Wait at least 1-2 minutes or more between repeat readings to avoid false highs. Compare readings obtained from electronic measuring device with that obtained using a sphygmomanometer each shift or per agency policy.
Oxygen saturation	Keep pulse oximeter unit plugged into electrical outlet when not in use. Put probe on digit/earlobe with adequate circulation to avoid false low readings. Consider measuring O_2 sat whenever client has a lung disorder or otherwise compromised respiratory status.

ISBN-13: 978-0-13-224078-9
ISBN-10: 0-13-224078-5

Prentice Hall

Areas to Auscultate Heart Sounds

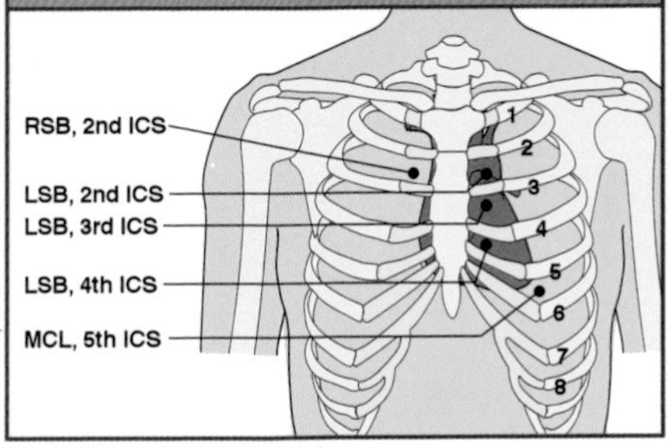
RSB, 2nd ICS
LSB, 2nd ICS
LSB, 3rd ICS
LSB, 4th ICS
MCL, 5th ICS
1
2
3
4
5
6
7
8

Sequence for Auscultating Lungs

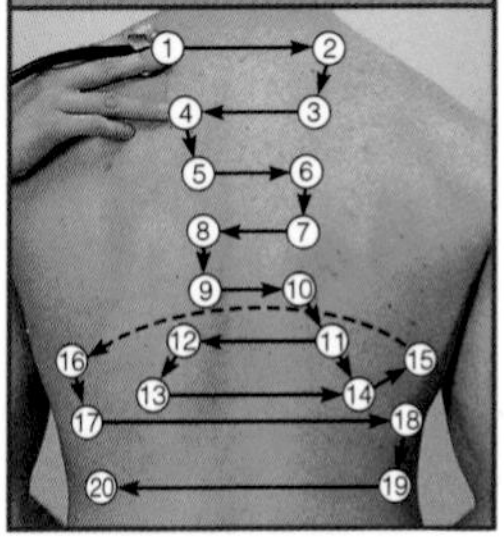
1
2
3
4
5
6
7
8
9
10
11
12
13
14
15
16
17
18
19
20

Adult Reference Ranges for Common Laboratory Tests

Coagulation Studies	*Prothrombin time (PT):* 10-13 seconds; 1.5-2.0 times the control in seconds for anticoagulant therapy *Activated partial thromboplastin time (APTT):* 20-35 seconds (1.5-2.5 times the control in anticoagulant therapy) *Partial thromboplastin time (PTT):* 60-70 seconds; 1.5-2.5 times the control in anticoagulant therapy *International normalized ratio (INR):* 2.0-3.0 for most anticoagulation needs
Electrolytes	*Sodium (Na^+):* 135-145 mEq/L; *Potassium (K^+):* 3.5-5.1 mEq/L *Chloride (Cl^-):* 95-105 mEq/L *CO_2 combining power:* 22-30 mEq/L; 22-30 mmol/L *Calcium, total (Ca^{++}):* 4.5-5.5 mEq/L, 9-11 mg/dL, 2.3-2.8 mmol/L *Calcium (ionized):* 4.25-5.25 mg/dL, 2.2-2.5 mEq/L, 1.1-1.24 mmol/L *Magnesium (Mg^{++}):* 1.5-2.5 mEq/L, 1.8-3.0 mg/dL
Glucose	*Fasting (FBS):* 70-110 mg/dL (serum, plasma); 60-100 mg/dL (whole blood); 70-120 mg/dL (elderly); panic values: < 40 or > 700 mg/dL *Fingerstick glucose (self-monitoring device):* 60-100 mg/dL
Hematology	*White blood cells (WBC):* 5,000-10,000 mm^3 or 4,500-11,500/mm^3 *Neutrophils:* 1,935-7,942 (absolute count) or 45-75% *Red blood cells (RBC):* 4.5-5.3 million or (10^6)/mm^3 (men), 4.1-5.1 million or (10^6)/mm^3 (women) *Hemoglobin (Hgb):* 13.0-18.0 grams/100mL (men), 12-16 grams/100mL (women) *Hematocrit (Hct):* 37-49 % (men), 36-46 % (women) *Platelet count:* 150,000-400,000/mm^3
Renal Function Studies	*Blood urea nitrogen (BUN):* 5-25 mg/dL *Serum creatinine:* 0.5-1.5 mg/dL
Therapeutic Drug Levels	*Digoxin (Lanoxin):* 0.5-2.0 ng/mL; *Phenytoin (Dilantin):* 10-20 mcg/mL *Theophylline derivatives:* 10-20 mcg/mL

Therapeutic Communication Techniques

Listening	Maintain eye contact and have open, receptive body posture
Broad Opening	"What would you like to talk about today?" "What brought you to the hospital?"
Restating	"You say the doctor told you that you will need surgery?" "What I hear you saying is…"
Clarification	"I'm not sure what you mean. Could you tell me again?"
Reflection	"You're feeling anxious and upset, and it's related to the conversation you just had with the cardiologist?"
Focusing	"Let's focus more on your relationship with your mother."
Sharing perceptions	"You look upset, but you are saying you don't mind that discharge from the hospital has been delayed."
Identifying themes	"I've noticed that in all the relationships you describe, you've been hurt by your partner. Do you think this is an underlying issue?"
Silence	Sitting with a client or group of clients and nonverbally communicating interest and presence

Center for Disease Control (CDC) Precautions

Tier 1: Standard Precautions (use for all clients)

Handwashing	Wash hands before contact with each client, during care as needed (even if wearing gloves) to prevent cross-contamination of body sites, and after touching blood, body fluids, secretions, excretions, and contaminated items (with or without gloves).
	Use a plain (nonantimicrobial) soap for routine handwashing; use an antimicrobial agent or a waterless antiseptic agent as per agency policy.
Gloves	Wear gloves (clean, nonsterile adequate) whenever contact is expected with blood, body fluids, secretions, excretions, mucous membranes and nonintact skin, and contaminated items.
	Always change gloves between clients and between tasks and procedures on the same client after contact with material that may contain a high concentration of microorganisms.
	Remove gloves promptly after use, before touching noncontaminated items and environmental surfaces, and before going to another client; wash hands.
Face protection (mask, goggles, face shield)	Wear a face shield, or wear goggles and a mask that covers both the nose and the mouth during procedures and client care activities that are likely to generate splashes or sprays of blood, body fluids, secretions, or excretions to provide protection of the mucous membranes of the eyes, nose, and mouth.
Gowns and other protective apparel	Wear a gown to prevent contamination of clothing and skin from blood and body fluid exposures.
	Gowns specially treated to make them impermeable to liquids and leg/shoe covers provide greater skin protection when splashes or large quantities of infective material are present or anticipated.
	Remove soiled gown as soon as possible, and wash hands to avoid transfer of microorganisms.
Others	Clean and reprocess reusable equipment before using it on another client.
	Follow agency procedure for routine cleaning and disinfection of surfaces and for handling spills of blood and body fluids.
	Avoid contamination of self with soiled linen by folding contaminated areas to the inside, holding linen away from the body, and placing it directly into the laundry receptacle.
	Avoid recapping needles; use scoop technique if recapping is necessary; discard used syringes and needles immediately into a puncture-proof container while holding the needle pointed away from self; do not bend or break needles.

Tier 2: Transmission Based Precautions (use when indicated)

Airborne Precautions: Use when small (<5 μm) pathogen-infected droplet nuclei may remain suspended in air over time and travel distances greater than 3 feet *Examples: varicella, measles, tuberculosis*	Use Standard Precautions.
	Place client in private room or with a client with the same infection but no other infection (cohorting).
	If possible, use room equipped with negative pressure ventilation, outside venting, and 6-12 air exchanges per hour.
	Keep the door to the room closed.
	Wear a special approved particulate filter mask (N95) whenever entering room of all clients with tuberculosis or when staff or visitors not exposed to rubeola or varicella must enter room.
	Limit visitors and caretakers to those already immune if chicken pox (varicella) or measles are involved.
	Keep client in room; place surgical mask on client if transport is necessary.
	Follow additional agency guidelines for preventing transmission of tuberculosis.
Droplet Precautions: Use with large (>5 μm) pathogen-infected droplets that travel 3 feet or less via coughing, sneezing, etc. or during procedures (suctioning) *Examples: Haemophilus influenzae, Neisseria meningitides, others*	Use Standard Precautions.
	Place client in private room or with a client with the same infection but no other infection (cohorting).
	When private room or cohorting is unavailable, keep a distance of 3 feet or more between the infected client and other clients or visitors.
	Special ventilation is not necessary and the door may remain open.
	Wear a mask when working within 3 feet of the client or entering the room according to agency policy.
	Limit the transport of the client from the room and then mask the client, if possible.
	Additional recommendations for specific pathogens may also apply.
Contact Precautions: Use with known or suspected microorganisms transmitted by direct hand-to-skin client contact or indirect contact with surfaces or care items in the environment *Examples: Clostridium difficile, diphtheria (cutaneous), herpes simplex (mucocutaneous or neonatal), impetigo, pediculosis, scabies, zoster (disseminated, immunocompromised host), viral/hemorrhagic infections (Ebola, Lassa, Marburg), others*	Use Standard Precautions.
	Place client in private room or use cohorting; consult agency infectious disease department as needed.
	Wear gloves when entering the room; change gloves after contact with infective material; remove gloves before leaving room and wash hands immediately with antimicrobial agent or waterless antiseptic agent; then ensure that hands do not touch potentially contaminated room surfaces or items.
	Wear a clean, nonsterile gown when entering room if clothing may have substantial contact with client, environmental surfaces or items, or if client is incontinent, or has diarrhea, ileostomy, colostomy, or wound drainage not contained by a dressing; remove gown before leaving the room; then ensure that clothing does not contact potentially contaminated environmental surfaces.
	Limit to essential purposes client transport from room; if transport needed, maintain precautions to minimize the risk of pathogen transmission to other clients and environmental surfaces or equipment.
	When possible, dedicate the use of noncritical client-care equipment to a single client or cohort colonized with the same pathogen; if use of common equipment or items is unavoidable, adequately clean and disinfect them before use on another client.
	Additional recommendations for specific pathogens may also apply.

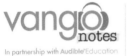
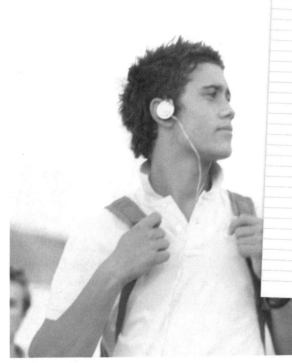

Prentice Hall Nursing Reviews & Rationales

Nursing Fundamentals

Second Edition

Series Editor
Mary Ann Hogan, MSN, RN

Clinical Assistant Professor
University of Massachusetts–Amherst
Amherst, Massachusetts

Consulting Editors
Sara Bolten, MSN, RN

Nursing Instructor
McKendree College
Louisville, Kentucky

Mary Jean Ricci, MSN, RN

Assistant Professor
Holy Family University
Bensalem, Pennsylvania

Donna Taliaferro, PhD

Associate Professor
University of Missouri–St. Louis
St. Louis, Missouri

PEARSON
Prentice Hall

Upper Saddle River, New Jersey 07458

Library of Congress Cataloging-in-Publication Data

Publisher: Julie Levin Alexander
Assistant to Publisher: Regina Bruno
Editor-in-Chief: Maura Connor
Editorial Assistants: Mary Ellen Ruitenberg and Marion Gottlieb
Developmental Editor: Danielle Doller
Managing Editor, Production: Patrick Walsh
Production Liaison: Anne Garcia
Production Editor: Jessica Balch, Pine Tree Composition
Manufacturing Manager: Ilene Sanford
Manufacturing Buyer: Pat Brown

Design Coordinator/Cover Designer: Mary Siener
Director of Marketing: Karen Allman
Senior Marketing Manager: Francisco Del Castillo
Marketing Coordinator: Michael Sirinides
Marketing Assistant: Anca David
Media Product Manager: John Jordan
New Media Project Manager: Stephen Hartner
Composition: Pine Tree Composition, Inc.
Printer/Binder: Courier Westford
Cover Printer: Phoenix Color Corp.

Pearson Education Ltd., *London*
Pearson Education Australia Pty. Limited, *Sydney*
Pearson Education Singapore, Pte. Ltd.
Pearson Education North Asia Ltd., *Hong Kong*
Pearson Education Canada, Ltd., *Toronto*

Pearson Educación de Mexico, S.A. de C.V.
Pearson Education—Japan, *Tokyo*
Pearson Education Malaysia, Pte. Ltd.
Pearson Education, Upper Saddle River, New Jersey

10   9   V013
ISBN-13: 978-0-13-224078-9
ISBN-10:   0-13-224078-5

Contents

Welcome to the Prentice Hall Nursing Reviews & Rationales Series!

This series has been specifically designed to provide a clear and concentrated review of important nursing knowledge in the following content areas:

- Anatomy & Physiology
- Nursing Fundamentals
- Nutrition & Diet Therapy
- Fluids, Electrolytes, & Acid-Base Balance
- Medical-Surgical Nursing
- Pathophysiology
- Pharmacology
- Maternal-Newborn Nursing
- Child Health Nursing
- Mental Health Nursing
- Physical Assessment
- Community Health Nursing
- Leadership & Management

The books in this series are designed for use either by current nursing students as a study aid for nursing course work, for NCLEX-RN® licensing exam preparation, or by practicing nurses seeking a comprehensive yet concise review of a nursing specialty or subject area.

This series is truly unique. One of its most special features is that it has been developed and reviewed by a large team of nurse educators from across the United States and Canada to ensure that each chapter is edited by a nurse expert in the content area under study. The series editor, Mary Ann Hogan, designed the overall series in collaboration with a core Prentice Hall team to take full advantage of Prentice Hall's cutting-edge technology. The consulting editors for each book, also experts in that specialty area, then reviewed all chapters and test questions submitted for comprehensiveness and accuracy. Finally, Mary Ann Hogan reviewed the chapters in each book for consistency, accuracy, and applicability to the NCLEX-RN® Test Plan.

All books in the series are identical in their overall design for your convenience. As an added value, each book comes with a comprehensive support package, including a bonus *NCLEX-RN® Test Prep* CD-ROM and a tear-out *NursingNotes* card for clinical reference and quick review.

Study Tips

Use of this book should help simplify your review. To make the most of your valuable study time, also follow these simple but important suggestions:

1. Use a weekly calendar to schedule study sessions.
   - Outline the timeframes for all of your activities (home, school, appointments, etc.) on a weekly calendar.
   - Find the "holes" in your calendar, which are the times in which you can plan to study. Add study sessions to the calendar at times when you can expect to be mentally alert and follow it!
2. Create the optimal study environment.
   - Eliminate external sources of distraction, such as television, telephone, etc.
   - Eliminate internal sources of distraction, such as hunger, thirst, or dwelling on items or problems that cannot be worked on at the moment.
   - Take a break for 10 minutes or so after each hour of concentrated study both as a reward and an incentive to keep studying.
3. Use pre-reading strategies to increase comprehension of chapter material.
   - Skim read the headings in the chapter (because they identify chapter content).
   - Read the definitions of key terms, which will help you learn new words to comprehend chapter information.

- Review all graphic aids (figures, tables, boxes) because they are often used to explain important points in the chapter.
4. Read the chapter thoroughly but at a reasonable speed.
   - Comprehension and retention are actually enhanced by not reading too slowly.
   - Do take the time to reread any section that is unclear to you.
5. Summarize what you have learned.
   - Use questions supplied with this book and the *NCLEX-RN® Test Prep* CD-ROM to test your application of chapter content.
   - Review again any sections that correspond to questions you answered incorrectly or incompletely.

Test-Taking Strategies

We added new test-taking strategies to the rationales for every question in the series. These strategies will enable you to select the correct answer by breaking down the question, even if you don't know the correct response. Use the following strategies to increase your success on nursing tests or examinations:

- Get sufficient sleep and have something to eat before taking a test. Take deep breaths during the test as needed. Remember, the brain requires oxygen and glucose as fuel. Avoid concentrated sweets before a test, however, to avoid rapid upward and then downward surges in blood glucose levels.
- Read the question carefully, identifying the stem, the 4 options, and any key words or phrases in either the stem or options.
  - Key words in the stem such as "most important" indicate the need to set priorities, since more than one option is likely to contain a statement that is technically correct.
  - Remember that the presence of absolute words such as "never" or "only" in an answer option is more likely to make that option incorrect.
- Determine who is the client in the question; often this is the person with the health problem, but it may also be a significant other, relative, friend, or another nurse.
- Decide whether the stem is a true response stem or a false response stem. With a true response stem, the correct answer will be a true statement, and vice-versa.

- Determine what the question is really asking, sometimes referred to as the issue of the question. Evaluate all answer options in relation to this issue, and not strictly to the "correctness" of the statement in each individual option.
- Eliminate options that are obviously incorrect, then go back and reread the stem. Evaluate the remaining options against the stem once more.
- If two answers seem similar and correct, try to decide whether one of them is more global or comprehensive. If the global option includes the alternative option within it, it is likely that the more global response is the correct answer.

The NCLEX-RN® Licensing Examination

The NCLEX-RN® licensing examination is a Computer Adaptive Test (CAT) that ranges in length from 75 to 265 individual (stand-alone) test items, depending on individual performance during the examination. Upon graduation from a nursing program, successful completion of this exam is the gateway to your professional nursing practice. The blueprint for the exam is reviewed and revised every three years by the National Council of State Boards of Nursing according to the results of a job analysis study of new graduate nurses practicing within the first six months after graduation. Each question on the exam is coded to a *Client Need Category* and an *Integrated Process*.

Client Need Categories. There are 4 categories of client needs, and each exam will contain a minimum and maximum percent of questions from each category. Each major category has subcategories within it. The *Client Needs* categories according to the NCLEX-RN® Test Plan effective April 2007 are as follows:

- Safe, Effective Care Environment
  - Management of Care (13–19%)
  - Safety and Infection Control (8–14%)
- Health Promotion and Maintenance (6–12%)
- Psychosocial Integrity (6–12%)
- Physiological Integrity
  - Basic Care and Comfort (6–12%)
  - Pharmacological and Parenteral Therapies (13–19%)
  - Reduction of Risk Potential (13–19%)
  - Physiological Adaptation (11–17%)

Integrated Processes. The integrated processes identified on the NCLEX-RN® Test Plan effective April 2007, with condensed definitions, are as follows:

- Nursing Process: a scientific problem-solving approach used in nursing practice; consisting of assessment, analysis, planning, implementation, and evaluation.
- Caring: client-nurse interaction(s) characterized by mutual respect and trust and that are directed toward achieving desired client outcomes.
- Communication and Documentation: verbal and/or nonverbal interactions between nurse and others (client, family, health care team); a written or electronic recording of activities or events that occur during client care.

- Teaching and Learning: facilitating client's acquisition of knowledge, skills, and attitudes that lead to behavior change

More detailed information about this examination may be obtained by visiting the National Council of State Boards of Nursing website at http://www.ncsbn.org and viewing the *NCLEX-RN® Examination Test Plan for the National Council Licensure Examination for Registered Nurses.*[1]

[1]Reference: National Council of State Boards of Nursing, Inc. *NCLEX Examination Test Plan for National Council Licensure Examination for Registered Nurses.* Effective April, 2007. Retrieved from the World Wide Web September 5, 2005 at http://www.ncsbn.org/RN_Test_Plan_2007_Web.pdf. Accessed January 16, 2007.

HOW TO GET THE MOST OUT OF THIS BOOK

Each chapter has the following elements to guide you during review and study:

Chapter Objectives describe what you will be able to know or do after learning the material covered in the chapter.

Objectives

➤ Discuss legal considerations related to maternity nursing.

➤ Delineate ethical issues that influence maternal-newborn nursing practice.

➤ Identify culturally diverse health beliefs that impact the maternity cycle.

➤ Describe a philosophy of care that maintains maternal–newborn safety and fosters family unity.

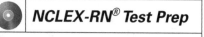

NCLEX-RN® Test Prep

Use the CD-ROM enclosed with this book to access additional practice opportunities.

Review at a Glance contains a glossary of key terms used in the chapter, with definitions provided up-front and available at your fingertips, to help you stay focused and make the best use of your study time.

Review at a Glance

belief something accepted as true, especially as a tenet or a body of tenets accepted by an ethnocultural group

cultural competency the awareness, knowledge and skills necessary to appreciate, understand and communicate with people of diverse cultural backgrounds

family a group of individuals related by blood, marriage, or mutual goals

family-centered maternity care maternity care that is family oriented and views childbirth as a vital, natural life event rather than an illness

scope of practice legally refers to permissible boundaries of practice for nurses and is defined by statute (written law), rules and regulations, or a combination of the two

Pretest provides a 10-question quiz as a sample overview of the material covered in the chapter and helps you decide in what areas you need the most—or the least—review.

PRETEST

1 The nurse performs a vaginal examination and determines that the fetus is in a sacrum anterior position. The nurse draws which conclusion from this assessment data?

1. The fetal sacrum is toward the maternal symphysis pubis.
2. The fetal sacrum is toward the maternal sacrum.
3. The fetal face is toward the maternal sacrum.
4. The fetal face is toward the maternal symphysis pubis.

Practice to Pass questions are open-ended, stimulate critical thinking, and reinforce mastery of the chapter information.

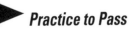

Practice to Pass

The client scheduled for a hysterosalpingogram reports an allergy to shellfish. What should the nurse do?

NCLEX Alert identifies concepts that are likely to be tested on the NCLEX-RN® examination. Be sure to learn the information highlighted wherever you see this icon.

Case Study, found at the end of the chapter, provides an opportunity for you to use your critical thinking and clinical reasoning skills to "put it all together." It describes a true-to-life client case situation and asks you open-ended questions about how you would provide care for that client and/or family.

Case Study

A 14-year-old primigravida is admitted in early labor with severe preeclampsia at 42 weeks gestation. The client's blood pressure is 168/102.

1. What other assessment data would you obtain?
2. Describe the complications this client is at risk for.
3. Discuss the medications you expect to administer to this client.
4. What concerns do you have for this fetus? Why?
5. What would you teach this client and her family about her condition?

For suggested responses, see page 343.

Posttest provides an additional 10-question quiz at the end of the chapter. It provides you with feedback about mastery of the chapter material following review and study. All pretest and posttest questions contain comprehensive rationales for the correct and incorrect answers, and are coded according to cognitive level of difficulty, NCLEX-RN® Test Plan category of client need and integrated process.

POSTTEST

1 A client who is a brittle diabetic is seeking to get pregnant. The nursing working in a primary care provider's office suggests that which of the following healthcare providers would be an optimal choice?

1. A certified nurse-midwife
2. A family nurse practitioner
3. An obstetrician
4. A maternal-fetal medicine specialist

NCLEX-RN® Test Prep CD-ROM

For those who want to practice taking tests on a computer, the CD-ROM that accompanies the book contains the pretest and posttest questions found in all chapters of the book. In addition, it contains 30 NEW questions for each chapter to help you further evaluate your knowledge base and hone your test-taking skills. We included some of the newly developed alternate NCLEX Test Items, so these items will give you valuable practice with different types of questions.

Prentice Hall NursingNotes Card

This tear-out card provides a reference for frequently used facts and information related to the subject matter of the book. These are designed to be useful in the clinical setting, when quick and easy access to information is so important!

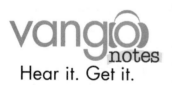

VangoNotes

Study on the go with VangoNotes. Just download chapter reviews from your text and listen to them on any mp3 player. Now wherever you are—whatever you're doing—you can study by listening to the following for each chapter of your textbook:

- **Big Ideas:** Your "need to know" for each chapter
- **Practice Test:** A gut check for the Big Ideas—tells you if you need to keep studying
- **Key Terms:** Audio "flashcards" to help you review key concepts and terms

VangoNotes are **flexible;** download all the material directly to your player, or only the chapters you need. And they're **efficient.** Use them in your car, at the gym, walking to class, wherever. So get yours today. And get studying.

About the Nursing Fundamentals Book

Chapters in this book cover "need-to-know" information about foundational concepts in nursing. The first three chapters of the book provide a review of core processes and skills, including nursing process, physical assessment, and communication. Next, a chapter on professional standards explores the roles of the nurse, ethical and legal considerations in practice, and principles of managing client care. Concepts related to health promotion throughout the lifespan are the focus of the next chapter. The remaining chapters in the book provide a review of key aspects of nursing practice, including the skills needed for safe practice, meeting basic human needs, managing pain, caring for clients with special needs or undergoing surgery and an overview of medication and IV therapy. Mastery of the information in this book and effective use of the test-taking strategies described will help the student be confident and successful in testing situations, including the NCLEX-RN®, and in actual clinical practice.

Acknowledgements

This book is a monumental effort of collaboration. Without the contributions of many individuals, this edition of *Nursing Fundamentals: Reviews and Rationales* would not have been possible. Thank you to all the contributors and reviewers who devoted their time and talents to the previous edition of this book. Their work will surely assist both students and practicing nurses alike to extend their knowledge in the area of nursing fundamentals.

I owe a special debt of gratitude to the wonderful team at Prentice Hall Nursing for their enthusiasm for this project, as well as their good humor, expertise, and encouragement as the series developed. Maura Connor, Editor-in-Chief for Nursing, was unending in her creativity, support, encouragement, and belief in the need for this series. Danielle Doller, Developmental Editor, devoted many long hours to coordinating different facets of this project, and tirelessly and cheerfully encouraged our efforts as well. Her high standards and attention to detail contributed greatly to the final "look" of this series. Editorial Assistants, Mary Ellen Ruitenberg and Marion Gottlieb, helped to keep the project moving forward on a day-to-day basis, and I am grateful for their efforts as well. A very special thank you goes to the designers of the book and the production team, led by Anne Garcia, Production Editor, and Mary Siener, Designer, who brought the ideas and manuscript into final form.

Thank you to the team at Pine Tree Composition, led by Project Coordinator Jessica Balch, for the detail-oriented work of creating this book. I greatly appreciate their hard work, attention to detail, and spirit of collaboration.

Finally, I would like to acknowledge and gratefully thank my children, who donated time that would have been spent with them, to bring this book to publication. Their love and support kept me energized and motivated.

Mary Ann Hogan

Contributors and Reviewers from First Edition

Contributors

Judy E. White, RNC, MA, MSN
Southern Union Community College
Opelika, Alabama
Consulting Editor

Donna Bowles, EdD, MSN, RN
Indiana University
New Albany, Indiana
Consulting Editor; Chapter 8

Ellise D. Adams, CNM, MSN, ICCE, CD (DONA)
Calhoun Community College
Decatur, Alabama
Chapter 5

Gina M. Ankner, MSN, RN, CS-ANP
University of Massachusetts-Dartmouth
North Dartmouth, Massachusetts
Chapter 1

Mary T. Boylston, RN, MSN, CCRN
Eastern College
St. Davids, Pennsylvania
Chapters 2 and 4

Ellen G. Christian, MS, RN
University of Massachusetts-Dartmouth
North Dartmouth, Massachusetts
Chapter 1

Arlene M. Coughlin, RN, MSN
Holy Name Hospital School of Nursing
Teaneck, New Jersey
Chapter 10

Lourdes A. D. de la Cruz, MSCHN, MHSc, RN
Sheridan College
Brampton, Ontario, Canada
Chapters 7 and 9

Jean Vanderbeek, MS, APRN, BC
Miami University Department of Nursing
Oxford, Ohio
Chapter 11

Heidi S. Walker, RN, BSN
Ashtabula, Ohio
Chapters 3 and 6

Marilyn L. Weitzel, MSN, RN
University of South Alabama
Mobile, Alabama
Chapter 9

Reviewers

Clara W. Boyle, PhD
Salem State College
Salem, Massachusetts

Carol Feingold, MS, RN
University of Arizona
Tucson, Arizona

Peggy L. Hawkins, RN, PhD
College of Saint Mary
Omaha, Nebraska

Beverly K. Hogan, MSN, RN, CS
University of Alabama
Birmingham, Alabama

Patricia Koller, MSN, RN
Milwaukee Area Technical College
Milwaukee, Wisconsin

Kenyann Lucas, RN, MS
Texarkana College
Texarkana, Texas

Terran R. Mathers, MSN, RN
Spring Hill College
Mobile, Alabama

Patricia Marrow, RN, BSN
Daytona Beach Community College
Daytona Beach, Florida

The Nursing Process

1

Chapter Outline

Objectives

- ➤ Outline the five steps of the nursing process.
- ➤ Identify characteristics of the nursing process.
- ➤ Identify three methods of problem solving.
- ➤ Discuss methods utilized to collect assessment data.
- ➤ Identify the steps used in the diagnostic process.
- ➤ Define the different categories of nursing diagnoses and collaborative problems.
- ➤ Describe the development of measurable client outcomes.
- ➤ Select nursing interventions that assist the client to achieve health outcomes.
- ➤ Identify ten responsibilities in implementing nursing care.
- ➤ List the steps necessary for the evaluation process.

NCLEX-RN® Test Prep

Use the CD-ROM enclosed with this book to access additional practice opportunities.

Review at a Glance

assessment the process of collecting, organizing, validating, and documenting information about a client's health status

collaborative problem physiological complication that the nurse monitors to detect the onset of changes in client status but for which the nurse cannot independently initiate definitive treatment

cue any piece of data/information that influences a decision

delegating transferring to a competent individual the responsibility and authority for performing a selected nursing task in a selected situation; the nurse retains accountability for the delegation and supervises the care provider

evaluation planned, ongoing, purposeful activity in which the client and nurse determine the client's progress toward achievement of outcome goals

goals aims or ends; expected outcomes

implementation phase of the nursing process in which the nursing care plan is put into action

inference the nurse's judgment or interpretation of cues, such as judging a blood pressure to be lower than normal

nursing diagnosis the nurse's clinical judgment about the client's responses to actual or potential health problems or state of wellness

nursing process a systematic, rational method of planning and providing nursing care

objective data includes measurable and observable data that can be detected by someone other than the client

planning a deliberate, systematic process that involves critical thinking, problem solving, and decision making

subjective data data that originates from the client, is not measurable, and includes the client's thoughts, beliefs, feelings, perceptions, and sensations

supervising provision by the nurse of guidance or direction, evaluation, and follow-up of assistive personnel for accomplishment of a delegated nursing task

PRETEST

1 A client comes to the walk-in clinic with reports of abdominal pain and diarrhea. While taking the client's vital signs, the nurse is implementing which phase of the nursing process?

1. Assessment
2. Diagnosis
3. Planning
4. Implementation

2 The nurse is measuring the client's urine output and straining the urine to assess for stones. Which of the following should the nurse record as objective data?

1. The client reports abdominal pain.
2. The client's urine output was 450 mL.
3. The client states, "I didn't see any stones in my urine."
4. The client states, "I feel like I have passed a stone."

3 When evaluating an elderly client's blood pressure (BP) of 146/78 mmHg, the nurse does which of the following before determining whether the BP is normal or represents hypertension?

1. Compare this reading against defined standards.
2. Compare the reading with one taken in the opposite arm.
3. Determine gaps in the vital signs data in the client record.
4. Compare the current measurement with previous ones.

4 Which of the following behaviors by the nurse demonstrates that the nurse is participating in critical thinking? Select all that apply.

1. Admitting not knowing how to do a procedure and requesting help
2. Using clever and persuasive remarks to support an opinion or position
3. Accepting without question the values acquired in nursing school
4. Finding a quick and logical answer, even to complex questions
5. Gathering three assistants to transfer the client to a stretcher after noting the client weighs 300 pounds.

5 The nurse has documented the following outcome goal in the care plan: "The client will transfer from bed to chair with two-person assist." The charge nurse tells the nurse to add which of the following to complete the goal?

1. Client behavior
2. Conditions or modifiers
3. Performance criteria
4. Target time

6 The nurse who documents on the client's care plan the outcome goal "Anxiety will be relieved within 20 to 40 minutes following administration of lorazepam (Ativan)" is engaged in which step of the nursing process?

1. Assessment
2. Planning
3. Implementation
4. Evaluation

7 When the client resists taking a liquid medication that is essential to treatment, the nurse demonstrates critical thinking by doing which of the following first?

1. Omitting this dose of medication and waiting until the client is more cooperative
2. Suggesting the medication can be diluted in a beverage
3. Asking the nurse manager about how to approach the situation
4. Notifying the physician regarding inability to give the client this medication

8 Which professionally appropriate response should the nurse make when a more stringent policy for the use of restraints is introduced on a surgical unit?

1. Use the previous, less restrictive policy conscientiously.
2. Express immediate disagreement with the new policy.
3. Ask for the rationale behind the new policy.
4. Obey the policy but continue to voice disapproval of it to co-workers.

9 The nurse assigned to care for a postoperative client has asked an unlicensed assistive person (UAP) to help the client ambulate in the hall. Before delegating this task, the nurse must do which of the following?

1. Assess the client to be sure ambulation with assistance is an appropriate care measure.
2. Ask the client if he or she is ready to ambulate.
3. Ask whether the UAP has time to assist the client.
4. Ask the charge nurse whether UAPs have ambulated the client during this shift.

10 The nurse makes the following entry on the client's care plan: "Goal not met. Client refuses to ambulate, stating, 'I am too afraid I will fall.'" The nurse should take which of the following actions?

1. Notify the physician.
2. Reassign the client to another nurse.
3. Reexamine the nursing orders.
4. Write a new nursing diagnosis.

➤ *See pages 23–25 for Answers and Rationales.*

I. OVERVIEW OF THE NURSING PROCESS

A. Definition of the nursing process

1. A systematic, rational method of planning and providing nursing care for individuals, families, groups, and communities
2. Requires critical thinking
3. Enables the nurse to identify a client's actual and potential healthcare needs, define **goals** (aims or ends; expected outcomes) with the client, establish a plan of care to meet those goals, implement the plan, and evaluate its effectiveness in improving the client's health
4. Provides a framework for a nurse's responsibility and accountability
5. Consists of five sequential and interrelated steps or phases: **A**ssessment, **D**iagnosis, **P**lanning, **I**mplementation, **E**valuation (ADPIE) (see Table 1-1 for an overview of the steps of the nursing process)

Table 1-1	**Overview of the Nursing Process**	
Component and Description	**Purpose**	**Activities**
Assessing Collecting, organizing, validating, and documenting client data	To establish a database about the client's response to health concerns or illness and the ability to manage healthcare needs	Establish a database: • Obtain a nursing health history • Conduct a physical assessment • Review client records • Review nursing literature • Consult support persons • Consult health professionals Update data as needed Organize data Validate data Communicate/document data
Diagnosing Analyzing and synthesizing data	To identify client strengths and health problems that can be prevented or resolved by collaborative and independent nursing interventions To develop a list of nursing diagnoses and collaborative problems	Interpret and analyze data: • Compare data against standards • Cluster or group data (generate tentative hypotheses) • Identify gaps and inconsistencies Determine client's strengths, risks, and problems Formulate nursing diagnoses and collaborative problem statements Document nursing diagnoses on the care plan
Planning Determining how to prevent, reduce, or resolve the identified client problems; how to support client strengths; and how to implement nursing interventions in an organized, individualized, and goal-directed manner	To develop an individualized care plan that specifies client goals/desired outcomes and related nursing interventions	Set priorities and goals/outcomes in collaboration with client Write goals/desired outcomes Select nursing strategies/interventions Consult with other health professionals Write nursing orders and nursing care plan Communicate care plan to relevant healthcare providers
Implementing Carrying out the planned nursing interventions	To assist the client to meet desired goals/outcomes; promote wellness; prevent illness and disease; restore health; and facilitate coping with altered functioning	Reassess the client to update the database Determine need for nursing assistance Perform or delegate planned nursing interventions Communicate what nursing actions were implemented: • Document care and client responses to care • Give verbal reports as necessary
Evaluating Measuring the degree to which goals/outcomes have been achieved and identifying factors that positively or negatively influence goal achievement	To determine whether to continue, modify, or terminate the plan of care	Collaborate with client and collect data related to desired outcomes Judge whether goals/outcomes have been achieved Relate nursing actions to client outcomes Make decisions about problem status Review and modify the care plan as indicated or terminate nursing care Document achievement of outcomes and modification of the care plan

Source: Berman, A. J., Snyder, S., Kozier, B. & Erb, G. (2008). *Fundamentals of nursing: Concepts, process, and practice* (8th ed.). Upper Saddle River, NJ: Pearson Education, p. 178.

B. Steps of the nursing process

1. **Assessment** (overview of components)

   a. A process of systematically collecting, organizing, validating and documenting data (information) about the health status of an individual, family, group, or community

   b. All phases of the nursing process rely on accurate and complete data

   c. A thorough assessment is an ongoing process that uses multiple sources and continues throughout the nurse-client relationship

2. **Diagnosis** (overview of components)

   a. May also be called "analysis"

   b. Involves critical analysis and interpretation of assessment data

   c. Identifies actual or potential health problems, risks, and strengths

   d. Provides a basis for selecting nursing interventions to achieve outcomes

   e. Is the process that results in formulating a **nursing diagnosis** (a statement representing a clinical judgment about the client's responses to actual or potential health problems or state of wellness) and creation or design of a care plan

3. **Planning** (overview of components)

   a. A deliberate, systematic process that involves decision making and problem solving

   b. Steps

   1) Prioritize problems

   2) Set outcome goals with client

   3) Identify interventions that will address client's health problem and achieve outcome goal(s)

   4) Document the care plan

   c. Involves formulating client goals and designing the nursing strategies (interventions) required to prevent, reduce, or eliminate the client's health problems

   d. Planning for discharge begins at the time of admission

   e. The nurse establishes a written care plan to use in client care

   f. Planning is an ongoing process

4. **Implementation** (overview of components)

   a. The phase of the nursing process in which the nursing care plan is put into action

   b. May also be called "intervention"

   c. Consists of carrying out the interventions or **delegating** nursing interventions, which involves assigning care for a client to another individual while retaining accountability for that care

   d. Nursing interventions are specific strategies designed to assist the client in achieving outcome goals

   e. Interventions are designed to prevent, reduce, or eliminate the client's health problem

   f. Includes documenting or recording nursing activities and the resulting client responses

5. **Evaluation** (overview of components)

    a. Is a planned, ongoing, purposeful activity in which the client and nurse determine the client's progress toward achievement of outcome goals

    b. Compares client response to the outcome goals to determine whether, or to what degree, goals have been met

    c. Based on evaluation, the care plan is either continued, modified, or terminated

    d. Evaluation may be:

        1) Ongoing: done while or immediately after carrying out the nursing intervention

        2) Intermittent: performed at specified intervals, such as twice a week

        3) Terminal: performed to indicate the client's condition at the time of discharge

C. Figure 1-1 illustrates the sequence and interrelationships among the steps of the nursing process

D. Characteristics of the nursing process

  1. Person-centered

    a. Process is open and flexible to meet the unique needs of client, family, group, and community

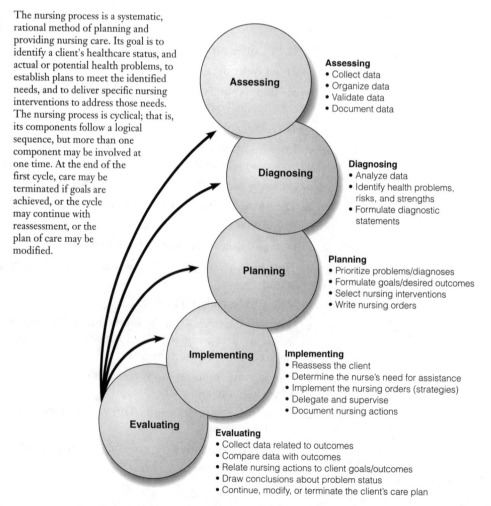

Figure 1-1

The Nursing Process in Action

The nursing process is a systematic, rational method of planning and providing nursing care. Its goal is to identify a client's healthcare status, and actual or potential health problems, to establish plans to meet the identified needs, and to deliver specific nursing interventions to address those needs. The nursing process is cyclical; that is, its components follow a logical sequence, but more than one component may be involved at one time. At the end of the first cycle, care may be terminated if goals are achieved, or the cycle may continue with reassessment, or the plan of care may be modified.

Assessing
- Collect data
- Organize data
- Validate data
- Document data

Diagnosing
- Analyze data
- Identify health problems, risks, and strengths
- Formulate diagnostic statements

Planning
- Prioritize problems/diagnoses
- Formulate goals/desired outcomes
- Select nursing interventions
- Write nursing orders

Implementing
- Reassess the client
- Determine the nurse's need for assistance
- Implement the nursing orders (strategies)
- Delegate and supervise
- Document nursing actions

Evaluating
- Collect data related to outcomes
- Compare data with outcomes
- Relate nursing actions to client goals/outcomes
- Draw conclusions about problem status
- Continue, modify, or terminate the client's care plan

      b. Emphasizes client problems rather than nursing problems

      c. The assessment process identifies unique characteristics of the client used to individualize the approach to care

  2. Emphasizes feedback

      a. Theoretically based in systems theory and uses feedback to:

        1) Reassess a problem or an outcome

        2) Identify the need to revise the care plan

      b. A cyclical and dynamic process rather than a static one

  3. Facilitates creativity

      a. Merges conscious, intuitive, and spontaneous thinking to solve nursing problems

      b. Encourages the nurse to bring together seemingly unrelated information, find the connections, and formulate an effective plan of care

      c. Develops solutions to problems in the rapidly changing healthcare environment

  4. Foundation of nursing practice

      a. Framework in which nurses use their knowledge and skill to assist clients to manage potential and/or actual health problems or maintain wellness

      b. Professionally recognized as the series of planned actions the nurse takes when planning and providing client care

II. CRITICAL THINKING AND PROBLEM SOLVING

A. Benner's model of skill acquisition applied to critical thinking

  1. Novice: uses rules to perform correctly in client care situations

  2. Advanced beginner: recognizes common patterns and benefits from assistance in setting priorities; begins to develop professional habits (see T.H.I.N.K. model in following section)

  3. Competent: recognizes own thinking and analyzes problems (often after 2 to 3 years of experience)

  4. Proficient: uses increasingly intuitive thinking; perceives a clinical situation "as a whole," rather than its individual aspects, with speed and accuracy (takes 3 to 5 years of experience generally)

  5. Expert: does not need analytical principles to understand a situation; intuition becomes prominent in thinking (usually takes 5 to 15 years of experience; this stage may or may not be achieved by all nurses)

B. Rubenfeld and Scheffer's T.H.I.N.K. model of critical thinking

  1. Consists of five modes or processes of thinking that occur in combination or simultaneously

  2. Applying this model to critical thinking and nursing process will enhance nursing assessment and nursing care

  3. T.H.I.N.K. modes (see Box 1-1)

C. Trial-and-error problem solving

  1. Problem solving in which a number of approaches are tried until a successful one is found

  2. Lacks precision and may be time consuming if failures occur

Box 1-1	T: Total recall (remembering essential or needed facts)
T.H.I.N.K. Model	H: Habits (behaviors that have been repeated many times and are "second nature")
	I: Inquiry (examining issues in depth; questioning situations or other things that seem obvious on the surface)
	N: New ideas and creativity (using new and different ways of looking at information to individualize client care)
	K: Knowing how you think (being able to recognize own patterns of logical reasoning)

3. Approaches are tried without carefully evaluating the situation, the options available, and the potential consequences of each option

4. Client may suffer harm if an approach is inappropriate

D. Scientific method as used in nursing for problem solving

1. Logical, organized, and systematic approach used to discover relationships between what is observed and its explanation

2. Follows a logical sequence of steps

  a. Identify the problem

  b. Define it carefully

  c. Review the literature

  d. Determine data-gathering methodology

  e. Collect data

  f. Generate solution(s)

  g. Execute solution(s)

  h. Evaluate results

3. Is most effective in controlled situations

4. The profession's unique use of the scientific method

  a. Involves the interaction between client and nurse as they work together

  b. Used to identify potential or actual healthcare needs, set goals, and devise a plan to meet the client's needs, and evaluate its effectiveness

5. Process is not always linear or sequential and the steps overlap

6. Critical thinking and decision making are important activities in the modified scientific method used in nursing

  a. Nurse applies nursing knowledge and knowledge from other disciplines to re-solve client problems

  b. Deals with stressful environments

  c. Creatively resolves nursing care dilemmas with a course of action

7. Evaluation and feedback are essential steps

8. A nurse who effectively uses nursing process must be proficient and comfortable with all the steps

III. ASSESSMENT *(see Figure 1-2)*

A. Collection of data: objective and subjective

1. Review of clinical record

  a. Client records contain information collected by many healthcare team members such as demographics, past medical history, diagnostic test results, and consultations

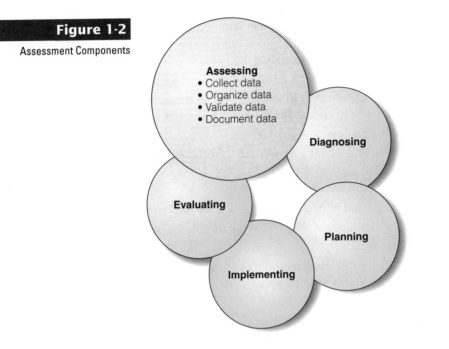

Figure 1-2

Assessment Components

Assessing
- Collect data
- Organize data
- Validate data
- Document data

Diagnosing

Evaluating

Planning

Implementing

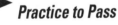

b. Reviewing the client's record before beginning an assessment prevents the nurse from repeating questions that the client has already been asked and identifies information that needs clarification

2. Interview

    a. The purpose of an interview is to gather and provide information, identify problems or concerns, and provide teaching and support

    b. The goals of an interview are to develop a rapport with the client and to collect data

    c. An interview has 3 major stages

        1) Opening: purpose is to establish rapport by creating goodwill and trust; this is often achieved through a self-introduction, nonverbal gestures (a handshake), and small talk about the weather, local sports team, or recent current event; the purpose of the interview is also explained to the client at this time

        2) Body: during this phase, the client responds to open- and closed-ended questions asked by the nurse

        3) Closing: either the client or the nurse may terminate the interview; it is important for the nurse to try to maintain the rapport and trust that was developed thus far during the interview process

    d. Types of questions

        1) Closed-ended questions used in directive interview

            a) Require short factual answers; e.g., "Do you have pain?"

            b) Often can be answered with a "yes" or "no"

            c) Answers usually reveal limited amounts of information

            d) Useful with clients who are highly stressed and/or have difficulty communicating

► **Practice to Pass**

The client says, "I have a pain in my chest." Write a closed-ended and an open-ended question the nurse could ask to find out more about this complaint.

> **2)** Open-ended questions used in nondirective interview
>> **a)** Encourage clients to express and clarify their thoughts and feelings; e.g., "How have you been sleeping lately?"
>> **b)** Specify the broad area to be discussed and invite longer answers
>> **c)** Useful at the start of an interview to encourage therapeutic communication or to encourage a descriptive or detailed answer
>
> **3)** Leading questions
>> **a)** Direct the client's answer; e.g., "You don't have any questions about your medications, do you?"
>> **b)** Suggest what answer is expected
>> **c)** Can result in client giving inaccurate data to please the nurse
>> **d)** Can limit client choice of topic for discussion

3. Nursing history

    a. Collection of information about the effect of the client's illness on daily functioning and ability to cope with the stressor (the human response)

    b. Subjective data

        1) Not measurable or observable

        2) Obtained from client (primary source), significant others, or health professionals (secondary sources)

        3) Includes client's thoughts, beliefs, feelings, perceptions, and sensations

        4) For example, the client states, "I have a headache"

        5) Refer to Table 1-2 for additional examples of subjective data

    c. Objective data

        1) Can be detected by someone other than the client

        2) Includes measurable and observable client behavior

        3) For example, a blood pressure reading of 190/110 mmHg

        4) Refer again to Table 1-2 for additional examples of objective data

4. Physical assessment

    a. Systematic collection of information about the body systems through the use of observation, inspection, auscultation, palpation, and percussion

    b. A body system format for physical assessment is found in Box 1-2

Table 1-2	Subjective	Objective
Examples of Subjective and Objective Data	"I feel weak all over when I exert myself."	Blood pressure 90/50 Apical pulse 104 Skin pale and diaphoretic
	Client states he has a cramping pain in his abdomen; states, "I feel sick to my stomach."	Vomited 100 mL green-tinged fluid Abdomen firm and slightly distended Active bowel sounds auscultated in all 4 quadrants
	"I'm short of breath."	Lung sounds clear bilaterally; diminished in right lower lobe
	"He doesn't seem so sad today," wife states.	Cried during interview
	"I would like to see the chaplain before surgery."	Holding open Bible Has small silver cross on bedside table

| **Box 1-2**

Suggested Format for Physical Assessment | ➤ General assessment
➤ Integumentary system
➤ Head, ears, eyes, nose, throat
➤ Breast and axillae
➤ Thorax and lungs
➤ Cardiovascular system
➤ Nervous system | ➤ Abdomen and gastrointestinal system
➤ Anus and rectum
➤ Genitourinary system
➤ Reproductive system
➤ Musculoskeletal system |

5. Psychosocial assessment
   a. Helpful framework for organizing data
   b. A suggested format for psychosocial assessment is found in Box 1-3
   c. The developmental theories of Erikson, Freud, Havighurst, Kohlberg, and Piaget may also be helpful for guiding data collection

6. Consultation
   a. The nurse collects data from multiple sources: primary (client) and secondary (family members, support persons, healthcare professionals, and records)
   b. Consultation with individuals who can contribute to the client's database is helpful in achieving the most complete and accurate information about a client
   c. Supplemental information from secondary sources (any source other than the client) can help verify information, provide information for a client who cannot do so, and convey information about the client's status prior to admission

7. Review of literature
   a. A professional nurse engages in continued education to maintain knowledge of current information related to health care and nursing practice
   b. Reviewing professional journals and textbooks can help provide additional data to support or help analyze the client database

B. **Patterns approach to assessment**
   1. Gordon's functional health patterns
      a. The 11 functional health patterns (FHPs) guide the collection of data about common patterns of behavior that contribute to health, quality of life, and achievement of human potential
      b. The 11 FHPs are applicable to all clients; see Box 1-4

| **Box 1-3**

Suggested Format for Psychosocial Assessment | ➤ Vocation/educational/financial
➤ Home and family
➤ Social, leisure, spiritual, and cultural
➤ Sexual | ➤ Activities of daily living
➤ Health habits
➤ Psychological |

Source: Berger, K. J. & Williams, M. B. (1999). *Fundamentals of nursing: Collaborating for optimal health* (2nd ed.). Stamford, CT: Appleton Lange, p. 346.

Box 1-4	➤ Health perception–health management	➤ Cognitive–perceptual
Gordon's Functional Health Problems	➤ Nutritional–metabolic	➤ Self-perception–self-concept
	➤ Elimination	➤ Role–relationship
	➤ Activity–exercise	➤ Sexuality–reproductive
	➤ Sleep–rest	➤ Coping–stress tolerance
		➤ Value–belief

2. Human response patterns
   a. Human responses are the biological, psychological, social, and spiritual reactions to an event or stressor
   b. The 9 human response patterns reflect the whole person in interaction with the environment (see Box 1-5)

IV. NURSING DIAGNOSIS

A. The nursing diagnosis step of the nursing process involves data analysis and identification of problems, risks, and strengths, and it leads to development of nursing diagnoses (see Figure 1-3)

B. Analysis and interpretation

1. The most common diagnostic system used is that of the North American Nursing Diagnosis Association International (NANDA-I)
2. Involves 3 activities that are sequential and continuous
   a. Compare data against standards, identifying significant **cues** (data that influences a decision)
   b. Cluster the cues and generate tentative hypotheses
   c. Identify gaps and inconsistencies

C. Making and validating inferences (the nurse's judgment or interpretation of cues)

1. Skillful assessment minimizes gaps and inconsistencies in data
2. Double-check to ensure data is complete and correct
3. Clarify all inconsistencies before making inferences

Box 1-5	1) **Exchanging:** mutual giving and receiving
Nine Human Response Patterns	2) **Communicating:** sending messages
	3) **Relating:** establishing bonds
	4) **Valuing:** assigning relative worth
	5) **Choosing:** selection of alternatives
	6) **Moving:** activity
	7) **Perceiving:** reception of information
	8) **Knowing:** meaning associated with information
	9) **Feeling:** subjective awareness of information

Source: Kozier, B., Erb, G., Berman, A. J., & Burke, K. (2000). *Fundamentals of nursing: Concepts process, and practice* (6th ed.). Upper Saddle River, NJ: Prentice Hall, p. 304.

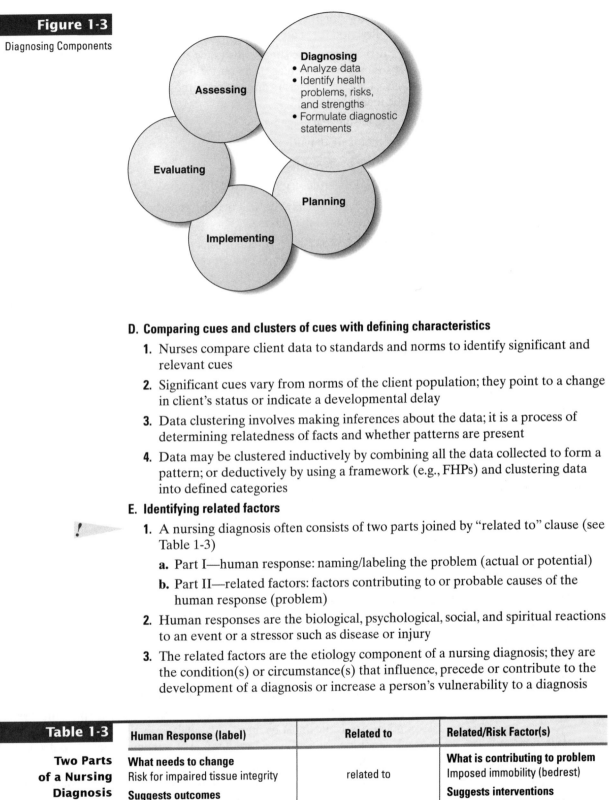

Figure 1-3

Diagnosing Components

D. Comparing cues and clusters of cues with defining characteristics

 1. Nurses compare client data to standards and norms to identify significant and relevant cues

 2. Significant cues vary from norms of the client population; they point to a change in client's status or indicate a developmental delay

 3. Data clustering involves making inferences about the data; it is a process of determining relatedness of facts and whether patterns are present

 4. Data may be clustered inductively by combining all the data collected to form a pattern; or deductively by using a framework (e.g., FHPs) and clustering data into defined categories

E. Identifying related factors

 1. A nursing diagnosis often consists of two parts joined by "related to" clause (see Table 1-3)

 a. Part I—human response: naming/labeling the problem (actual or potential)

 b. Part II—related factors: factors contributing to or probable causes of the human response (problem)

 2. Human responses are the biological, psychological, social, and spiritual reactions to an event or a stressor such as disease or injury

 3. The related factors are the etiology component of a nursing diagnosis; they are the condition(s) or circumstance(s) that influence, precede or contribute to the development of a diagnosis or increase a person's vulnerability to a diagnosis

Table 1-3	**Human Response (label)**	**Related to**	**Related/Risk Factor(s)**
Two Parts of a Nursing Diagnosis	**What needs to change** Risk for impaired tissue integrity	related to	**What is contributing to problem** Imposed immobility (bedrest)
	Suggests outcomes Client will remain free of pressure ulcers throughout hospitalization.		**Suggests interventions** Reposition client every 2 hours.

4. Related factors identify one or more probable causes of the health problem and provide direction for required nursing interventions

5. Some nursing diagnostic statements that pertain to actual (not risk) nursing diagnoses may be written as three-part statements and contain the human response, the related factors and end with the clause "as evidenced by (client's specific manifestations)"

! ▸ F. Documenting the nursing diagnosis

1. Parts of a nursing diagnosis

   a. *Label:* the name for the diagnosis

   b. *Definition:* clear description of the diagnosis

   c. *Defining characteristics:* critical behaviors and signs and symptoms that are manifestations of the diagnosis

   d. *Related factors/risk factors:* conditions or circumstances that contribute to development of a diagnosis or factors that increase one's vulnerability to a diagnosis

2. A nursing diagnosis should be concise, related to only one problem, and written clearly

3. Document the nursing diagnosis on the client's care plan

4. Follow agency policy and guidelines

G. Types of Nursing Diagnoses

1. Actual

   a. Client demonstrates defining characteristics of a problem

   b. Nurse intervenes to resolve or help client cope with the problem

2. High-risk

   a. A problem is likely to develop based on assessment of risk factors

   b. Nurse intervenes to reduce risk factors or increase protective factors

   c. Example: encourages smoking cessation

3. Wellness

   a. Client is presently healthy but wishes to achieve a higher level of function

   b. Nurse intervenes to promote growth or maintenance of the healthy response

H. Collaborative problems

1. Definition: a potential problem the nurse manages using both independent and interdependent interventions

2. Example: potential complication of head injury: loss of consciousness, epidural or subdural hematoma, seizures

3. Usually occurs when a disease is present or a treatment is prescribed

4. Clients with similar disease or treatments will have the same potential for complications, which must be managed collaboratively; however, their responses to the condition will vary, so a broad range of nursing diagnoses will apply

   a. Example: a client with asthma will always be at risk for lowered oxygen saturation; however the client's response to this condition will be unique based on his/her developmental level, past experiences and family configuration

   b. Refer to Table 1-4 for examples of collaborative problems

---

▶ **Practice to Pass**

Write a diagnostic statement for each of the following clients.

• A client with type 2 diabetes who states that she hasn't been taking her medication because it doesn't make her feel any better and she has difficulty remembering when to take it.

• A 90-year-old client with left-sided hemiparesis who has a red, broken area on the skin over his coccyx and cannot turn himself in bed.

Table 1-4	Disease/Situation	Complication	Related to	Etiology
Collaborative Problems	Potential complication of childbirth	Hemorrhage	Related to	1. Uterine atony 2. Retained placental fragments 3. Bladder distention
	Potential complication of diuretic therapy	Dysrhythmia	Related to	Low serum potassium

V. PLANNING

A. Consists of developing the plan of care that will assist the client in the identified area of concern (nursing diagnosis)

B. Has three components (see Figure 1-4)

   1. The identified problems/nursing diagnoses must be prioritized according to level of importance; frequently Maslow's hierarchy, physiological condition, and client preference are taken into account when setting priorities; psychological condition of client may also be considered when setting prioritites

   2. Goals or desired outcomes must be formulated; these are necessary to determine whether the plan of care is effective, once implemented

     a. Outcomes are derived from the nursing diagnosis

     b. Outcomes should identify desirable human responses

     c. Outcomes define specific behaviors that demonstrate that the problem has been reduced, prevented, or eliminated

     d. Outcome goals must include client behavior, target time, conditions/modifiers, and performance criteria

     e. Outcomes should be *SMART* (specific, measurable, appropriate, realistic, timely) (Table 1-5)

     f. Example: client will ambulate in hall with a walker by 11/3/07

   3. Nursing interventions or nursing orders (a nursing intervention that has all the specificity of a physician order) must be written to guide the actions of healthcare providers when implementing care

Practice to Pass

Write expected outcomes for the following nursing diagnosis: Risk for fluid volume deficit related to decreased oral intake and increased insensible losses secondary to tachypnea and fever.

Figure 1-4

Planning Components

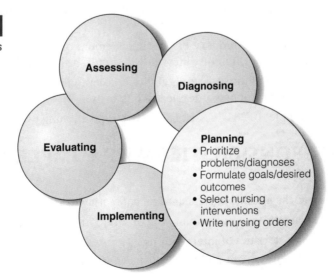

Table 1-5	S	Specific	Indicate how the nurse will know that the client's response has changed.
Outcomes Should Be SMART	M	Measurable	Address what the client will do, when this will be accomplished, and to what extent.
	A	Appropriate	Include client in formulating outcomes.
	R	Realistic	Consider client's present and potential capabilities.
	T	Timely	Include a time estimate for outcome attainment.

VI. IMPLEMENTATION

A. Types of nursing interventions

1. Independent

   a. Interventions that nurses are licensed to implement for a client by virtue of their education and experience; they may be broad statements that indicate the action to be taken; some interventions are called nursing orders when they are very specific (see Section B that follows)

   b. May be performed by a nurse without a physician's order

   c. Example: assess for decreased skin integrity/pressure ulcers

2. Interdependent

   a. Also called *collaborative* interventions

   b. Are carried out by a nurse in cooperation with other healthcare team members

   c. Example: carrying out a physician's activity order to assist client with ambulating in hall; this may be accomplished in collaboration with physical therapists on the healthcare team

B. Components of a correctly written nursing order

1. Date

   a. Nursing orders are dated when they are written

   b. Orders are reviewed periodically depending on the client's needs

2. Specific action verb

   a. An action verb starts the nursing order

   b. The verb should be precise

3. Prescribed activity: the content of the order is the where and what of the order or prescribed activity

4. Time units or frequencies: the time element of the order indicates when, how long, or how often the intervention should be implemented

5. Signature of nurse: accountability is accepted when the nurse signs name and title to the nursing order he/she has written

6. Example: 10/28/07 Assist client with repositioning every 1–2 hours N. Nurse, RN

VII. NURSING RESPONSIBILITIES WHILE IMPLEMENTING CARE *(Figure 1-5)*

A. Review the planned interventions for appropriateness

1. Focus strategies on eliminating or modifying the cause of the nursing diagnosis

2. Characteristics of interventions

   a. Realistic, safe, and consider the client's age, health status, and condition

   b. Achievable with available resources

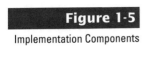

Figure 1-5

Implementation Components

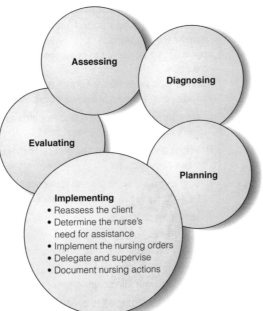

c. Congruent with client's values, beliefs, and culture, and acceptable to the client

d. Based on nursing science and knowledge or rationale from other sciences

e. Lies within established standards of care, the state Nurse Practice Act, professional organizations, and policies of institution

B. Scheduling and organizing

1. Time management and organizational skills facilitate effective nursing care

a. Plan to get organized before caregiving begins

b. Put time management down in written form when beginning to coordinate care

c. Plan the day around the most complex client

d. Identify the busiest times on the unit; do not plan treatments or interventions at those times

2. Assess the capabilities of the staff and make assignments that fit corresponding strengths

3. Use assertive communication techniques (direct and honest but without impeding the rights of others)

4. Plan time for documentation

C. Collaboration

1. Complexity of care planning necessitates working with others to provide quality client care and improve outcomes

2. Table 1-6 outlines the dimensions of nurses' collaboration with clients, peers, other healthcare professionals, professional nursing organizations, and legislators

3. Is increasingly important as boundaries of healthcare professions change

4. Key elements

a. Establish trusting relationships

b. Use effective communication

c. Develop mutual respect

Table 1-6	With Clients	Acknowledges, supports, and encourages clients' active involvement in healthcare decisions
The Nurse as a Collaborator		Encourages a sense of client autonomy and an equal position with other members of the healthcare team
		Helps clients set mutually agreed-upon goals and objectives for health care
		Provides client consultation in a collaborative fashion
	With Peers	Shares personal expertise with other nurses and elicits the expertise of others to ensure quality client care
		Develops a sense of trust and mutual respect with peers that recognizes their unique contributions
	With Other Healthcare Professionals	Recognizes the contribution that each member of the interdisciplinary team can make by virtue of his or her expertise and view of the situation
		Listens to each individual's views
		Shares healthcare responsibilities in exploring options, setting goals, and making decisions with clients and families
		Participates in collaborative interdisciplinary research to increase knowledge of a clinical problem or situation
	With Professional Nursing Organizations	Seeks out opportunities to collaborate with and within professional organizations
		Serves on committees in state (or provincial) and national nursing organizations or specialty groups
		Supports professional organizations in political action to create solutions for professional and healthcare concerns
	With Legislators	Offers expert opinions on legislative initiatives related to health care
		Collaborates with other healthcare providers and consumers on healthcare legislation to best serve the needs of the public

   d. Demonstrate good decision-making skills

   e. Manage conflict

   5. To fulfill a collaborative role, nurses must assume accountability and authority in their practice areas

D. Supervising/delegating

   1. Delegating and **supervising** (providing guidance or direction, evaluation and follow-up after delegation) are integrated processes

   a. Once the nurse delegates, he/she must supervise

   b. Need to know the delegation rules and regulations of the Nurse Practice Act in the state in which employed

   c. Review the delegation policies of the institution and the job descriptions of nursing team members

   d. Assess the client to be sure delegation is appropriate for his or her care

   2. Check that the person to whom the task is delegated has the knowledge and skill to carry it out safely and effectively

   a. The registered nurse is legally responsible for seeing that delegated tasks are performed properly

   b. Appropriate delegation involves assigning people duties within the scope of their practice

   c. Set expectations clearly and verify that the person understands the instructions

   d. Offer and receive feedback effectively

   e. Adequate supervision of licensed practical/vocational nurses (LPN/LVN) and unlicensed personnel is a responsibility of the registered nurse

E. Provide direct care

   1. Nurses use three major types of interventions in providing direct care to the client

   a. Interpersonal: verbal and nonverbal activities involved in communication

   b. Technical/psychomotor: "hands-on" skills or procedures

   c. Cognitive: involves critical thinking and problem solving to provide safe care

   2. The nurse is responsible to act in a reasonable and prudent manner using the nursing process

F. Provide counseling

   1. Help clients recognize and cope with stressful psychological or social problems

   2. Develop and improve interpersonal relationships and promote personal growth

   3. Provide emotional, intellectual, and psychological support

   4. The nurse primarily counsels healthy clients with adjustment difficulties

G. Involve the client

   1. Nurses do not plan *for* the client but partner *with* the client and family to formulate a plan of care

   a. Consider client's health and mental status

   b. Protect client's right to autonomy in decision making supported in Patient's Bill of Rights

   c. Assess client's readiness to learn and participate in care

   2. Clients are more motivated and successful in meeting goals they consider important

H. Teach client/family

   1. Client education is an essential aspect of nursing practice and an independent nursing function

   2. Patient's Bill of Rights mandates client education as a right of all clients

   3. Develop and carry out a teaching plan to promote, protect, and maintain health after assessing each client's individual learning needs

I. Make referrals

Practice to Pass

The nurse is working with a nursing assistant to care for an elderly man who has had a stroke but is now stable. He is very thin and immobile. In shift report, the nurse heard that he has a reddened area on his coccyx. If the nurses decides to delegate the bedbath and hygiene measures to the nursing assistant, what instructions should the nurse provide?

   1. Help clients use resources to meet their healthcare needs

   2. Requires knowledge of community resources and the ability to solve problems

   3. Referrals should present a clear picture of the client and his or her healthcare needs

J. Document

   1. Nurses must accurately document each step of the nursing process in the client's record

   a. Documentation must be legible, in ink, and include time, date, and appropriate signature

   b. Medications and treatments should be documented immediately to safeguard the client against duplication and provide accurate, up-to-date information available to all healthcare professionals

   c. The nurse is accountable for using the healthcare agency's designated documentation system appropriately

2. Documentation is a legal nursing responsibility

   a. Client's record is a legal document and admissible in court

   b. Confidentiality is important as the American Nurses Association (ANA) Code of Ethics describes the nurse's responsibility to maintain the client's right to privacy by judiciously protecting information of a confidential nature

VIII. EVALUATION

A. Is the final step of the nursing process

B. May or may not be an end point; if problem is not resolved, then reassessment needs to occur

C. Has various components (see Figure 1-6)

D. Refer back to client's planned outcomes

E. Evaluate client's condition, comparing to outcomes

1. Compare the client's current health status with the outcomes defined on the care plan

2. Determine if the outcome was or was not achieved

   a. If the client's current human response is consistent with the desired outcome, the goal was met

   b. If the client's current human response is not consistent with the desired outcome, the goal was not met

3. Evaluation is systematic and ongoing, helping to revise the diagnosis, interventions, and/or outcome goals

F. Summarize results

1. Write an evaluation statement that provides a conclusion (the goal was or was not met) and supporting data (human responses to support the conclusion)

2. Example: 11/3/07 Goal met. Client ambulated 80 feet in hall with walker.

Figure 1-6

Evaluation Components

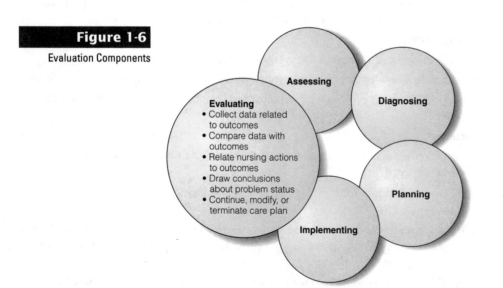

G. Identify reasons outcomes not achieved

1. The outcome goal was not appropriate
2. Collection of new assessment data may reveal that the outcome was not specific, measurable, appropriate, realistic, or timely
3. The client may need more time to achieve the desired outcome
4. It may be more appropriate to set outcomes at increasing levels of difficulty; example: client states pain is ≤ 6/10 on day 1, ≤ 4/10 on day 2, ≤ 2/10 on day 3

H. Corrective action to modify plan

1. Reassess client for additional or incomplete data
2. Make a judgment about the problem status and use new data to analyze whether the diagnosis is appropriate for the client
3. The outcome goals may need to be revised to be more realistic and attainable
4. Nursing interventions should be examined to ensure the best interventions were selected to move the client toward a more optimal level of functioning
5. A revised diagnosis will require new interventions
6. The manner in which the nursing interventions were implemented may have interfered with achieving the outcome
7. The diagnosis, outcome(s), and/or interventions may need to be changed or additional diagnoses, outcomes, and/or interventions may need to be added

I. Document

1. Client's responses to interventions and any changes made to the care plan should be documented according to agency policy
2. To discontinue a diagnosis once it has been resolved, follow agency documentation procedures, which can include: highlight it with yellow highlighter/marker, then write initials and date; some forms may require the nurse to put date and initials in "Date Resolved" column

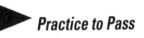

Practice to Pass

The nurse has formulated the nursing diagnosis, "Disturbed sleep pattern related to cough, pain, orthopnea, and fever." The identified outcome is, "Client will sleep for at least 5 uninterrupted hours and report feeling rested in the morning." What criteria will the nurse use for outcome evaluation? Be specific.

Case Study

A client has just arrived on the nursing unit from the postanesthesia care unit (PACU) following a hysterectomy this morning. She is complaining of pain and nausea. You are the nurse assigned to care for her.

1. What critical assessment data do you need to identify and collect?
2. Formulate a nursing diagnosis based on your assessment data.
3. Write two outcome goals for the nursing diagnosis.
4. Describe three nursing interventions to assist the client in achieving the outcome goal.
5. What criteria would you use to evaluate the effectiveness of the nursing interventions?

For suggested responses, see page 335.

POSTTEST

1 In developing a plan of care for a client with chronic hypertension, which nursing activity would be most important?

1. Set incremental goals for blood pressure reduction.
2. Instruct the client to make dietary changes by reducing sodium intake.
3. Include the client and family when setting goals and formulating the plan of care.
4. Assess past compliance to medication regimens.

2 Which nurse is demonstrating the assessment phase of the nursing process?

1. The nurse who observes that the client's pain was relieved with pain medication
2. The nurse who turns the client to a more comfortable position
3. The nurse who asks the client how much lunch he or she ate
4. The nurse who works with the client to set desired outcome goals

3 The client states, "My chest hurts and my left arm feels numb." The nurse interprets that this data is of which type and source?

1. Subjective data from a primary source
2. Subjective data from a secondary source
3. Objective data from a primary source
4. Objective data from a secondary source

4 The nurse feels a client is at risk for skin breakdown because he has only had clear liquids for the last 10 days (and essentially no protein intake). The nurse would formulate which diagnostic statement that would best reflect this problem?

1. Risk for malnutrition related to clear liquid diet
2. Impaired skin integrity related to no protein intake
3. Risk for impaired skin integrity related to malnutrition
4. Impaired nutrition related to current illness

5 The nurse would place which correctly written nursing diagnostic statement into the client's care plan?

1. Cancer related to cigarette smoking
2. Impaired gas exchange related to aspiration of foreign matter as evidenced by oxygen saturation of 91%
3. Imbalanced nutrition: more than body requirements related to overweight status
4. Impaired physical mobility related to generalized weakness and pain

6 Which of the following outcome goals has the nurse designed correctly for the postoperative client's plan of care? Select all that apply.

1. Client will state pain is less than or equal to a 3 on a zero to ten pain scale
2. Client will have no pain
3. Client will state pain is less than or equal to a 3 on a zero to ten pain scale within 24 hours
4. Client will state pain is less than or equal to a 5 on a zero to ten pain scale by time of discharge
5. Client will be medicated every 4 hours by the nurse

7 The nurse questions if the dosage of a medication is unsafe for the client because of the client's weight and age. The nurse should take which of the following actions?

1. Administer the medication as ordered by the prescriber.
2. Call the prescriber to discuss the order and the nurse's concern.
3. Administer the medication, but chart the nurse's concern about the dosage.
4. Give the client half of the dosage, and document accordingly.

8 Which activity would be appropriate for the nurse to delegate to an unlicensed assistive person (UAP)?

1. Taking vital signs of clients on the nursing unit
2. Assisting the physician with an invasive procedure
3. Adjusting the rate on an infusion pump
4. Evaluating achievement of client outcome goals

9 In giving a change-of-shift report, which type of client information communicated by the nurse is most appropriate?

1. Vital signs are stable
2. Client is pleasant, alert, and oriented to time, place, and person
3. The chest x-ray results were negative
4. Client voided 250 mL of urine 2 hours after urinary catheter removal

10 Twenty minutes after administering pain medication to the client, the nurse returns to ask if the client's level of pain has decreased. The nurse documents the client's response as part of which phase of the nursing process?

1. Diagnosis
2. Planning
3. Implementation
4. Evaluation

ANSWERS & RATIONALES

Pretest

1 **Answer: 1** The first step in the nursing process is assessment, the process of collecting data. All subsequent phases of the nursing process (options 2, 3, and 4) rely on accurate and complete data.
Cognitive Level: Comprehension **Client Need:** Physiological Integrity: Basic Care and Comfort **Integrated Process:** Nursing Process: Assessment **Content Area:** Fundamentals **Strategy:** The critical words are *vital signs.* Recall that vital signs give information or assessment data about the client to choose correctly, or recall that a basic nursing assessment of any ill client will include measurement of vital signs. **Reference:** Kozier, B., Erb, G., Berman, A., & Snyder, S. J. (2004). *Fundamentals of nursing: Concepts, process and practice* (7th ed.). Upper Saddle River, NJ: Pearson Education, p. 260.

2 **Answer: 2** Objective data is measurable data that can be seen, heard, or verified by the nurse. The objective data is the measurement of the urine output. A client's statements and reports of symptoms are documented as subjective data, such as the data found in options 1, 3, and 4.
Cognitive Level: Application **Client Need:** Physiological Integrity: Basic Care and Comfort **Integrated Process:** Communication and Documentation **Content Area:**

Fundamentals **Strategy:** The critical words are *objective data.* Recall that objective data must be measurable and then determine that only option 2 would meet that criterion. **Reference:** Kozier, B., Erb, G., Berman, A., & Snyder, S. J. (2004). *Fundamentals of nursing: Concepts, process and practice* (7th ed.). Upper Saddle River, NJ: Pearson Education, p. 262.

3 **Answer: 1** Analysis of the client's BP requires knowledge of the normal BP range for an older adult. The nurse compares the client's data against identified standards to determine whether this reading is normal or abnormal. Measuring the BP in the other arm (option 2) and comparing the reading to previous ones (option 4) will give additional client data, but the comparison alone will not determine whether the BP is normal. Gaps in the record (option 3) will not aid in interpreting the current measurement.
Cognitive Level: Application **Client Need:** Physiological Integrity: Basic Care and Comfort **Integrated Process:** Nursing Process: Analysis **Content Area:** Fundamentals **Strategy:** Knowledge of the analysis phase of the nursing process would direct you to compare data collected in the assessment process (in this case the BP) against established standards or norms before drawing a

conclusion about the significance of this data. **Reference:** Kozier, B., Erb, G., Berman, A., & Snyder, S. J. (2004). *Fundamentals of nursing: Concepts, process and practice* (7th ed.). Upper Saddle River, NJ: Pearson Education, p. 250.

4 **Answer: 1, 5** Critical thinking in nursing is self-directed, supporting what nurses know and making clear what they do not know. It is important for nurses to recognize when they lack the knowledge they need to provide safe care for a client (option 1). Nurses must also utilize their resources to acquire the support they need to care for a client safely (option 5). Options 2, 3, and 4 do not demonstrate critical thinking. **Cognitive Level:** Application **Client Need:** Safe, Effective Care Environment: Safety and Infection Control **Integrated Process:** Nursing Process: Analysis **Content Area:** Fundamentals **Strategy:** Critical words in the question are *critical thinking.* Recall that critical thinking is a process involving problem solving and evaluation to eliminate the incorrect options. **Reference:** Kozier, B., Erb, G., Berman, A., & Snyder, S. J. (2004). *Fundamentals of nursing: Concepts, process and practice* (7th ed.). Upper Saddle River, NJ: Pearson Education, p. 245.

5 **Answer: 4** The outcome goal does not state the target timeframe for when the nurse should expect to see the client behavior ("transfer"). The condition or modifier is present ("with two assists"). The performance criterion is "from bed to chair." **Cognitive Level:** Application **Client Need:** Safe, Effective Care Environment: Management of Care **Integrated Process:** Communication and Documentation **Content Area:** Fundamentals **Strategy:** Recall that outcome statements would include four essential elements (client behavior, target time, condition/modifier, and performance criteria). Analyze the goal as it is written and use the process of elimination to determine that only the target time was omitted from this statement. **Reference:** Kozier, B., Erb, G., Berman, A., & Snyder, S. J. (2004). *Fundamentals of nursing: Concepts, process and practice* (7th ed.). Upper Saddle River, NJ: Pearson Education, p. 299.

6 **Answer: 2** The planning step of the nursing process involves formulating client goals and designing the nursing interventions required to prevent, reduce, or eliminate the client's health problems. Outcome goals are documented on the client's care plan. Assessment data (option 1) is used to help identify a client's human response, and once a plan is established, the interventions are implemented (option 3) and evaluated (option 4). **Cognitive Level:** Application **Client Need:** Safe, Effective Care Environment: Management of Care **Integrated Process:** Nursing Process: Planning **Content Area:** Fundamentals **Strategy:** The critical words are *outcome goal.* Use the process of elimination and recall that client goals/outcomes are stated in the planning phase. **Reference:** Kozier, B., Erb, G., Berman, A., & Snyder, S. J. (2004). *Fundamentals of nursing: Concepts, process and practice* (7th ed.). Upper Saddle River, NJ: Pearson Education, p. 293.

7 **Answer: 2** Diluting the medication in a beverage may make the medication more palatable. Using critical thinking skills, the nurse should try to problem-solve in a situation such as this before asking for the assistance of the nurse manager. Suggesting an alternative method of taking the medication (provided that there are no contraindications to diluting the medication) should improve the likelihood of the client taking the medication. **Cognitive Level:** Application **Client Need:** Safe, Effective Care Environment: Safety and Infection Control **Integrated Process:** Nursing Process: Implementation **Content Area:** Fundamentals **Strategy:** The critical word is *first.* Options 3 or 4 may ultimately be necessary, but not until option 2 has been tried without success. **Reference:** Kozier, B., Erb, G., Berman, A., & Snyder, S. J. (2004). *Fundamentals of nursing: Concepts, process and practice* (7th ed.). Upper Saddle River, NJ: Pearson Education, p. 250.

8 **Answer: 3** Understanding the rationale behind a decision helps the nurse analyze the proposed change and understand its purpose. Options 1, 2, and 4 represent unprofessional behavior. Option 1 also places a client's safety at risk. **Cognitive Level:** Application **Client Need:** Safe, Effective Care Environment: Management of Care **Integrated Process:** Communication and Documentation **Content Area:** Fundamentals **Strategy:** The critical words are *professionally appropriate response.* Eliminate each of the incorrect options systematically by recalling that the initial response should be to understand the rationale for the change. This gives the nurse insight about how to proceed professionally if there is disagreement about a new policy or procedure. **Reference:** Kozier, B., Erb, G., Berman, A., & Snyder, S. J. (2004). *Fundamentals of nursing: Concepts, process and practice* (7th ed.). Upper Saddle River, NJ: Pearson Education, p. 11.

9 **Answer: 1** Prior to delegating any client care responsibilities, the nurse must assess the client to assure that the delegation is appropriate to his or her care. Options 2, 3, and 4 would not constitute an assessment of the client's current status. **Cognitive Level:** Application **Client Need:** Safe, Effective Care Environment: Management of Care **Integrated Process:** Nursing Process: Implementation **Content Area:** Fundamentals **Strategy:** The critical word is *delegating.* Recall principles of appropriate delegation in nursing practice to select the care measures that can be safely delegated. **Reference:** Kozier, B., Erb, G., Berman, A., & Snyder, S. J. (2004). *Fundamentals of nursing: Concepts, process and practice* (7th ed.). Upper Saddle River, NJ: Pearson Education, p. 54.

10 Answer: 3 The plan needs to be reassessed whenever goals are not met. Nursing interventions should be examined to ensure the best interventions were selected to assist the client achieve the goal. The goal may be appropriate, but the client may need more time to achieve the desired outcome. The manner in which the nursing interventions were implemented may have interfered with achieving the outcome.
Cognitive Level: Application **Client Need:** Safe, Effective Care Environment: Management of Care **Integrated Process:** Nursing Process: Evaluation **Content Area:** Fundamentals **Strategy:** Recall that the evaluation phase of the nursing process involves reassessing the client, the outcome goals, and nursing interventions for appropriateness whenever goals are not met. **Reference:** Kozier, B., Erb, G., Berman, A., & Snyder, S. J. (2004). *Fundamentals of nursing: Concepts, process and practice* (7th ed.). Upper Saddle River, NJ: Pearson Education, p. 320.

Posttest

1 Answer: 3 In developing a plan of care, nurses engage in a partnership with the client and family. Nurses do not plan care *for* clients; instead they plan care *with* clients and families. Assessment (option 4), goal setting (option 1), and interventions (option 2) will be most accurate and effective when carried out in partnership with the client and family. The other options represent other actions to take, but they will have less overall effectiveness if the client and family are not part of the plan.
Cognitive Level: Application **Client Need:** Safe, Effective Care Environment: Management of Care **Integrated Process:** Nursing Process: Planning **Content Area:** Fundamentals **Strategy:** The critical phrases are *most important* and *developing a plan of care.* Recall elements of the Patient's Bill of Rights to assist in making client-centered care decisions. **Reference:** Kozier, B., Erb, G., Berman, A., & Snyder, S. J. (2004). *Fundamentals of nursing: Concepts, process and practice* (7th ed.). Upper Saddle River, NJ: Pearson Education, p. 304.

2 Answer: 3 Assessment involves collecting, organizing, validating, and documenting data about a client. Option 1 represents the evaluation phase. Option 2 represents the implementation phase. Option 4 represents the planning phase.
Cognitive Level: Application **Client Need:** Safe, Effective Care Environment: Management of Care **Integrated Process:** Nursing Process: Assessment **Content Area:** Fundamentals **Strategy:** Look for the answer that involves acquiring or collecting data that can be used to formulate a diagnosis. Assessment consists of collecting, organizing, validating, and documenting data.
Reference: Kozier, B., Erb, G., Berman, A., & Snyder, S. J. (2004). *Fundamentals of nursing: Concepts, process and practice* (7th ed.). Upper Saddle River, NJ: Pearson Education, p. 262.

3 Answer: 1 Subjective data is apparent only to the person affected and cannot be measured, seen, felt, or heard by the nurse. The client is always considered the primary source. Secondary sources of data include the family, other health personnel, and client records.
Cognitive Level: Comprehension **Client Need:** Safe, Effective Care Environment: Management of Care **Integrated Process:** Nursing Process: Assessment **Content Area:** Fundamentals **Strategy:** The critical words in the question are *the client states.* Recall that subjective data is reported (not observed) behavior and that primary sources are original sources (the client). **Reference:** Kozier, B., Erb, G., Berman, A., & Snyder, S. J. (2004). *Fundamentals of nursing: Concepts, process and practice* (7th ed.). Upper Saddle River, NJ: Pearson Education, pp. 262, 264.

4 Answer: 3 This is a risk diagnosis, and the diagnostic statement has two parts: the human response (impaired skin integrity) and the related/risk factor (malnutrition). Options 1 and 2 do not have related factors that are under the control of the nurse (i.e., type of diet ordered). The diagnosis in option 4 does not specify the type of impairment (greater than or less than body requirements) and is therefore incomplete. It also does not provide direction for development of goals and interventions.
Cognitive Level: Analysis **Client Need:** Safe, Effective Care Environment: Management of Care **Integrated Process:** Nursing Process: Analysis **Content Area:** Fundamentals **Strategy:** The critical phrase is *at risk for skin breakdown.* To eliminate options 1 and 2, use knowledge that nursing diagnoses are developed to address client responses that are amenable to nursing intervention. Note that the diagnosis in option 4 is incomplete, and choose option 3. **Reference:** Kozier, B., Erb, G., Berman, A., & Snyder, S. J. (2004). *Fundamentals of nursing: Concepts, process and practice* (7th ed.). Upper Saddle River, NJ: Pearson Education, p. 279.

5 Answer: 2 A nursing diagnosis consists of two parts joined by *related to.* The first part (the human response) names/labels the problem. The second part (related factors) includes the factors that either contribute to or are probable etiologies of the human response. Some formats include a third part to the statement for actual (not risk) diagnoses; this third part consists of the client's signs or symptoms and is joined to the statement with the label *as evidenced by.* This type of statement is the most complete. Option 1 is not a nursing diagnosis but is a medical diagnosis. Options 3 and 4 are vague. **Cognitive Level:** Application **Client Need:** Safe, Effective Care Environment: Management of Care **Integrated Process:** Communication and Documentation **Content Area:** Fundamentals **Strategy:** Recall that the diagnosis statement is an actual or potential problem that is evidenced by signs and symptoms that are related to contributing risk factors. **Reference:** Kozier, B., Erb, G., Berman, A., & Snyder, S. J. (2004). *Fundamentals of nursing: Concepts, process and practice* (7th ed.). Upper Saddle River, NJ: Pearson Education, pp. 279–281.

6 **Answer: 3, 4** An outcome goal should be SMART: specific, measurable, appropriate, realistic, and timely. Options 3 and 4 are SMART goals. Options 1 and 2 have no timeframe to achieve the goal and are therefore incomplete. Option 2 is also unrealistic; the nurse cannot expect a postoperative client to be pain free. Option 5 is not a client goal. **Cognitive Level:** Analysis **Client Need:** Safe, Effective Care Environment: Management of Care **Integrated Process:** Communication and Documentation **Content Area:** Fundamentals **Strategy:** Recall the mnemonic SMART to recall that an outcome goal should be SMART: specific, measurable, appropriate, realistic, and timely. **Reference:** Kozier, B., Erb, G., Berman, A., & Snyder, S. (2004). *Fundamentals of nursing; concepts, process, and practice* (7th ed.). Upper Saddle River, NJ: Pearson/Education, p. 303.

7 **Answer: 2** Client safety is of the utmost importance when implementing any nursing intervention. If the nurse feels that an order is unsafe or inappropriate for a client, the nurse must act as a client advocate and collaborate with the appropriate healthcare team member to determine the rationale for the order and/or modify the order as necessary. A nurse accepts accountability for his or her actions. Options 1, 3, and 4 are inappropriate and unsafe. **Cognitive Level:** Application **Client Need:** Safe, Effective Care Environment: Safety and Infection Control **Integrated Process:** Nursing Process: Implementation **Content Area:** Fundamentals **Strategy:** The critical phrase is *unsafe for the client.* The nurse's first priority is client safety, so all other listed options would be immediately ruled out. Whenever the nurse believes there is a questionable order, the nurse should advocate for the client by discussing concerns with the physician. **Reference:** Kozier, B., Erb, G., Berman, A., & Snyder, S. J. (2004). *Fundamentals of nursing: Concepts, process and practice* (7th ed.). Upper Saddle River, NJ: Pearson Education, pp. 62, 81.

8 **Answer: 1** Part of the professional nurse's role is to delegate responsibility for activities while maintaining ac-

countability. The nurse must match the needs of the client with the skills and knowledge of UAPs. Certain skills and activities, such as those in options 2, 3, and 4, are not within the legal scope of practice for a UAP. **Cognitive Level:** Application **Client Need:** Safe, Effective Care Environment: Management of Care **Integrated Process:** Nursing Process: Implementation **Content Area:** Fundamentals **Strategy:** Recognize what is within the scope of practice of an RN, LPN, and UAP. Client needs and activities delegated must be matched to the skill level of health personnel. Knowledge of the Nurse Practice Act and the institution's polices will assist the nurse in making appropriate decisions regarding delegation of care activities. **Reference:** Kozier, B., Erb, G., Berman, A., & Snyder, S. J. (2004). *Fundamentals of nursing: Concepts, process and practice* (7th ed.). Upper Saddle River, NJ: Pearson Education, p. 472.

9 **Answer: 4** A change-of-shift report should include significant changes (good or bad) in a client's condition. The information should be accurate, concise, clear, and complete. Options 1 is vague and options 2 and 3 are normal data and are therefore of lesser importance to convey in the change-of-shift report. **Cognitive Level:** Analysis **Client Need:** Safe, Effective Care Environment: Management of Care **Integrated Process:** Communication and Documentation **Content Area:** Fundamentals **Strategy:** Recall that communications that are clear and accurate provide the best information. Recall also that priority information in a change-of-shift report includes changes in the client's condition. **Reference:** Kozier, B., Erb, G., Berman, A., & Snyder, S. J. (2004). *Fundamentals of nursing: Concepts, process and practice* (7th ed.). Upper Saddle River, NJ: Pearson Education, p. 345.

10 **Answer: 4** Evaluating is the process of comparing client responses to the outcome goals to determine whether, or to what degree, goals have been met. Diagnosing identifies health problems, risks, and strengths. Planning is the formulation of client goals and nursing strategies (interventions) required to prevent, reduce, or eliminate the client's health problems. Implementing is carrying out or delegating the nursing interventions. **Cognitive Level:** Application **Client Need:** Safe, Effective Care Environment: Management of Care **Integrated Process:** Nursing Process: Evaluation **Content Area:** Fundamentals **Strategy:** Use basic knowledge of the steps of the nursing process to identify common activities carried out in each phase. **Reference:** Kozier, B., Erb, G., Berman, A., & Snyder, S. J. (2004). *Fundamentals of nursing: Concepts, process and practice* (7th ed.). Upper Saddle River, NJ: Pearson Education, p. 320.

References

Berman, A. J., Snyder, S., Kozier, B., & Erb, G. (2008). *Fundamentals of nursing: Concepts process, and practice* (8th ed.). Upper Saddle River, NJ: Pearson Education, pp. 251–364.

Craven, R. & Hirnle, C. (2006). *Fundamentals of nursing: Human health and function* (5th ed.). Philadelphia: Lippincott Williams & Wilkins.

Gordon, M. (1994). *Nursing diagnosis: Process and application* (3rd ed.). St. Louis: Mosby, p. 70.

Harkreader, H. Hogan, M. & Thobaben, M. (2004). *Fundamentals of nursing: Caring and clinical judgment* (3rd ed.). St. Louis, MO: Elsevier Science, pp. 76–255.

Potter, P. & Perry, A. (2005). *Fundamentals of nursing* (6th ed.). St. Louis, MO: Mosby, Inc., pp. 476–499.

Taylor, C., Lillis, C., & LeMone, P. (2005). *Fundamentals of nursing: The art and science of nursing care* (5th ed.). Philadelphia: Lippincott Williams & Wilkins pp. 193–369.

Wilkinson, J. (2005). *Prentice Hall nursing diagnosis handbook: With NIC interventions and NOC outcomes.* Upper Saddle River, NJ: Prentice Hall.

2

Overview of Health Assessment

Chapter Outline

The Health History
Preparing for the Physical Assessment
Conducting the Physical Assessment

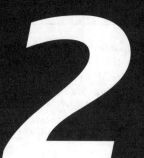

NCLEX-RN® Test Prep

Use the CD-ROM enclosed with this book to access additional practice opportunities.

Objectives

➤ Verbalize the process utilized in obtaining a health history.
➤ Identify the preparation required for physical assessment.
➤ Describe the process used to complete a physical assessment.

Review at a Glance

auscultation utilizes the sense of hearing and a stethoscope to detect normal and abnormal sounds produced by the body, including the gastrointestinal tract, arteries, heart, and lungs

health history a process used by healthcare professionals to obtain complete relevant information about a client's physical, psychosocial, and spiritual health

inspection utilizes the sense of sight to visually observe all areas of the body to assess pathology, color, level of comfort, anxiety, and any visual signs that provide clues to the client's health status; determining odor is also included under inspection

palpation utilizes the sense of touch to examine the client's body, using the pressure of the hands and fingers to as-

sess masses, elevations, temperature, organ position, and any abnormal findings; palpation can be deep or light depending on the area being examined; the ulnar surfaces of the hands and fingers are most commonly used for palpation

percussion utilizes pressure from the hands and fingers to generate sounds that will elicit clues about the density of underlying tissues or organs

PRETEST

1 When taking a health history, the nurse should focus on which of the following?

1. Completing the process in a timely manner
2. Using therapeutic communication skills to identify the client's healthcare status
3. Documenting objective data using the client's own words
4. Attempting to have no interruptions from family members who are present

2 Before palpating the abdomen during an assessment, the nurse should perform which of the following actions?

1. Put on clean gloves.
2. Auscultate bowel sounds.
3. Elevate the client's head.
4. Percuss all four quadrants.

3 The nurse would attempt to gather which of the following information while obtaining a health history from a client? Select all that apply.

1. Who lives with the client and the client's support systems
2. Annual household income
3. Use of vitamins and herbal supplements
4. History of past illnesses and surgeries
5. Religious preference and beliefs that might relate to healthcare issues

4 The nurse would document which of the following in the medical record as objective data obtained during client assessment?

1. Detailed description of pain in an extremity
2. Loss of hair on lower legs bilaterally
3. Report of numbness of the right hand
4. Description of scalp itching, which occurs each evening

5 What action should the nurse take to increase the likelihood of obtaining quality data when doing a complete physical assessment?

1. Provide adequate lighting and a comfortably warm room for the interview and physical assessment.
2. Outline the process in detail prior to beginning the examination.
3. Ask all family members or significant others to wait outside the room.
4. Identify each piece of equipment used with the appropriate medical term.

6 The nurse would use which method of examination to assess for the presence of a bruit in the abdomen?

1. Auscultation
2. Percussion
3. Palpation
4. Inspection

7 In order to examine the ocular mobility of a client who recently experienced a stroke, the nurse should examine which of the following cranial nerves? Select all that apply.

1. Cranial nerves I and VII
2. Cranial nerves II and V
3. Cranial nerves III and IV
4. Cranial nerve VI
5. Cranial nerve IX

8 Which statement made by the client indicates an understanding of how the nurse will perform the Romberg test?

1. "You want me to bend over so you can inspect my spine for curvature."
2. "I need to touch my toes without bending my knees if possible."
3. "I am going to walk five or six steps on my toes only, then on my heels only."
4. "You want me to stand with my feet together and eyes closed for a short time."

9 A client who is alert and responsive was admitted directly from the physician's office with a diagnosis of "rule out acute myocardial infarction." Of the following alterations found on the initial assessment, which is of greatest concern to the nurse?

1. Blood pressure supine is 138/76.
2. Respirations are 28 and labored.
3. Temperature is 99.8°F.
4. There are infrequent missed apical beats.

10 A nurse has conducted a physical examination on a client and notes that the thyroid gland is normal. How would the nurse document this in the medical record?

1. Thyroid slightly deviated to the left, no nodules palpated
2. Thyroid midline, smooth, with no nodules palpated
3. Thyroid midline, with parathyroid glands easily palpated bilaterally
4. Thyroid slightly deviated to the right, with pea-size nodules at the base

➤ *See pages 57–59 for Answers and Rationales.*

I. THE HEALTH HISTORY

A. A health history is a collection of data about the client's present and past health status

B. Purposes of a health history

1. To obtain all relevant information about a client's physical, psychosocial, and spiritual health in an organized manner using communication skills and interviewing techniques; the health history gathers *subjective* information

2. An added benefit is that it provides a forum for the nurse to develop a therapeutic relationship with the client

C. Sources of data

1. Primary: the client, who is the best source of data unless confused, too young, or too ill to participate in the interview

2. Secondary: family members/caregivers/support people, old medical or other health records, and results of laboratory and diagnostic tests

D. Principles of history taking

1. Provide privacy: draw the curtains or close the door to the room to eliminate distractions; assure the client that all information is for the records and to generate a complete picture of the client's overall health status; immediately document the data in the chart for information security; do not keep any data on a loose piece of paper

2. Maintain confidentiality: assure the client that all information will remain confidential; do not discuss the client or his/her family with anyone else who is not part of the health team; do not discuss confidential information in the corridors, on the elevator, or in any public area; keep client records away from unofficial personnel

3. Plan an appropriate time frame: may require up to 1 hour or longer; allot enough time to take the health history; do not rush through the interview because important clues to the client's health status could be missed; pace the interview so as not to overtire the client; if the client is tired or ill, ask the most critical questions first

4. Develop trust

   a. Approach the client and family in a professional manner; explain your role and the rationale for the interview

   b. If the interview takes place during a nonemergent situation, try to find something in common with the client; this will relax the client so he or she will feel more at ease

   c. Tell the client that if he/she becomes ill during the interview to alert you right away

   d. Use good communication skills; listen with diligence, demonstrating active listening techniques; be aware of own nonverbal behavior; maintain good eye contact if consistent with client's cultural preference

   e. Ask appropriate follow-up questions to gather complete data

   f. Be careful with your choice of words; avoid using overly technical language or excessive medical terminology; avoid overreacting to comments made by the client or family

   g. Remain relaxed during interview

   h. Use touch sparingly and only as appropriate

5. Note nonverbal cues about client's demeanor, posture, and overall appearance

   a. Physical appearance: including cleanliness, body odor, personal grooming, hygiene, client's eye contact

   b. Signs of physical discomfort: diaphoresis, tremors, grimaces, and frequent changes in position

   c. Client stress: tears, skin blotching, nervous movements, inability to concentrate, arms folded, diaphoresis; if client wants to end the interview, respect this request and terminate the interaction

6. Assess client's reliability

   a. Client answers questions with authority and does not change data reported

   b. Client uses proper terminology or words that indicate an understanding of health status; offers pertinent information about health status; refers to previous illnesses and their treatments; does not change the subject during the discussion of an issue; is oriented to person, place, time, and event

   c. If client's family is present, they concur that the data is accurate

7. Use an interpreter consistent with agency policy if the nurse and client cannot communicate in the same language; an increasing number of hospitals are using special telephone numbers answered by certified interpreters

8. Conduct the interview in a logical, orderly manner and focus the discussion

   a. Ask open-ended questions to determine the most important issues

   b. Ask pertinent follow-up questions; for example, if a client mentions feeling "jumpy" since beginning a medication, ask what is meant by the word *jumpy*

   c. Closed-ended questions should yield "yes/no" responses; closed-ended questions clarify previous statements made by the client or family

   d. Closed-ended questions should be used when asking clients for specific additional information; for example, "Since your last heart attack have you experienced any chest pain?"

9. Clarify discrepancies: elaborate on questionable statements and use active communication skills

   a. Ask questions in a clear manner; phrase all questions after determining the intellectual level of the client or family; if a client does not understand the question, rephrase it or use different terms

   b. Probing questions help yield accurate information if several explanations for a symptom are offered; do not use leading questions

   c. Connect a client's explanations with the symptoms; seek a logical explanation for the client's descriptions and symptoms

   d. Provide feedback to convey to the client that his or her communication is being understood; paraphrase the client's descriptions in order to clarify accuracy of statements; summarize the data collected during the interview

   e. Thank the client and family for their assistance through this process

   f. Allay the client's fears and maintain open communication; be forthright with additional information

   g. Confirm that the client understands the next aspect of care

10. See Box 2-1 for tips on conducting a successful interview; also see Chapter 3 for further information about general communication techniques

E. **Components of the health history**

   1. Format used may vary slightly depending on the client's age, associated developmental considerations, and whether the reason for the visit is routine care or to address an acute problem

   2. Biographical data includes name, address, telephone number, gender, marital status, religion, occupation, health insurance information, and possibly name and contact information for primary care healthcare provider (physician/nurse practitioner)

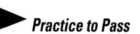

Practice to Pass

The nurse needs to interview a client. What approaches should the nurse take to obtain information most effectively?

Box 2-1	
Tips for Conducting a Successful Client Interview	➤ Maintain poise and exude warmth during the history; the client and/or family may be tense and afraid.
	➤ Use a nonthreatening and nonjudgmental attitude as you begin the interview.
	➤ Address the client in the manner of his or her choosing.
	➤ Be polite and respectful of the client and family.
	➤ Once the client offers the reason for his or her visit, then proceed in a logical, orderly fashion.
	➤ Pace the interview to obtain as much data as possible without overtiring the client or rushing the interview; if the interview proceeds too quickly, important information may be overlooked.

3. Chief complaint: the problem or reason for which the client is currently seeking treatment

   a. Ask the client/family to describe the reason for seeking treatment

   b. Do a symptom analysis, getting data about each of the following:

      1) Location: be as specific as possible in obtaining and recording the part(s) of the body involved

      2) Quantity: sometimes referred to as *severity* or *intensity;* a numerical rating scale (0 to 10) or some type of visual analog scale is often useful in obtaining this data; frequent examples of symptoms assessed this way are pain and dyspnea

      3) Quality: description of the symptoms; various adjectives are frequently used, such as *burning, stabbing, pressure,* etc.; some disorders tend to be described in similar ways by clients, which can aid in diagnosing the current problem

      4) Setting: location of the client when the symptom(s) began and a description of the events going on at that time

      5) Timing or chronology: notation of when the symptom first began; slow onset versus sudden; constant versus intermittent; whether the symptom disturbs the client's sleep

      6) Aggravating or alleviating factors: factors that make the symptom worse or better (such as eating, resting, use of medication, among others)

      7) Associated factors: other symptoms that accompany the primary symptom (such as diaphoresis or shortness of breath with chest pain, as an example)

   c. Document the findings verbatim, using the client's or family's own words

   d. Previous state of health and physical capabilities and how current symptom(s) has/have impacted physical, emotional, and psychosocial functioning

4. History of present illness (useful if the problem has occurred more than once)

   a. When the symptoms originally started

   b. How frequently exacerbations occur, and whether they are gradual or sudden in onset

   c. The client's understanding of the nature of the health problem

   d. Medications and/or other therapies used to treat the problem and their degree of success (or lack of success)

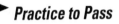

Practice to Pass

The chief complaint of the client provides multiple clues and helps to focus the interview. What would these clues typically include?

5. Past health history: sometimes referred to as "past history" or "medical history"

   a. Includes other health problems that a client may have; a checklist is useful to obtain this information; focused (more detailed) assessment can be done on areas that are still currently problematic for the client; it is increasingly common for clients to seek treatment for one health problem while having an active history of other health problems, called comorbidities, that require ongoing management

   b. Immunizations: includes childhood immunizations and date of last tetanus prophylaxis; may also include influenzae and pneumonia vaccines

   c. Childhood illnesses: such as measles, mumps, rubella (German measles), rubeola, chickenpox, rheumatic fever, scarlet fever, streptococcal infections, or other major illnesses

   d. Prior hospitalizations: including dates, reasons (includes accidents and injuries as well as illnesses), surgical procedures, outcomes, and any complications experienced (such as reactions to anesthesia or blood products)

e. Allergies

1) Medication allergies: reaction and symptoms; includes prescription, over-the-counter (OTC), and herbal products

2) Food allergies

3) Seasonal allergies (and their treatment)

4) Allergy to dyes used in diagnostic procedures (often determined by asking about allergy to iodine or shellfish)

f. Pregnancy history and menstrual history as appropriate for female clients

g. Current medications: prescribed dose, rationale and duration of drug therapy, date and time of last dose; OTC medications; herbal remedies; home remedies; complementary or adjunctive health care (if so, have the client explain the remedies used and effects)

6. Family health history

a. Includes identification of the overall state of health of parents and relatives, any significant and chronic illnesses, cause of death, and age at time of death

b. The family history is an important assessment; it can highlight genetically transmitted traits or disorders; keep in mind that ethnic background also plays a role in the risk of developing certain disorders

c. Often if a client has a strong family history for a specific disorder, the health-care team is likely to focus its efforts on disease prevention and health promotion to lower the client's risk in that area; for example, if a client's parent died at the age of 47 from a myocardial infarction, health promotion would focus on cardiac health and healthy living

d. Establish whether there is a history of hereditary disorders such as coronary heart disease, diabetes mellitus, stroke, high blood pressure, cancer, obesity, arthritis, bleeding disorders, or mental health disorders

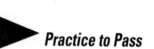

Practice to Pass

The family history provides the nurse with a clear direction to follow during the health assessment. Why is the family history so significant?

7. Personal/social history: includes social data and lifestyle assessment

a. Diet: foods eaten on a usual day; number of meals and snacks; who does the shopping and cooking; food preferences and patterns based on culture and/or religion; usual fluid intake; intake of caffeine (such as coffee, tea, cola)

b. Activity and exercise: type, frequency and duration of exercise; ability to perform activities of daily living or ADLs (eating, bathing, elimination, dressing, grooming), ability to move about at will (locomotion)

c. Sleep and rest: usual number of hours of sleep, sleep hygiene practices (all lights off, no television, no late-day caffeine), sleep problems, and effectiveness of any sleep aids used (prescription, OTC, or herbal)

d. Tobacco use: the number of packs per day (cigarettes) and the number of years of smoking; the type, frequency, and duration of use for other tobacco products

e. Substance use: the amount, frequency, and duration of alcohol or recreational drug use

f. Living arrangements: include location, type of dwelling, number of stairs to climb, home safety information, ability to access neighborhood or community resources/services

g. Family relationships or friendships: who is/are the support person(s) in times of need; effects of illness on client and family roles and relationships (dynamics); identification of next of kin

h. Psychological data: major lifestyle changes or stressors experienced and how the client dealt with them; client's usual coping patterns; general communication style and ability; appropriateness of verbal and nonverbal behavior; whether client is seeing a mental health professional; significance of current illness to the client; effect of the current illness on self-esteem or body image

i. Occupation: presence of occupational hazards, such as exposure to carcinogens, (such as asbestos, other chemicals); distance and length of time the client commutes to work each day and associated concerns; amount of time missed from work due to illness; history of a need to change jobs in the past because of illness

j. Travel (out of country): when, where, and amount of time; military service abroad

k. Health resources used: current and past use of healthcare providers (generalists and specialists), dentists, folk healers; satisfaction with care; accessibility to care

8. Review of systems (ROS): in a medically oriented assessment, this section includes questions about the past and current health status in each system reviewed (see below); it is used to obtain subjective data; in many situations, nursing assessments use a nursing model instead of the ROS to obtain this information, such as Gordon's Typology of 11 Functional Health Patterns, Orem's Self-Care Model, or Roy's Adaptation Model; healthcare agencies generally have a specific form to gather this data (forms based on nursing models may blend gathering of subjective data [history] and objective data [physical assessment or examination])

a. Skin: skin disease (eczema, psoriasis, hives), changes in moles, skin dryness or moisture, itching, bruising, rashes or other lesions, changes in hair or nails, sun exposure and use of sunscreen (SPF strength, frequency of use)

b. Head: headaches (frequency, type, and effectiveness of treatments), dizziness (vertigo) or fainting (syncope), head injury

c. Eyes: vision problems (blurring, blind spots, reduced acuity), double vision (diplopia), glaucoma, cataracts, eye pain, redness, discharge or watering, swelling, method of vision correction being used

d. Ears: hearing loss, hearing aid use, tinnitus, vertigo, earaches, infections, discharge and characteristics

e. Nose/sinuses: frequency and severity of colds, sinus pain or obstruction, discharge, nosebleeds (epistaxis), allergies, reduced sense of smell

f. Mouth/throat: pain or lesions in mouth (or tongue), toothaches, change in sense of taste, frequency of sore throats, bleeding gums, dysphagia, hoarseness, history of tonsillectomy, frequency of dental care and presence of any dental prostheses

g. Neck: pain, mobility, enlarged or tender lymph nodes, goiter, lumps or other swelling

h. Breasts: history of breast disease or surgery, pain, lumps, rashes, nipple discharge, knowledge and performance of breast self-examination (BSE); date of last mammogram

i. Axilla: rash, lumps, tenderness, or swelling

j. Respiratory: history of lung disease (tuberculosis, pneumonia, asthma, chronic obstructive pulmonary disease [COPD]), shortness of breath (amount and triggering factors, such as activity level), wheezes or other noises associated with respiration, cough (frequency and characteristics), sputum production (color, amount, and if relevant, timing), pain associated with breathing, hemoptysis, and exposure to pollutants or other inhaled toxins

k. Cardiovascular: history of heart disease, murmur, hypertension, or anemia; chest pain (precordial or retrosternal, radiation, and other pain characteristics); dyspnea on exertion (specify amount); orthopnea (head elevation or number of pillows needed), paroxysmal nocturnal dyspnea (PND); edema, nocturia

l. Peripheral vascular: discoloration of extremities (especially feet and ankles; note whether associated with activity); coolness, numbness or tingling of lower limbs (note relationship to activity and time of day); history of intermittent claudication, ulcerations, thrombophlebitis, or varicose veins

m. Gastrointestinal (GI): appetite, nausea and vomiting, constipation or diarrhea, frequency of bowel movements and any recent changes, tarry or bloody stools, history of rectal conditions (such as hemorrhoids), food intolerances, dysphagia, heartburn, (frequency, triggers, and effectiveness of treatments used), pyrosis (upper-GI burning with sour eructation), indigestion, abdominal pain (with or without eating), history of GI disorder, antacid use, and prescribed diet

n. Urinary: frequency, urgency, or dysuria; nocturia (number of trips to bathroom nightly); polyuria or oliguria; characteristics of stream (narrowed, hesitancy, straining); cloudy urine or hematuria; incontinence; history of urinary disorder (renal disease or calculi, urinary tract infections); pain in back, flank, suprapubic area, or groin

o. Male genital: lumps, hernia, penile lesions or discharge, pain in testicles or penis, knowledge and performance of testicular self-examination (TSE), sexual health practices (contraceptive method and prevention of sexually transmitted diseases)

p. Female genital: menstrual history (age of menarche, last monthly period, duration of cycle, premenstrual pain, intermenstrual spotting or metrorrhagia, dysmenorrhea, amenorrhea, menorrhagia), vaginal itching or discharge, age at menopause, menopausal manifestations, postmenopausal bleeding, last Pap test and gynecological exam, sexual health practices

q. Musculoskeletal: joint pain, stiffness, or swelling; history of arthritis or gout; limited movement, noise with joint movement, obvious deformity; muscle pain, weakness, or cramping; difficulty with gait or activities; back pain or stiffness, history of back pain or disease; use of mobility aids and satisfaction with ability to perform ADLs

r. Neurologic: weakness, tics or tremors, paralysis, problems with coordination, paresthesias (numbness and tingling), recent or distant memory disorder, nervousness, mood changes, history of depression or other mental health problem, hallucinations, history of stroke, fainting or blackouts, seizure disorder

s. Hematologic: easy bruising or bleeding, swollen lymph nodes, history of blood transfusion and reactions, exposure to radiation or other toxins

t. Endocrine: history of diabetes, thyroid disease, adrenal disease, abnormal hair distribution, change in skin (pigmentation, texture), excessive sweating, relationship between appetite and weight, hormone therapy

II. PREPARING FOR PHYSICAL ASSESSMENT

A. Purpose

1. Determine the following: objective data (both normal and abnormal); the level of a client's health; possible anomalies and whether they are life-altering or life-threatening; whether findings are considered normal for the client; comparison of findings with client's personal and family history

2. Regular physical assessments: evaluate the client's health and offer a baseline for comparison

3. Provides the healthcare professional with data for planning intervention

B. Equipment needed (see Box 2-2)

C. Techniques

1. Use the senses of vision, hearing, smell, and touch when conducting a physical assessment; the skills needed include the four listed below which should be practiced until mastery occurs

2. Inspection

   a. **Inspection** is a physical assessment technique that utilizes observation to obtain important information about a client's state of health

   b. Ensure adequate lighting to visually inspect the body without distortions or shadows; lighting can be sunlight or artificial

   c. Assess the following items using the skill of inspection:

      1) Overall appearance

      2) Demeanor, eye contact

      3) Interactions with other healthcare professionals and family

      4) Skin color, hair, nail beds, skeletal deformities

      5) Clothing appropriate for weather conditions

      6) Congruence of verbal and nonverbal behavior

      7) Sense of smell: does the client have a peculiar odor?

3. Palpation

   a. **Palpation** is a physical assessment technique that utilizes touch to obtain important information about a client's state of health

   b. It uses the sensation of touch and pressure of the hands and fingers to determine masses, elevations, temperature, organ position, and any abnormal findings

▶ *Practice to Pass*

The client will not remove clothing for the physical assessment. What can the nurse do to alleviate the client's discomfort?

Box 2-2			
Equipment That May Be Used for Physical Examination	Blood pressure cuff	Near vision charts	Strabismoscope
	Clean disposable gloves	Neurologic hammer	Tape measure
	Cotton ball	Ophthalmoscope	Thermometer
	Doppler	Otoscope	Tongue depressor/blade
	Drape	Penlight	Tuning fork
	Goniometer	Reflex hammer	Tympanometer
	Hammer	Skin calipers	Vaginal speculum
	Lubricant	Snellen visual acuity chart	Watch with a second hand
	Nasal speculum	Stethoscope	Weight scale

Table 2-1	Tone	Quality	Pitch	Example
Percussion Notes	Tympany	Drum-like	High	Gastric bubble
	Resonance	Hollow	Low	Healthy lungs
	Hyperresonance	Booming	Very low	Emphysemic lung tissue
	Flatness	Very dull	High	Muscle, bone
	Dullness	Thud-like	Medium	Liver, spleen, heart

    c. The ulnar surfaces of the hands and fingers are the most common areas used for palpation; the hands should be warm and gentle; follow standard precautions as appropriate

    d. Palpation can be light or deep depending on the area of the body being examined; the examiner controls amount of pressure

      1) Light palpation is 1 cm in depth

      2) Deep palpation is about 4 cm in depth; should occur after light palpation

  4. Percussion

    a. **Percussion** is a skill in which the finger of one hand touches or taps a finger of the other hand to generate vibration, which in turn produces a specific, diagnostic sound; the sound changes as the practitioner moves from one area to the next

    b. To become proficient, the novice should practice this skill and listen to the change in sounds as various areas of the body are percussed

    c. Sounds can be classified as tympanic, hyperresonant, resonant, dull, or flat; see Table 2-1 for further description and examples of percussion notes

  5. Auscultation

    a. **Auscultation** uses the sense of hearing to identify sounds produced by the body; some sounds can be heard and identified without a stethoscope; others can only be identified in a quiet environment with a stethoscope

    b. Allot enough time to listen carefully to auscultated sounds; if in doubt, consult another healthcare professional for a second opinion

    c. Place stethoscope over bare skin to eliminate changes in sound caused by clothing

    d. Listen to the sound, including the duration, pitch, intensity

    e. Isolate the sounds; if the client has a large amount of chest or back hair, flatten the hair by wetting it to diminish extra sounds

D. Promoting comfort during physical assessment

  1. Provide a comfortable room with appropriate temperature and adequate lighting

  2. Minimize distractions

  3. Ensure client privacy

III. CONDUCTING THE PHYSICAL ASSESSMENT

A. Vital signs

  1. Are important indicators of a client's overall health status; compare current findings to identified norms for age and to client's previously identified baseline values

2. Temperature: average is 37°C or 98.6°F; normal range is 35.8°C to 37.3°C or 96.4°F to 99.1°F; varies slightly depending on age, time of day, phase of menstrual cycle, exercise level, and method of measurement (rectal higher, oral lower); measure using the oral, rectal, axillary, or otic (tympanic membrane) route

3. Pulse: adult average is 68 to 78 beats per minute (bpm) with a range of 60 to 100; newborn average is 140 bpm (range of 120 to 160) and decreases with increasing age

   a. Radial: count the rate, rhythm, and note amplitude

    b. Apical: listen for a full minute and compare to radial pulse; place stethoscope over the chest at the left fifth intercostal space, midclavicular line (apex of the heart)

   c. Rhythm should be regular; if the pulse is irregular, assess whether it is regularly irregular or irregularly irregular and alert appropriate healthcare personnel

   d. If irregular, assess for pulse deficit by measuring apical and radial rates simultaneously (requires 2 people) and note if radial rate is lower (apical and radial rates should be equal)

4. Respiration: normal adult rate is 12 to 20 breaths/minute; can be higher at younger age levels (e.g., 30 to 40 per minute is normal in the newborn); count the rate, rhythm, and depth of respiration; note comfort level as client breathes; normal respirations are relaxed, silent, automatic, and regular

5. Blood pressure (BP): normal adult range is 100/60 mmHg to 130/85 mmHg; varies with age (lower pressures may be normal in childhood), gender, weight, exercise, emotion, stress, and diurnal rhythm (early morning low and late afternoon/early evening high)

   a. Select the proper type and size of cuff; there are six sizes ranging from newborn to extra-large adult, a cone-shaped cuff for obese arm, and a thigh cuff

   b. Have person sit or lie down with arm supported at heart level; allow a 5-minute rest period with no activity, smoking, eating, or drinking before measuring BP

   c. Locate the brachial artery by palpation (above the antecubital fossa and medial to the biceps tendon) for arm BP; locate the popliteal artery (behind the knee) to measure thigh BP

   d. Wrap and tighten the cuff around the selected limb; arm is most commonly used but the thigh can be used when necessary

   e. Inflate the cuff by pumping the hand bulb while palpating the artery to determine when the pulse disappears; this is the expected systolic BP

   f. Deflate the cuff and wait 15 to 30 seconds for venous blood to dissipate

   g. Relocate the brachial pulse and place the diaphragm of the stethoscope over this area; inflate the cuff to a point 20 to 30 mm above where the pulse disappeared to ensure measuring the true systolic pressure

   h. Watch the sphygmomanometer and listen for the first sound, which indicates systolic pressure

   i. Deflate the cuff slowly and listen carefully for the last audible sound, which indicates diastolic pressure (the range of Korotkoff sounds from tapping to silence will be heard during this process)

   j. Record the systolic and diastolic BP

    k. If there is a question about either of the sounds, wait 1 to 2 minutes before taking the BP again to avoid falsely high diastolic readings

l. If unable to hear the BP take a palpated BP by placing the index finger over the brachial artery, inflating the cuff, deflating the cuff while palpating, and noting when the pulsation disappears; the systolic pressure is noted and recorded as palpated (i.e., 90/palpated)

m. If the client has poor circulation, the BP sounds may be faint; in this case or if BP cannot even be palpated, use a doppler to hear the sounds; the systolic pressure is noted and recorded as a doppler BP

B. Height and weight

1. Height

    a. Using a balance scale, raise the headpiece on the measuring pole and align it with the top of the head while the client is shoeless, standing erect, and looking straight ahead

    b. From birth until age 2, use a horizontal measuring board to measure length; avoid using a tape measure because the readings are often inaccurate; extend an infant's legs to obtain true length since infants tend to flex the legs while at rest

    c. A wall-mounted ruler can be used to measure the height of small children if they have difficulty standing erect on a scale

2. Weight

    a. Use a platform scale for adults if they can stand without assistance; electronic scales, wheelchair scales, and bed scales are also available if needed

    b. Measure infants on a platform-type balance scale, making sure that it is calibrated by noting that the beam is balanced when the weight is set to zero

3. Use professionally authorized charts to determine if the client's height and weight fall within the normal limits for age; also compare readings to client's own previous measurements to detect changes

C. General appearance

1. Includes the client's grooming and attire, and personal hygiene

2. Includes gait and posture, general body build, and behavior

D. Mental status

1. A short mental status assessment usually is obtained in the context of the health history interview; assess the client for overt signs of mental distress, crying, sullen demeanor, and comments appropriate to the situation

2. Four key areas of functioning

    a. Appearance: as noted in section above

    b. Behavior: level of consciousness (LOC), awake, alert, aware of and responding to internal and external stimuli; lethargic and drowsy, stuporous, or unresponsive (use Glasgow coma scale for additional information), facial expression, speech (quality, pace, articulation of words, word choice), aphasia (receptive/Wernicke's, motor/expressive/Broca's, global, or mixed), mood and affect, apraxia (inability to carry out previously known behavior, such as tooth brushing)

    c. Cognition: orientation (to time, place, person, and events), attention span, recent memory, remote memory, new learning (four unrelated words test), judgment

    d. Thought processes: includes thought content (logical, consistent), client's perceptions (reality-based, congruent with others), and absence/presence of suicidal thoughts/ideation

    e. Remember these areas (appearance, behavior, cognition, and thought processes) by memorizing the abbreviation "A, B, C, T"

    f. The Mini-Mental State Exam (Folstein) may be used to gather this data; requires 5 to 10 minutes to administer; highest score is 30 (average people score 27)

    g. A full mental status examination may be done if indicated, and other tests can be added to gather more data when problems exist (brain lesions or stroke, aphasia, mental illness, memory changes, alcoholism, and others)

E. Integument (skin)

1. Skin provides the first layer of protection for the body, protecting against infection and trauma and preventing fluid loss

2. It also regulates body temperature, provides sensory perception, produces vitamin D, excretes sweat and impurities, and is a barometer of emotions

3. Inspection of skin

    a. Assess the skin for color; look at entire body, including areas that are not usually exposed

    b. Daylight is the best light to detect jaundice (yellowing of skin, sclera); use good lighting for best illumination; flashlights/penlights are also very helpful for general inspection

    c. Scan the body for skin color, texture, tone, distribution of lesions, skin symmetry, differences between body areas, evidence of rashes or eruptions, and hygiene

    d. Inspect the body for color; compare areas that are exposed to the sun and those that are not

    e. Assess moles (pigmented nevi) for defining features such as symmetry, elevation, color, and texture

    f. Normal findings: range of skin color varies from person to person, color should be uniform, sun exposed areas will be darker, calluses appear yellow, nevi (moles) can be normal findings

    g. Abnormal findings: color changes in moles (could indicate cancer); pale, shiny skin of the lower extremities (may indicate decreased peripheral circulation or diabetes mellitus); localized hemorrhages into cutaneous tissues (petechiae less than 0.5 cm in diameter or purpura greater than 0.5 cm in diameter) that appear purple red (could indicate injury, steroid use, or vasculitis)

4. Palpation of skin

    a. Note moisture, temperature, texture, turgor, and mobility; gently pinch skin to test turgor; skin should immediately return to normal but will be altered if edema or dehydration is present

    b. Normal findings: skin should be cool to warm, dry, and smooth under normal conditions; in stressful situations, the skin may feel cool and clammy; assess the skin by touching bilaterally and comparing findings

    c. Abnormal findings: lesions (provide descriptions of size, shape, color, texture, elevation/depression, pedunculation, exudates, configuration, location and distribution)

5. Inspection of nails

    a. Inspect the nails for color, contour, texture, configuration, symmetry, and cleanliness

    b. Nails offer a quick assessment of the individual and cleanliness; note whether they are clean and well-manicured, bitten down, yellow and tobacco-stained;

color should be pink with a brisk capillary refill (3 seconds or less) when depressed (blanch test)

    c. Normal findings: nail plate is smooth and flat or slightly convex; nail base angle is 160 degrees

    d. Abnormal findings

        1) Sudden appearance of white bands can indicate melanoma

        2) Yellow: psoriasis, fungal infections, and chronic respiratory diseases

        3) Diffuse darkening of the nail: malaria medication, candidal infection, hyperbilirubinemia, chronic trauma

        4) Green black: pseudomonas infection or nail bed trauma (subungual hematoma)

        5) White spots: cuticle manipulation or trauma

  6. Palpation of nails: should be hard and smooth with uniform thickness

    a. Squeeze nail; if it separates from the nail bed can indicate psoriasis or trauma

    b. A clubbed boggy nail can indicate infection with candida or pseudomonas

F. Head and neck

  1. Inspection

    a. Head should be erect and still with symmetrical facial features

    b. Assess the structure, conjunctiva, sclera, cornea, and iris of each eye

    c. Assess position, alignment, skin condition, and external meatus of ears

    d. Inspect external nose

    e. Inspect inside of mouth and throat (mucosa, tongue, teeth and gums, floor of mouth, palate, uvula)

    f. Assess for tics, spasms, lesions, and facial paralysis

    g. Neck should be symmetrical without masses

  2. Palpation: palpate from front to back assessing for smoothness and symmetry of cranium, scalp and hair; palpate temporal artery; palpate salivary glands; palpate temporomandibular joint; palpate maxillary and frontal sinuses; push on tragus of ear for tenderness; palpate thyroid gland (for size, shape, tenderness, and presence of nodules) by standing behind client and use two fingers of each hand on sides of trachea, then displace trachea to left and ask client to swallow (thyroid should feel smooth, small, and free of nodules); palpate for midline position of trachea

  3. Inspect and palpate cervical lymph nodes

  4. Special testing

    a. Eyes: test visual fields (confrontation), extraocular movements (EOMs), pupil size, equality, roundness, and response to light and accommodation (PERRLA); check ocular fundus (with an ophthalmoscope) for red reflex, condition of optic disc, blood vessels, and background of retina; may be documented under neurological exam

    b. Ears: use an otoscope to inspect the ear canal and tympanic membrane (should be movable, intact, and pearly white-gray in color); use tuning fork to do the Rinne and Weber tests to check for bone and air conduction in hearing (see section on neurological exam for further information); may be documented under neurological exam

    c. Nose: use a nasal speculum to check the nasal mucosa, septum, and turbinates

G. Breasts and axillae

1. With client in a sitting position, inspect breasts for symmetry, contour, and shape; should be rounded and generally symmetrical

2. Look for areas of discoloration, hyperpigmentation, dimpling or retraction, swelling or edema; should be uniform in color, smooth, and elastic

3. Detect any areas of retraction by asking client to do three maneuvers: raise arms above the head, push hands together with elbows flexed, and press hands down on hips

4. Observe areola for size, shape, symmetry, color, general surface characteristics, lesions or masses; should be round or oval, and color may vary from individual to individual, from light pink to dark brown

5. Inspect nipples for size, shape, position, color, and presence of any discharge or lesions; should be round, everted, and equal in size

6. Palpate axillary, subclavicular, and supraclavicular lymph nodes using palmar surface of the fingertips in the following four areas: edge of greater pectoral muscle in the anterior axillary line, thoracic wall in midaxilla, upper portion of humerus, anterior edge of latissimus dorsi muscle in posterior axillary line

7. Palpate breast for masses and tenderness, using one of three patterns: hands-of-the-clock, spokes-on-a-wheel, concentric circles (see Figure 2-1); there should be no masses or tenderness

8. Palpate areola and nipples for masses; there should be none

H. Chest

1. Lungs

   a. Function is to provide oxygen to the blood and to assist in maintaining acid-base and water balance

   b. Use standard thoracic landmarks when performing respiratory assessment

   c. Inspection: note overall appearance, nutritional status (dyspnea can impair oral intake), ability to breathe, respirations (bradypnea, tachypnea, shortness of breath, dyspnea), contour and movement of chest (should be symmetrical); note presence of retractions and the color of skin, nail beds, and lips

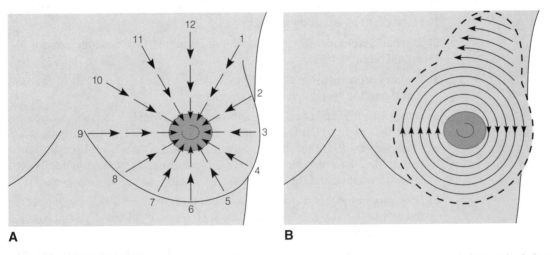

A   B

 Figure 2-1   Breast Palpation A. Hands-of-the-clock or spokes-on-a-wheel pattern; B. Concentric circle pattern

d. Palpation: assess posterior aspect of chest for masses, bulges, muscle tone, subcutaneous emphysema (crepitus), and areas of tenderness

    1) Respiratory expansion: place hands on 8th to 10th ribs (posterior); place thumbs close to the vertebrae; slide hand medially and grasp a small fold of skin between thumbs; ask client to take a deep breath; thumbs should move evenly away from vertebrae during inspiration; note any delay in expansion

    2) Tactile fremitus: is a palpable vibration whereby sounds generated in the larynx are transmitted via patent bronchi to lung parenchyma and chest wall; to assess this, place the ulnar surface of the hand or balls of the fingers (palmar base) on the outer chest wall; ask the client to speak the words "ninety-nine" or "blue moon"; begin palpating at lung apices and work from one side to the other moving down the posterior chest (but not over the scapula)

        a) Vibration should be equal on both sides in any location

        b) Decreased fremitus occurs with conditions that obstruct transmission of vibrations (such as pleural effusion, pneumothorax, and others)

        c) Increased fremitus occurs with consolidation or compression of lung tissue (such as in extensive lobar pneumonia with patent bronchus)

e. Percussion

    1) General procedure: have client lean forward slightly; begin by percussing over apex of left lung; then move hands systematically and compare percussion notes lobe to lobe and side to side

    2) Determine excursion: at 7th intercostal space, percuss downward along the scapular line to the diaphragm level; mark the line where resonance changes to dullness; have client take a deep breath and hold; mark the second line; the distance should be between 3 and 6 cm

f. Auscultation: use the flat diaphragm of the stethoscope to listen systematically to the posterior and anterior chest; begin posteriorly and listen from apices (at C7 level) to the bases (at about T10), and laterally from axilla to 7th or 8th rib; assess the actual sounds being heard with those expected in each location to determine the presence of adventitious breath sounds; compare findings side to side while working downward over the posterior chest

    1) Have client sit up straight/erect

    2) Trachea: listen over the trachea with diaphragm of stethoscope; sounds should be bronchial

    3) Primary bronchi: listen at the T3 to T5 level to the right and left of the vertebral line for bronchovesicular sounds

    4) Lungs: begin at apex and move symmetrically from left to right, down a level, then right to left (repeat sequence down entire chest); compare sides; listen for vesicular breath sounds (normal) and adventitious breath sounds (see Table 2-2 for description of various adventitious breath sounds); note location, quality, and time of occurrence during the respiratory cycle

    5) Bronchophony: assess quality of voice sounds by asking client to repeat the words "ninety-nine"; sound should be faint or unidentifiable; if it can be heard clearly, it indicates lung density in that area

    6) Egophony: occurs over dense lung tissue; ask client to say "ee-ee-ee-ee" during auscultation; sound should be heard through the stethoscope; the sound changes to a long "aaaa" sound in areas of consolidation or compression

Table 2-2	Sound	Characteristics	Timing and Occurrence
Adventitious Breath Sounds	Crackles (coarse)	Popping, frying sound, moist, low-pitched	Inspiration, some expiration
	Crackles (medium)	Not as loud as coarse crackles	Middle of inspiration
	Crackles (fine)	Non continuous, popping, high-pitched	End of inspiration
	Rhonchi or gurgles	Continuous, low-pitched, prolonged	Expiration
	Wheezes	Continuous, high-pitched, musical	Inspiration Expiration
	Pleural friction rub	Low-pitched, dry, grating	Inspiration Expiration

▶ **Practice to Pass**

While performing a respiratory assessment, the nurse notes that the client has adventitious breath sounds. What would the nurse do next to complete the assessment?

7) Whispered pectoriloquy: have the client say "one-two-three" during auscultation; the sound should be faint or muffled and almost inaudible, but will be faint yet clear and distinct with small amounts of consolidation

8) Pleural friction rub: may be heard over inflamed areas of parietal and visceral pleura; it sounds like a grating, creaking or groaning noise, and is often more noticeable on inspiration

   g. Repeat the entire assessment process with the anterior chest

2. Neck vessels

   a. Palpate the carotid arteries *one at a time* in the area medial to the sternomastoid muscle; avoid the area higher in the neck to prevent stimulating the baroreceptors and triggering bradycardia from vagus nerve stimulation; note the pulse contour and amplitude and compare findings side to side

   b. Auscultate over carotid arteries for bruits using bell of stethoscope; sound should be absent; if bruit is present, note whether it sounds like a buzzing, swishing, or blowing sound; a bruit indicates turbulent blood flow from obstruction (i.e., atherosclerotic narrowing of the carotid vessel)

   c. Assess jugular vein distention (head of bed at 30 to 45 degrees; turn head slightly away; highest pulsation should be no more than 1.5 inches above sternal notch; see Figure 2-2)

Figure 2-2

Assessment of Jugular Vein Distention (JVD)

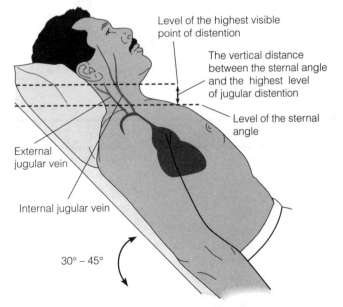

Level of the highest visible point of distention

The vertical distance between the sternal angle and the highest level of jugular distention

Level of the sternal angle

External jugular vein

Internal jugular vein

30° – 45°

3. Heart
    a. Inspection: general appearance of client and color of skin and nail beds; observe for symmetry of movement, anatomical defects, retractions, pulsations, and heaves; locate point of maximal impulse (PMI) if visible (usually at the apex, 5th left intercostal space, midclavicular line)
    b. Palpate PMI (not visible in all clients) with ball of hand, then fingertips; next assess for abnormal pulsations in the sternoclavicular, aortic, pulmonic, tricuspid, and epigastric areas; palpate for thrills (over areas of turbulent blood flow)
    c. Auscultate for S_1, S_2, extra heart sounds (S_3 and S_4) and murmurs; see Table 2-3 for heart sounds; place client in three positions for complete assessment: lying on back with head of bed at 30 degrees, sitting up, and lying on left side; use the stethoscope's diaphragm to detect higher-pitched sounds and then the bell to detect lower-pitched sounds
        1) Listen in a predetermined sequence; sounds are not heard over the valves themselves but in the area to which blood flows distal to the valve; one frequently used sequence is to listen in the following areas (see Figure 2-3):
            a) Second right intercostal space (aortic valve area)
            b) Second left intercostal space (pulmonic valve area)
            c) Left lateral sternal border of the fifth intercostal space (tricuspid valve area)
            d) Left fifth intercostal space, mid-clavicular line (mitral valve area)
        2) Identify pattern of sounds heard; listen first to the overall rate and rhythm; next identify S_1 and S_2 separately (one sound at a time); then listen for S_3 and/or S_4; finally, listen for murmurs
        3) S_1: first heart sound, often called "lub"; heard best in pulmonic and mitral areas; indicates closure of the mitral and tricuspid valves; sounds are low-pitched and dull, occurring at the beginning of ventricular systole
        4) S_2: second heart sound, often called "dub"; heard best over aortic area at the end of systole; indicates closure of the pulmonic and aortic valves; is short and high-pitched; a split S_2 occurs when pulmonic valve closes later than aortic valve during inspiration
        5) S_3: normal in children and clients with high cardiac output; in adults is called a ventricular gallop; is heard best over apex; is low-pitched sound that is often characterized as sounding like "Ken-tuck-y"; occurs immediately after the S_2 heart sound in conditions when ventricles fill rapidly; is

Table 2-3	Sound	Location	Description	Character	Cardiac Manifestation
Heart Sounds	S_1	Apex	Lub	Low pitched and dull	Closure of mitral and tricuspid valves
	S_2	Base	Dub	Shorter, more high pitched than S_1	Closure of pulmonic and aortic valves
	S_3	Apex	"Ken-tuck-y"	Low pitched	Ventricles filling rapidly
	S_4	Tricuspid or mitral areas	"Ten-nes-see"	Occurs just before S_1 after atrial contraction	Increased resistance to ventricular filling
	Pericardial friction rub	Left sternal border	Grating, leathery	Muffled, high-pitched, and transient	Pericardial inflammation

Figure 2-3

Sites for Auscultation
of the Heart

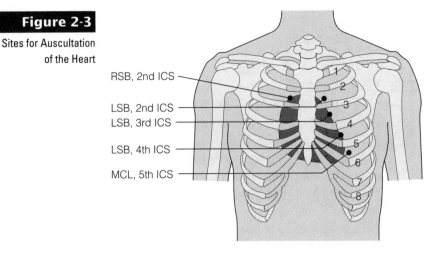

RSB, 2nd ICS

LSB, 2nd ICS

LSB, 3rd ICS

LSB, 4th ICS

MCL, 5th ICS

associated with congestive heart failure, pulmonary edema, atrial septal
defect, and acute myocardial infarction

6) S_4: atrial gallop; is best heard over tricuspid or mitral areas; is often characterized as sounding like "Ten-nes-see"; occurs just before S_1 after the atrial
contraction

7) Murmurs: generally labeled as systolic or diastolic, with many variations
of each; may be described by nature of the sound (e.g., blowing); are typically described according to timing, loudness or intensity, pitch, pattern,
quality, location, radiation, and posture (body position); Table 2-4 provides additional information about murmurs; intensity is graded on a scale
of 1 to 6 and is often documented as a fraction, with 6 being the denominator (e.g., $\frac{3}{6}$)

Table 2-4

**Overview
of Cardiac Murmurs**

Murmur	Type	Sound	Location	Pathology
Aortic stenosis	Midsystolic	Low-pitched	Right sternal border 2nd intercostal space	Calcification or restricted blood flow
Pulmonic stenosis	Midsystolic	Medium-pitched and harsh	Left sternal border 2nd to 3rd intercostal space	Calcified pulmonic valve with restricted right ventricular flow
Aortic insufficiency	Diastolic	High-pitched, blowing decrescendo diastolic	Erb's point (left sternal border 3rd intercostal space)	Backflow of blood into the pulmonic valve
Pulmonic insufficiency	Diastolic	High-pitched, blowing	3rd intercostal space, left sternal border	Incomplete valve closure
Mitral stenosis	Diastolic	Low-pitched, rumbling	Apex	Turbulent blood flow across stiffened valve
Mitral insufficiency	Systolic	High-pitched blowing	Apex	Regurgitation of blood into the atrium
Tricuspid stenosis	Diastolic	Low rumbling	Tricuspid area, lower left sternal border	Calcification of tricuspid valve
Tricuspid insufficiency	Systolic	High-pitched blowing; louder during inspiration	4th intercostal space, left sternal border	Blood regurgitation into right atrium

       a) Grade 1: very faint

       b) Grade 2: quiet

       c) Grade 3: moderately loud

       d) Grade 4: loud

       e) Grade 5: very loud, may be heard with stethoscope partly off chest

       f) Grade 6: extremely loud; may be heard with stethoscope entirely off chest

    8) Pericardial friction rub: ask client to sit up, lean forward, and exhale; listen with diaphragm of stethoscope over 3rd intercostal space on the left side of the chest; if present, friction rub feels like scratching or sandpaper; client may have accompanying chest pain, pulsus paradoxus, and/or fever

    9) Percussion: can be done to locate cardiac border, where sound changes from resonance to dullness; not often performed, since chest x-ray used to determine cardiac size

I. Abdomen

1. Preparation: ask client to empty the bladder before beginning the exam; have the client lie supine with a small pillow under the head; have the client bend the knees or place a pillow under them; expose the abdomen fully; place arms at sides or across chest (not over head because it tenses abdominal muscles); warm the hands and stethoscope and ensure that fingernails are short; keep the room warm to prevent chilling; use distraction techniques as needed

2. Inspection: four quadrants for contour, symmetry, bumps, bulges, or masses; note the skin color (redness, jaundice) and condition (striae, scars), umbilicus, hair distribution, and any abdominal pulsations or movements

    a. A bulge may indicate a distended bladder or hernia; look at shape and contour

    b. Midline umbilicus: to assess for umbilical hernia, have client lift arms over head; if umbilicus protrudes, hernia may be present

    c. Abdominal movements: slight, wavelike movements are normal, especially in a thin person; visible rippling waves may indicate obstruction

3. Auscultation: must auscultate before palpation and percussion to avoid increasing the frequency of bowel sounds

    a. Place diaphragm of stethoscope lightly against the skin in the right lower quadrant, where bowel sounds are most frequent (the location of the ileocecal valve)

    b. Listen in a clockwise fashion for at least 2 minutes

    c. Note character and quality; normal sounds are high-pitched and gurgling at a rate of 5 to 34 times per minute

    d. Sounds are classified as normal, hypoactive (heard infrequently), hyperactive (loud high pitched, more frequent than normal)

    e. Use bell of stethoscope to detect vascular sounds over iliac, aortic, renal, and femoral arteries; listen for bruits, venous hums, and friction rubs

4. Percussion: do not percuss if abdominal aortic aneurysm is present or suspected

    a. Detects size and location of abdominal organs

    b. Percuss in all four quadrants

    c. Tympany: indicates an area of empty stomach or bowel or air in a cavity

      d. Dullness: is normally heard over liver (used to estimate size), kidney, full bladder, feces-filled intestines, or possibly a solid mass

  5. Palpation: with warm hands, palpate lightly (about 1 cm deep with four fingers positioned close together) using a rotary motion in all areas to assess skin surface and superficial musculature; then repeat the sequence deeply (about 4 to 6 cm) to determine size, shape, position and tenderness of organs

      a. Light palpation will help detect superficial masses and fluid accumulation; a normal finding is an abdomen that is soft and nontender

      b. Deep palpation: can identify masses, tenderness, pulsations, organ enlargement (liver, spleen, kidneys)

      c. If a mass is found, note its location, size, shape, consistency (whether hard, firm, or soft), type of surface (smooth vs. nodular), mobility, pulsatility, and tenderness

      d. If a mass is noted to be pulsatile, stop palpating in that area to avoid rupture

      e. Identify rebound tenderness: if an area was tender to light palpation or if client reports pain in an area, move the hand to an area away from the painful site, and position the hand perpendicular (at a 90-degree angle) in relation to the abdomen; push down slowly and deeply and then lift up quickly; normally there is no pain or tenderness, but if present (often severe and accompanied by muscle rigidity), it indicates peritoneal inflammation, possibly appendicitis or peritonitis from another disorder

      f. Abdominal pain: indicates possible ulcers, intestinal obstruction, cholecystitis, peritonitis

      g. Ascites: use a tape measure at fullest site on abdomen, usually at or near the umbilicus

      h. Inguinal area: palpate each groin for femoral pulse and inguinal nodes

J. Extremities

  1. Inspect bilaterally for symmetry, skin characteristics, and distribution of hair; trophic changes (hair loss, thin shiny skin, and thickened toenails) in older adults are often due to decreased circulation from peripheral arterial disease caused by atherosclerosis

  2. Palpate peripheral pulses; upper extremity pulses include radial and ulnar pulses; lower extremity pulses include the popliteal, dorsalis pedis, and posterior tibial pulses

  3. Palpate the skin for pretibial or other edema and to note temperature of extremities; compare side-to-side bilaterally

  4. Separate toes and inspect for dryness, scaliness, maceration, or infection

K. Musculoskeletal

  1. Inspect each joint for size, contour, masses, and deformity; measure any discrepancies in extremity (leg) length

  2. Palpate each joint for musculature, bony articulations, and crepitation; assess for heat, swelling, or tenderness

  3. Test range of motion (ROM) of joints of upper extremities (shoulders, elbows, wrists, and fingers) and lower extremities (hips, knees, ankles, and toes); describe any physical limitations; if less than full ROM is present, use a goniometer to measure joint angles more precisely

  4. Note the size, tone, and any involuntary movements of major muscle groups; compare findings bilaterally

Box 2-3	
Muscle Strength Grading Scale	Grade 5: full ROM against gravity and full resistance (100% of normal, "normal")
	Grade 4: full ROM against gravity and some resistance (75% of normal, "good")
	Grade 3: full ROM with gravity (50% of normal, "fair")
	Grade 2: full ROM with gravity eliminated; called passive ROM (25% of normal, "poor")
	Grade 1: slight contraction (10% of normal, "trace")
	Grade 0: no contraction (0% of normal, "zero")

5. Test the strength of major muscle groups that control joints in upper and lower extremities by asking the client to resist attempts to put the joint through ROM; use the grading scale in Box 2-3

6. Test ROM in spine by asking client to bend forward and touch the toes (flexion should be 75 to 90 degrees with no curvature side-to-side; if curvature present, suspect and further assess for scoliosis), bend sideways (35 degrees of flexion normal), bend backward (hyperextension of 30 degrees normal), and twist shoulders from one side to the other (rotation of 30 degrees bilaterally normal)

7. Straight leg-raising (with knee straight) should not be painful; if it is, suspect herniated nucleus pulposus

8. Note any musculoskeletal pain that is present during assessment; pain description should be very specific
   a. Bone pain: pain unrelated to movement unless fracture is present, deep, aching, and continuous; it also causes insomnia
   b. Muscle pain: cramps or spasms with possible relationship to posture or movement; tremors, twitches or weakness may be manifested; muscle tension may produce referred pain
   c. Joint pain: joint may be tender to palpation; referred pain can be present; nerve root irritation may produce radiculitis (pain is distal); mechanical joint pain is worse with movement and worsens throughout the day

L. Neurologic

1. Assess cranial nerves; see Table 2-5 for a summary of normal and abnormal findings
   a. Olfactory nerve, cranial nerve (CN) I: not tested routinely but use items with different smells (alcohol, coffee, vanilla, peppermint, etc.) to detect abnormalities in sense of smell; test one nostril at a time if performed; sense of smell normally diminishes with aging
   b. Optic nerve, CN II: test visual acuity with Snellen chart, test visual fields by confrontation, and use an ophthalmoscope to examine the fundus of the eye (refer back to section on examination of head and neck)
   c. Oculomotor, trochlear, and abducens nerves (CN III, IV, VI): assess pupils for size (in mm), equality, roundness, reactivity to light, accommodation (PERRLA); assess extraocular movements by asking the client to visually follow a finger through the cardinal fields of gaze; observe for nystagmus (rapid back-and-forth oscillating movements of eyes in a horizontal or vertical plane, rotary direction, or combination)
   d. Trigeminal nerve (CN V)
      1) Assess motor function by palpating temporal and masseter muscles while asking client to clench the teeth and by trying to separate jaws by pushing down on chin

Table 2-5 Cranial Nerve Assessment	Cranial Nerve	Assessment	Normal	Abnormal
	CN I	Smell	Can identify common substances	Difficulty detecting common substances
	CN II	Visual acuity	Able to read Visual fields intact	Visual field defects
	CN III, IV, VI	Extraocular movements/ elevation of eyelids/pupil constriction	Can elevate eyes PERRLA, eyeball movement present	Drooping of the eye, ptosis, unequal pupils
	CN V	Sensory: corneas, nasal and oral mucosa, facial skin Motor: jaw and chewing muscles	Sensory: able to detect both sharp and dull sensations when face touched with pointed or blunt object Motor: clenches teeth while palpating temporal and masseter muscles	Inability to feel or identify facial stimuli Muscle weakness
	CN VII	Sensory: taste on anterior portion of tongue Motor: facial muscles	Sensory: can discriminate sweet, sour, and salty tastes Motor: facial symmetry present at rest and when frowning and smiling	If neurological impairment: entire side of face could be immobile
	CN VIII	Hearing and equilibrium	Cochlear (hearing): cover one ear with hand and whisper into other; client can repeat what was said Vestibular (equilibrium): normal balance, absence of nystagmus	Sensorineural loss
	CN IX, X	Swallowing, salivating, taste perception, voice quality	Client swallows Gag reflex present With tongue depressor against posterior pharynx, client says "ah"; movement of soft palate and uvula present	Soft palate does not rise Deviation of soft palate and uvula, no gag reflex, dysphagia, hoarseness, taste abnormalities
	CN XI	Strength of sternocleido-mastoid muscles and upper portion of trapezius	Client shrugs with equal strength bilaterally	Drooping shoulders, asymmetric muscle contraction
	CN XII	Tongue movement in swallowing and speech	Tongue protrudes in midline; client pushes tongue against cheek while nurse offers resistance	Tongue atrophy and fasciculation, deviation

2) Assess sensory function by touching client's face bilaterally in the three divisions of the nerve (ophthalmic, maxillary, and mandibular) and asking client to say "now" when face is touched with a wisp of cotton

3) Test corneal reflex if necessary (may be omitted in a screening exam) by lightly touching cornea with a wisp of cotton brought in from the side of the client's face

e. Facial nerve (CN VII): test motor function by asking client to smile, frown, close eyes tightly (while examiner tries to keep them open), lift the eyebrows, puff the cheeks, and show the teeth; test sensory function (not done routinely) by asking client to identify salty, sweet, or sour solutions applied to the tongue

f. Acoustic or vestibulocochlear nerve (CN VIII)

   1) Use voice test (whispered words from 1 to 2 feet away) to determine hearing ability

   2) Do the Weber test by placing a vibrating tuning fork on the midline of the skull and ask whether sound is heard equally, or is better in one ear than the other; test each ear separately; with conductive hearing loss, sound lateralizes to "bad" ear; with sensorineural loss, sound lateralizes to "good" ear

   3) Do the Rinne test by placing a vibrating tuning fork on the client's mastoid process and have client indicate when the sound disappears; quickly invert the tuning fork and place the vibrating end near the ear canal and ask the client to indicate when sound disappears; normally sound is heard twice as long by air conduction (AC) as bone conduction (BC); with conductive loss, AC is equal to or less than BC; with sensorineural loss, the ratio of AC to BC is normal but is reduced overall

g. Glossopharyngeal and vagus nerves (CN IX and X): using a tongue blade, note pharyngeal movement when the client says "ahh" or yawns; watch for the uvula and soft palate to rise in the midline, and for the tonsilar pillars to move medially; test the gag reflex by touching the posterior pharyngeal wall with the tongue blade; note voice quality (should be smooth with no straining)

h. Spinal accessory nerve (CN XI): ask client to rotate head forcibly against resistance applied to other side of chin; ask client to shrug shoulders against resistance (all findings should be equal bilaterally); examine sternomastoid and trapezius muscles for size

i. Hypoglossal nerve (CN XII): inspect tongue; ask client to protrude tongue (should stay in midline); ask client to say words such as "light, dynamite, tight" to determine that lingual speech (the letters l, t, d, n) is clear

2. Assess motor system: inspect and palpate muscles as described in previous section

3. Assess cerebellar function

a. Observe gait after asking client to walk 10 to 20 feet, turn, and return to starting point; efforts should be rhythmic, smooth, and without effort; step length should be about 15 inches (heel to heel); next ask client to walk heel-to-toe in a straight line (should be able to do this and maintain balance)

b. Romberg test: ask client to stand with feet together with arms at sides; have client close the eyes and hold this position for 20 seconds; client should be able to maintain posture with minimal to no swaying, but stand close by to catch client to prevent falls

c. Other tests of cerebellar function include hopping on one leg, rapid alternating movements test (patting knees with palms of hands and then back of hands quickly) or touching each finger to thumb (one hand at a time), finger-to-finger test (touching examiner's finger and then own nose); finger-to-nose test (touching own nose with eyes closed after stretching out arm, and heel-to-shin test (placing the heel of one foot on the other knee and running it down the leg to the heel); these movements should be done smoothly or in a straight line, depending on the test

4. Assess the sensory system

    a. Requires client to be alert, cooperative, have an adequate attention span, and be in a comfortable position

    b. Test client's ability to discriminate light pain (with a sharp object such as a pin) and touch (with a dull object such as a cotton wisp or pencil eraser), to detect temperature (warm water versus cold), vibration (placement of a vibrating tuning fork on various points of the body), stereognosis (recognition of objects placed in the hand while eyes are closed), graphesthesia (ability to determine a number that is traced on the palm of the hand) with eyes closed, two-point discrimination (ability to detect two separate stimuli, normally varies depending on the area of the body; fingertips are most sensitive at 2 to 8 mm, and upper arms, thighs, and back are least sensitive at 40 to 75 mm)

5. Assess deep tendon reflexes using a reflex hammer

    a. Have limb relaxed and muscle partly stretched; strike the reflex hammer on the insertion tendon of biceps (C5 to C6), triceps (C7 to C8), brachioradialis (C5 to C6), quadriceps or "knee jerk" (L2 to L4), and Achilles or "ankle jerk" (S1 to S2)

    b. Reflexes are graded using the scale in Box 2-4

6. Assess superficial reflexes

    a. Abdominal (upper T8 to T10; lower T10 to T12): stroke skin with a smooth object from one side of abdomen toward the midline; the abdominal muscle contracts on the side of the stimulus (ipsilateral response) and the umbilicus deviates toward the stroke); perform at both the upper and lower end of the abdomen

    b. Cremasteric reflex (L1 to L2): lightly stroke inner aspect of the thigh of a male client with a reflex hammer or tongue blade and watch for elevation of ipsilateral testicle

    c. Plantar reflex or Babinski reflex (L4 to S2): use same object to stroke upward on the lateral sole of the foot and across the ball of the foot; the normal (negative) response in the adult is flexion of the toes and possibly the whole foot; an abnormal or positive response (that is normal in infants) is dorsiflexion of the big toe and fanning of the other toes

    d. Normal reflexes in infants (see Table 2-6)

M. Genitals/rectum

1. Perianal region

    a. Put on gloves and spread buttocks to visualize site

    b. Inspect for hemorrhoids, blood, fissures, scars, lesions, rectal prolapse, discharge

Practice to Pass

The neurological system controls many functions of the body. Identify them.

Box 2-4	4 + = Very brisk, hyperactive with clonus (rhythmic contraction with stretching of a muscle), indicates disease
Reflex Grading Scale	3 + = Brisker than usual, possibly indicates disease
	2 + = Average or normal
	1 + = Diminished or low normal
	0 = No response

Table 2-6	Reflex	Description
Normal Reflexes in Infants	Rooting	Infant turns head toward side of face where cheek is touched; disappears at 3 to 4 months
	Sucking	Infant suckles when object is placed in mouth; disappears at 10 to 12 months
	Palmar grasp	Infant grasps finger of examiner; strongest at 1 to 2 months and disappears at 3 to 4 months
	Plantar grasp	Infant's toes curl down when thumb is touched to ball of foot; present at birth and disappears at 8 to 10 months
	Babinski	Infant's great toe dorsiflexes and other toes fan out
	Tonic neck	When the infant's head is turned to one side while supine and relaxed or sleeping, the ipsilateral arm and leg extend and the opposite arm and leg flex (also called the fencing position; appears by 2 to 3 months, decreases at 3 to 4 months, and disappears by 4 to 6 months
	Moro (startle)	Infant responds to a jarring or noisy stimulus by motions that look like hugging a tree; is present at birth and disappears by 1 to 4 months
	Placing	Infant flexes hip and knee to place foot on table when dorsal aspect of that foot is touched to the underside of a table; tested while holding infant upright under the arms; appears at 4 days after birth
	Stepping	When infant is held upright under the arms with feet on a flat surface, makes alternating regular steps; disappears before voluntary walking begins

    c. Palpation: lubricate a gloved index finger; ask client to take a deep breath; explain that the purpose of the exam is to palpate for rectal masses and assess stool for blood

        1) Insert finger into rectum gently and smoothly following the posterior wall of the rectum; rotate finger to follow curve of rectal wall, which should feel smooth and soft

        2) In males palpate the prostate gland on the anterior wall, noting size (should be 2.5 to 4 cm and not protrude into rectum by more than 1 cm), shape (heart shape with palpable central groove), surface (smooth), consistency (elastic or rubbery), mobility (slight), sensitivity (nontender)

        3) In females, palpate the cervix through the anterior wall; should feel like a small round mass

    d. After withdrawing finger, check for stool on glove and note color and consistency (brown, soft); note presence of any frank blood and test stool for occult blood (guaiac, hematest)

  2. Male genitalia

    a. Inspection

        1) Hair distribution in pubic region

        2) Penis: assess presence of dorsal vein; retract foreskin if client uncircumcised; urethral meatus appears slit-like; note bumps, blisters, redness, lesions, and masses; assess underlying skin after moving the pubic hair

        3) Scrotum: loose, wrinkled, deeply pigmented pouch at base of penis; two compartments house testicles (oval, suspended vertically and slightly forward in the scrotum); may appear asymmetrical because the left testicle has a longer spermatic cord

    b. Palpation: use thumb and first two fingers; area is sensitive to gentle compression; penis should feel smooth, semi-firm, and nontender; testicles should feel smooth, rubbery, and movable with no nodules, lumps, swelling, soreness, masses, or lesions

  3. Female genitalia

    a. Inspect external genitalia: mons pubis, labia majora, labia minora, clitoris, vagina, urethra, and Skene's and Bartholin's glands; with gloved hands, spread labia and assess the urethral meatus; it should be a pink, slit-like opening that is midline; labia majora and minora should be moist and free from lesions; discharge should be odorless; examine vestibule for swelling, lesions, discharge and unusual odors

    b. Palpate external genitalia: spread labia and palpate; should feel smooth

    c. Internal genitalia: vagina, uterus, ovaries, and fallopian tubes

    d. Inspect internal genitalia: need speculum, examination table, stirrups, good lighting; insert speculum after client takes a deep breath and tries to relax abdominal muscles; thin, white, odorless discharge should line the vaginal walls; assess cervix for color, position, size, shape, and discharge

    e. Palpate with lubricated index and middle fingers; note tenderness and nodules; palpate cervix; should feel smooth, firm and protrude 1.3 to 3 cm into vagina

    f. Rectovaginal palpation: with gloved lubricated finger, insert into rectum and assess for rectal sphincter, masses, tenderness, and nodules; palpate posterior wall of uterus for size, shape, tenderness, and masses

N. Postexamination responsibilities

  1. Provide tissues or assist client to cleanse lubricant/secretions as needed

  2. Remove drape

  3. Allow client opportunity or assistance to get dressed

  4. Leave client in comfortable position

  5. Document data clearly, thoroughly, and immediately

    a. Compare findings to established norms and to previous findings

    b. Note specimens obtained during examination

  6. Handle specimens collected during the screening in a manner consistent with standard precautions

    a. Label specimens completely and send to laboratory with requisition attached

    b. Use special plastic bag with red biohazard label and follow hospital, office, or agency protocol for disposition of specimens

Case Study

A client who is a married 56-year-old female secretary has decided to retire after working for 30 years in an office located in an old warehouse in the city. She has five children who have moved out of the house. The youngest is preparing to leave for college in another state. The client is 5' 8" tall and weighs 184 pounds. She has smoked one pack of cigarettes per day since she was 15 years old. Her husband is a bus driver in the inner city.

She has come to the clinic to see her primary healthcare provider. She has had some difficulty sleeping at night and has had to use two pillows to breathe comfortably. She has noticed some respiratory congestion and has treated it with cough syrup. She has been afebrile but cannot seem to comfortably catch her breath. She has also noticed that her rings and shoes are a bit tight, but she attributes this to her recent weight gain. The client states, "I have not been eating much, but I seem to be gaining some weight. I no longer have the energy that I once had. Maybe I am getting old."

1. What would the nurse do first to gain the client's confidence?

2. How would the nurse approach the health history?

3. The client's symptoms "cross over" several body systems. Describe how the nurse can link the symptoms and develop appropriate nursing diagnoses.

4. The client's husband has entered the room, and he wants to take the client home. He seems angry and agitated. She begins to get dressed even though the health assessment and history are not yet completed. Describe how his agitation can impact the client's symptoms.

5. The client begins to breathe heavily and appears to be in respiratory distress. She states that she feels "one of her spells coming on." What are the next steps that the nurse should take?

For suggested responses, see page 335.

POSTTEST

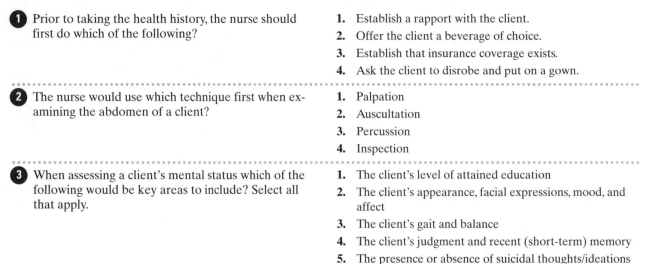

1 Prior to taking the health history, the nurse should first do which of the following?

1. Establish a rapport with the client.
2. Offer the client a beverage of choice.
3. Establish that insurance coverage exists.
4. Ask the client to disrobe and put on a gown.

2 The nurse would use which technique first when examining the abdomen of a client?

1. Palpation
2. Auscultation
3. Percussion
4. Inspection

3 When assessing a client's mental status which of the following would be key areas to include? Select all that apply.

1. The client's level of attained education
2. The client's appearance, facial expressions, mood, and affect
3. The client's gait and balance
4. The client's judgment and recent (short-term) memory
5. The presence or absence of suicidal thoughts/ideations

4 When taking health history, the first action the nurse should perform after the client describes the chief complaint is to:

1. Document verbatim what the client has said about the problem.
2. Paraphrase in the nurse's own words what the problem is.
3. Refrain from note-taking to appear focused.
4. Ask the client to repeat the data to ensure reliability.

5 The nurse selects which of the following pieces of equipment to test for a cremasteric reflex?

1. Blood pressure cuff
2. Cotton applicator
3. Sharp end of a needle
4. Percussion hammer

6 The nurse preparing to assess for jugular venous distention (JVD) places the client into which position?

1. Supine with head of bed elevated 30 degrees
2. Supine with neck placed downward on chest
3. High Fowler's with head elevated upward
4. Side-lying with no pillows under the head

7 The nurse selects which of the following as the highest priority nursing diagnosis for a 70-year-old male client with an absence of hair on the lower left leg?

1. Imbalanced nutrition: less than body requirements
2. Risk for infection
3. Deficient fluid volume
4. Impaired peripheral tissue perfusion

8 The nurse is preparing to assess for the first time the pulse of a client who has heart disease and a history of cardiac dysrhythmias. What would be the best technique for the nurse to use?

1. Auscultate the apical pulse for one full minute while another nurse palpates the radial pulse.
2. Auscultate the apical pulse for 30 seconds and multiply the rate by 2 to obtain an accurate heart rate.
3. Auscultate the apical pulse over the 2nd intercostal space at the midclavicular line.
4. Auscultate the apical pulse for one full minute and then palpate the radial pulse during the next minute.

9 In which position should the nurse place the client to best inspect and palpate the Bartholin glands?

1. Semi-Fowler's
2. Sim's
3. Lithotomy
4. Prone

10 To adequately inspect the external ear canal of an adult client, the nurse should do which of the following prior to inserting the otoscope?

1. Require that all earrings be removed for safety purposes.
2. Pull the pinna up and back.
3. Use a cotton-tipped applicator to remove cerumen.
4. Have the client lie down to promote comfort.

➤ *See pages 59–61 for Answers & Rationales.*

ANSWERS & RATIONALES

Pretest

1 **Answer: 2** A nurse must focus on using therapeutic communication skills, which will enhance the interview. In addition, the ability to interpret nonverbal communication is paramount in achieving the goals of history taking. The history should be done at a comfortable pace and should not be rushed. The nurse must document carefully, but it is subjective data, not objective, that is recorded using the client's own words. The client can have family in the room if they do not distract the client or nurse in the interview; in many instances family members are helpful in the process.
Cognitive Level: Application **Client Need:** Safe, Effective Care Environment: Management of Care **Integrated Process:** Communication and Documentation **Content Area:** Fundamentals **Strategy:** The critical word is *focus*.

POSTTEST
ANSWERS & RATIONALES

Recall that the purpose of the health history is to obtain accurate and complete information from the client; use the process of elimination to make a selection. **Reference:** Kozier, B., Erb, G., Berman, A., & Snyder, S. J. (2004). *Fundamentals of nursing: Concepts, process and practice* (7th ed.). Upper Saddle River, NJ: Pearson Education, p. 266.

2 Answer: 2 Before palpating the abdomen, the nurse should first listen to all four quadrants for bowel sounds. Palpating and percussing the abdomen first can alter bowel sounds, making the assessment less reliable. It is unnecessary to use sterile gloves unless there is an open wound or lesion. The client should be in a supine position if tolerated by the medical condition.
Cognitive Level: Application **Client Need:** Health Promotion and Maintenance **Integrated Process:** Nursing Process: Assessment **Content Area:** Fundamentals **Strategy:** The critical phrase is *before palpating*. Recalling that bowel sounds can be altered by pressure from palpation or percussion will help you to choose correctly. **Reference:** Kozier, B., Erb, G., Berman, A., & Snyder, S. J. (2004). *Fundamentals of nursing: Concepts, process and practice* (7th ed.). Upper Saddle River, NJ: Pearson Education, p. 593.

3 Answer: 1, 3, 4, 5 The nurse seeks to obtain data from the client using a holistic approach. The nurse focuses on physical, psychosocial, and spiritual concerns (options 1, 3, 4, and 5). Information regarding a client's personal finances (option 2) is not appropriate or necessary to inquire about in the interview.
Cognitive Level: Application **Client Need:** Health Promotion and Maintenance **Integrated Process:** Communication and Documentation **Content Area:** Fundamentals **Strategy:** Recall the purpose of the health history and select options that collect pertinent information without unduly invading the client's privacy. **Reference:** Kozier, B., Erb, G., Berman, A., & Snyder, S. J. (2004). *Fundamentals of nursing: Concepts, process and practice* (7th ed.). Upper Saddle River, NJ: Pearson Education, p. 263.

4 Answer: 2 Subjective data is only apparent to the person affected and can be described or verified only by that person. Itching, pain, and feelings of worry are examples. In addition, the client's sensations, feelings, values, beliefs, and attitudes are regarded as subjective. Objective data is detectable by an observer or can be measured against accepted standards. Objective data can be seen, heard, felt, or smelled during physical examination.
Cognitive Level: Application **Client Need:** Safe, Effective Care Environment: Management of Care **Integrated Process:** Communication and Documentation **Content Area:** Fundamentals **Strategy:** The core issue of the question is the ability to distinguish between objective data and subjective data. Recall that objective data is mea-

surable or observable, and use the process of elimination to make a selection. **Reference:** Kozier, B., Erb, G., Berman, A., & Snyder, S. J. (2004). *Fundamentals of nursing: Concepts, process and practice* (7th ed.). Upper Saddle River, NJ: Pearson Education, pp. 263–264.

5 Answer: 1 A comfortable environment puts the client at ease and increases the likelihood that the nurse will be able to obtain necessary data. The family may be able to provide additional data through the assessment process (option 3). As the nurse proceeds with the more intimate components of the assessment, the family may be asked to leave. Inform the client immediately prior to assessing each system (rather than before the examination) what is entailed to facilitate understanding (option 2). Using lay terms for medical equipment (e.g., *blood pressure cuff* versus *sphygmomanometer*) is appropriate (option 4).
Cognitive Level: Application **Client Need:** Health Promotion and Maintenance **Integrated Process:** Nursing Process: Assessment **Content Area:** Fundamentals **Strategy:** The critical words are *increase the likelihood*. Recall the elements of preparing for the physical assessment process to select the item that maintains an appropriate environment for the exam. **Reference:** Kozier, B., Erb, G., Berman, A., & Snyder, S. J. (2004). *Fundamentals of nursing: Concepts, process and practice* (7th ed.). Upper Saddle River, NJ: Pearson Education, p. 526.

6 Answer: 1 Auscultation uses the sense of hearing to identify sounds that are normal and abnormal during the assessment. A bruit is an abnormal sound of the venous/arterial system that is only detectable by listening with a stethoscope. A bruit cannot be detected by percussion or inspection. The turbulent blood flow that is heard as a bruit would be palpated as a thrill.
Cognitive Level: Application **Client Need:** Health Promotion and Maintenance **Integrated Process:** Nursing Process: Assessment **Content Area:** Fundamentals **Strategy:** The critical word in the question is *bruit*. Use knowledge of common assessment terminology and findings to identify common alterations. **Reference:** Kozier, B., Erb, G., Berman, A., & Snyder, S. J. (2004). *Fundamentals of nursing: Concepts, process and practice* (7th ed.). Upper Saddle River, NJ: Pearson Education, p. 595.

7 Answer: 3, 4 Evaluation of ocular motility provides information about the extraocular muscles; the orbit; cranial nerves III, IV, and VI; their brain stem connections; and the cerebral cortex. Cranial nerves I, VII, and IX, respectively, assess smell, facial movement, swallowing, and the tongue.
Cognitive Level: Analysis **Integrated Process:** Nursing Process: Assessment **Client Need:** Health Promotion and Maintenance **Content Area:** Fundamentals **Strategy:** Recall that assessment of cranial nerves is performed when

there is an identified deficit and that cranial nerves III, IV, and VI are responsible for extraocular movements, elevation of eyelids, and pupillary constriction. **Reference:** Nettina, S. (2005). *Lippincott manual of nursing practice* (8th ed.). Philadelphia, PA: Lippincott, Williams, & Wilkins, p. 77.

8 **Answer: 4** The Romberg test is performed to test motor function. The client is asked to stand with feet together, arms resting at the sides and then to close the eyes. The nurse watches for the presence of swaying, which is considered normal if it is only slight. However, if the client cannot maintain foot stance, it is documented as a positive Romberg's sign.
Cognitive Level: Analysis **Client Need:** Physiological Integrity: Reduction of Risk Potential **Integrated Process:** Nursing Process: Assessment **Content Area:** Fundamentals **Strategy:** The critical term is *Romberg test.* Use knowledge of neurologic assessment measures to select the statement that best explains the test. **Reference:** Kozier, B., Erb, G., Berman, A., & Snyder, S. J. (2004). *Fundamentals of nursing: Concepts, process and practice* (7th ed.). Upper Saddle River, NJ: Pearson Education, p. 606.

9 **Answer: 2** Using the principles of the ABCs (airway, breathing, and circulation), an alteration in respiration is always a primary concern. A disturbance in normal ventilation (rate 16–20) is occurring secondary to the medical diagnosis of myocardial infarction. The blood pressure remains in acceptable range, and the slight temperature elevation is likely related to the overall inflammatory response of the body. Infrequent abnormalities of cardiac rhythm are common and should be of concern when appearing frequently or with longer duration.
Cognitive Level: Analysis **Client Need:** Physiological Integrity: Reduction of Risk Potential **Integrated Process:** Nursing Process: Analysis **Content Area:** Fundamentals **Strategy:** The critical phrase is *of greatest concern.* This tells you that more than one option may be partially correct and you must choose the best option. Use knowledge of normal assessment parameters and etiologies of common deviations to recognize abnormalities that would require further care. **Reference:** Kozier, B., Erb, G., Berman, A., & Snyder, S. J. (2004). *Fundamentals of nursing: Concepts, process and practice* (7th ed.). Upper Saddle River, NJ: Pearson Education, p. 508.

10 **Answer: 2** The thyroid should be midline, smooth, and free of nodules. The parathyroid glands are too small to be manually palpated. Any other assessment finding is considered an abnormality.
Cognitive Level: Application **Client Need:** Health Promotion and Maintenance **Integrated Process:** Communication and Documentation **Content Area:** Fundamentals **Strategy:** Knowledge of normal assessment findings will allow the nurse to describe findings using appropriate terminol-

ogy. **Reference:** Kozier, B., Erb, G., Berman, A., & Snyder, S. J. (2004). *Fundamentals of nursing: Concepts, process and practice* (7th ed.). Upper Saddle River, NJ: Pearson Education, p. 570.

Posttest

1 **Answer: 1** In order to gain as much insight and information from the client as possible, the nurse should establish a level of trust or rapport with the client. The client will be best able to relax and answer questions if he or she is asked in a nonthreatening manner. Offering the client food and drink is not appropriate. The nurse should not ask the client about health insurance or finances, as other personnel determine this. The client does not need to wear an examining gown to answer questions.
Cognitive Level: Application **Client Need:** Health Promotion and Maintenance **Integrated Process:** Nursing Process: Assessment **Content Area:** Fundamentals **Strategy:** Use knowledge of basic interviewing techniques to choose the option that represents the best approach to the client. **Reference:** Kozier, B., Erb, G., Berman, A., & Snyder, S. J. (2004). *Fundamentals of nursing: Concepts, process and practice* (7th ed.). Upper Saddle River, NJ: Pearson Education, p. 268.

2 **Answer: 4** During inspection, the nurse scrutinizes and evaluates by sight any clues of pathology that may be present. By first performing the other assessment techniques (auscultation, percussion, and palpation), the nurse could alter the findings.
Cognitive Level: Application **Client Need:** Health Promotion and Maintenance **Integrated Process:** Nursing Process: Assessment **Content Area:** Fundamentals **Strategy:** The critical word in the question is *first.* Recall that it is important to visualize the area being examined as the initial step in assessment to make the correct selection. Auscultation is then secondary to inspection of the abdomen. Percussion and palpation may falsely generate bowel sounds. **Reference:** Kozier, B., Erb, G., Berman, A., & Snyder, S. J. (2004). *Fundamentals of nursing: Concepts, process and practice* (7th ed.). Upper Saddle River, NJ: Pearson Education, p. 593.

3 **Answer: 2, 4, 5** Four key areas of functioning to be addressed in the mental status exam are appearance, behavior (option 2), and cognition and thought processes (options 4 and 5). Educational level is unrelated to mental status. Gait and balance are assessed as part of the neurological exam.
Cognitive Level: Application **Client Need:** Health Promotion and Maintenance **Integrated Process:** Nursing Process: Assessment **Content Area:** Fundamentals **Strategy:** The core issue of the question is knowledge of the components of the mental status exam. Recall the four key areas of the

mental status exam using the abbreviation A, B, C, T (appearance, behavior, cognition, and thought processes). **Reference:** Kozier, B., Erb, G., Berman, A., & Snyder, S. J. (2004). *Fundamentals of nursing: Concepts, process and practice* (7th ed.). Upper Saddle River, NJ: Pearson Education, pp. 531, 534.

4 Answer: 1 The chief complaint offers the nurse an indication of what the problem is and how health care should proceed. The nurse can continue to probe during the interview to identify contributing factors to the client's chief complaint. The client's statements must be documented using his or her own phrases and terminology. **Cognitive Level:** Application **Client Need:** Health Promotion and Maintenance **Process:** Communication and Documentation **Content Area:** Fundamentals **Strategy:** Recall that in order to increase accuracy of documentation the nurse should document the history immediately. **Reference:** Kozier, B., Erb, G., Berman, A., & Snyder, S. J. (2004). *Fundamentals of nursing: Concepts, process and practice* (7th ed.). Upper Saddle River, NJ: Pearson Education, p. 263.

5 Answer: 2 The cremasteric reflex is tested in men only. The nurse uses a cotton-tipped applicator or other smooth object to stimulate the inner thigh. The normal reaction is contraction of the cremaster muscle and elevation of the testicle on the side stimulated. **Cognitive Level:** Application **Client Need:** Health Promotion and Maintenance **Integrated Process:** Nursing Process: Assessment **Content Area:** Fundamentals **Strategy:** The critical words are *cremasteric reflex.* Recall that gloves and a smooth object or cotton-tipped applicator should be used to stroke the inner thigh of a male to elicit the reflex. **Reference:** Kozier, B., Erb, G., Berman, A., & Snyder, S. J. (2004). *Fundamentals of nursing: Concepts, process and practice* (7th ed.). Upper Saddle River, NJ: Pearson Education, p. 620.

6 Answer: 1 To assess for jugular venous distention (which indicates fluid volume overload), the client should be lying supine with the head elevated to 30 degrees (low Fowler's). The nurse assesses the highest point of distention of the internal jugular vein in centimeters in relation to the sternal angle, the point at which the clavicles meet. The other positions listed would not aid in this physical assessment technique. **Cognitive Level:** Application **Client Need:** Health Promotion and Maintenance **Integrated Process:** Nursing Process: Assessment **Content Area:** Fundamentals **Strategy:** Recall that elevation of the head of the bed places the vessels above the level of the heart and that if vessels are distended, the client has fluid overload. **Reference:** Kozier, B., Erb, G., Berman, A., & Snyder, S. J. (2004). *Fundamentals of nursing: Concepts, process and practice* (7th ed.). Upper Saddle River, NJ: Pearson Education, p. 585.

7 Answer: 4 During physical assessment, the nurse inspects the client's legs for hair distribution. The most common reason for shiny skin and a complete absence of hair is poor circulation related to peripheral vascular disease (PVD). Thus the nursing diagnosis of impaired peripheral tissue perfusion applies. The other nursing diagnoses do not relate to or affect hair distribution. **Cognitive Level:** Analysis **Client Need:** Physiological Integrity: Physiological Adaptation **Integrated Process:** Nursing Process: Assessment **Content Area:** Fundamentals **Strategy:** The critical phrase is *absence of hair on legs.* Recall common abnormalities encountered in the client assessment and their usual etiologies to make the correct selection. Remember, one must have circulation in order to have hair growth. **Reference:** Kozier, B., Erb, G., Berman, A., & Snyder, S. J. (2004). *Fundamentals of nursing: Concepts, process and practice* (7th ed.). Upper Saddle River, NJ: Pearson Education, p. 587.

8 Answer: 1 The apical pulse should be auscultated for one full minute with the stethoscope at the 5th intercostal space in the midclavicular line (apex of the heart). While auscultating the apical pulse, the radial pulse should be palpated simultaneously to detect discrepancies caused by dysrhythmias. One radial pulse should be felt for each apical beat heard, but with some dysrhythmias, the radial pulsation is absent with early beats because of reduced stroke volume. Options 2 and 4 would not allow for simultaneous assessment of the apical and radial pulses. Option 3 is an incorrect location for cardiac auscultation. **Cognitive Level:** Application **Client Need:** Health Promotion and Maintenance **Integrated Process:** Nursing Process: Assessment **Content Area:** Fundamentals **Strategy:** Use knowledge of cardiac anatomy and basic assessment techniques to select the appropriate assessment technique. **Reference:** Kozier, B., Erb, G., Berman, A., & Snyder, S. J. (2004). *Fundamentals of nursing: Concepts, process and practice* (7th ed.). Upper Saddle River, NJ: Pearson Education, p. 503.

9 Answer: 3 The Bartholin glands are part of the female anatomy located on the posterior aspect of the vaginal orifice. Therefore, if the medical condition allows, having the client in a lithotomy position (on her back, knees flexed, legs apart, with feet supported on a surface or in stirrups) will provide the best opportunity for examination. The other responses do not allow for assessment of the female genitalia. **Cognitive Level:** Application **Client Need:** Health Promotion and Maintenance **Integrated Process:** Nursing Process: Assessment **Content Area:** Fundamentals **Strategy:** The core issue of the question is knowledge of what the Bartholin glands are and then determining the proper position for physical assessment. Recall that lithotomy

is the position of choice for examination of female genitalia except in the elderly, who may be placed in a side-lying position due to musculoskeletal deformities.
Reference: Kozier, B., Erb, G., Berman, A., & Snyder, S. J. (2004). *Fundamentals of nursing: Concepts, process and practice* (7th ed.). Upper Saddle River, NJ: Pearson Education, p. 615.

10 Answer: 2 In order to facilitate visualization of the ear canal and tympanic membrane, the pinna should be pulled up and back for an adult client. If earrings are attached to the lobe, there should not be a safety issue; however, they may be removed if they are large in size or are causing the client discomfort during the examination. The nurse should not remove cerumen with an applicator because of the risk of pushing it further into the canal or rupturing the tympanic membrane. Generally, the ear and eye physical assessment are performed with the client sitting upright.
Cognitive Level: Application **Client Need:** Health Promotion and Maintenance **Integrated Process:** Nursing Process: Assessment **Content Area:** Fundamentals **Strategy:** The adult is tall, so pull the pinna up and back, and children are short, so pull the pinna down and back.
Reference: Kozier, B., Erb, G., Berman, A., & Snyder, S. J. (2004). *Fundamentals of nursing: Concepts, process and practice* (7th ed.). Upper Saddle River, NJ: Pearson Education, p. 557.

References

Berman, A., Snyder, S., Kozier, B. & Erb, G. (2008). *Fundamentals of nursing: Concepts, process, and practice* (8th ed.) Upper Saddle River, NJ: Prentice Hall, pp. 526–665, 1196–2002.

Harkreader, H. & Hogan, M. (2004). *Fundamentals of nursing: Caring and clinical judgment* (2nd ed.). St. Louis, MO: Elseview Science, pp. 105–175.

Jarvis, C. (2004). *Physical examination and health assessment* (4th ed.). St. Louis, MO: pp. 83–105, 161–765.

LeMone, P. & Burke, K. (2004). *Medical surgical nursing: Critical thinking in client care* (3rd ed). Upper Saddle River, NJ: Prentice Hall, pp. 54–76.

Lewis, S., Heikkemper, M., & Dirksen, S. (2004). *Medical-surgical nursing; Assessment and management of clinical problems* (6th ed.). St. Louis, MO: Mosby, pp. 1–15, 30–43, 416–487, 688–697, 756–777, 946–969, 1152–1172, 1248–1268, 1339–1360, 1464–1491, 1635–1650.

Potter, P. & Perry, A. (2005). *Basic nursing: A critical thinking approach* (5th ed.). St. Louis, MO: Mosby, pp. 566–585.

ANSWERS & RATIONALES

3

Overview of Communication

Chapter Outline

Overview of Communication

Documenting and Reporting

Teaching and Learning

Objectives

➤ Describe the elements, levels, and forms of communication.

➤ Contrast effective and ineffective techniques of communication.

➤ Identify the purposes of maintaining a client's healthcare record.

➤ Discuss the purpose of documentation and legal guidelines used to document a client's health care.

➤ Review various methods used by nurses to record and report a client's healthcare status.

➤ Identify the standards and purposes associated with client teaching and learning.

➤ Identify the basic principles of teaching and learning.

➤ Describe teaching methods used based on the client's developmental level.

Review at a Glance

affective domain *learning in this domain involves feelings, emotions, interest, and attitudes*

charting by exception *a form of documentation in which only unanticipated client responses and events are documented; format is organized by problem (P), intervention (I), and evaluation (E)*

cognitive domain *learning in this domain involves processing information by listening or reading facts and descriptions; learning is a mental, intellectual, or thinking process*

communication *a two-way process involving the sending and receiving of messages*

critical pathways *multidisciplinary guidelines for client care based on specified medical diagnoses and designed to achieve predetermined outcomes*

documentation *information about a client recorded in the medical record either manually or using a computer*

feedback *the response or message that the receiver returns to the sender during communication*

focus charting *a method of charting that focuses on client strengths or on problems or needs*

health beliefs *concepts about health that an individual believes to be true*

health practice *an activity that a person carries out as a result of his or her health beliefs and definition of health*

Kardex *the trade name for a method that makes use of a series of cards to concisely organize and record client demographic data and instructions for daily nursing care*

narrative charting *a descriptive record of client data and nursing interventions, written in sentences and paragraphs*

nonverbal communication *communication other than words, including posture, gestures, and facial expressions*

problem-oriented medical record (POMR) *a record in which data about the client is written and arranged according to the client's problem, rather than according to the source of the information*

progress notes *chart entries using a variety of methods made by all health professionals involved in a client's care, for the purpose of describing client's problems, treatments, and progress toward desired outcomes*

psychomotor domain *learning in this domain involves learning by doing*

standards of care *detailed guidelines describing the minimal nursing care that can reasonably be expected to ensure high-quality care in a defined situation*

variance *a deviation from expected goal achievement using a critical pathway*

verbal communication *communication that involves the use of words in either written or oral form*

PRETEST

1 A nurse enters the room of a female client and asks how she is doing. The client states, "I'm a little nervous this morning." What would be the nurse's best reply?

1. "What is making you feel nervous?"
2. "You do look as if you are feeling nervous."
3. "Can I give you a backrub for your nerves?"
4. "Can you tell more about how you are feeling?"

2 A client tells the nurse that her husband is an alcoholic and hasn't worked for the last 3 months. The nurse's best initial response would be which of the following?

1. "Have you tried Al-Anon meetings?"
2. "I'm really sorry to hear that."
3. "You sound worried; perhaps you should talk to the chaplain."
4. "What have you done before to cope with his problem?"

3 Which of the following care approaches would be the most appropriate for the nurse to use when caring for an unresponsive comatose client?

1. Keep radio or TV on at a moderate volume at all times.
2. Avoid verbal communication while client appears unresponsive; focus instead on gentle touch and physical care measures.
3. Speak normally and as if client can hear and understand what is being said.
4. Direct verbal communication to family members at the bedside, providing them realistic updates on client's condition.

4 Using a mannequin, a nurse has demonstrated wound care for a client. To validate client learning, which of the following would be the best nursing action at this time?

1. Complete wound care on the client, explaining the procedure while performing it.
2. Show video explaining the sterile technique to be used for the client's wound care.
3. Have client perform wound care with the nurse present to supervise.
4. Ask client to review written client education literature and perform wound care at the next scheduled time.

5 Which of the following methods would be most effective for an ambulatory care nurse to use when trying to determine the priority health-related learning needs of a client?

1. Carefully review physician's orders.
2. Conduct a thorough nursing assessment.
3. Determine the amount of time required to present information.
4. Ask client what learning needs he or she has regarding current state of health.

6 An acute care nurse has to discharge to home a client who needs services from a home health nurse. What discharge information is most important for the acute care nurse to give to the referral agency nurse so that a plan of care can be developed?

1. Surgical report
2. Client's current self-care abilities
3. Vital signs on discharge
4. Time of last dose for medications administered

7 Which of the following items of information would be important for the nurse to include in an intershift report? Select all that apply.

1. Client still needs to demonstrate that he/she can do a dressing change before being discharged.
2. Client has had several family members in to visit today.
3. Client is on bed rest with bathroom privileges.
4. Diet was changed from NPO (nothing by mouth) to clear liquids two hours ago.
5. Client was transported to radiology in a wheelchair for a chest x-ray at 10 A.M.

8 Which of the following statements heard by a nurse during preparation of an intershift report provides the most useful information related to priority setting for the upcoming shift?

1. A client who had catheter removed eight hours ago has not urinated.
2. A client is alert and oriented to person and place.
3. A client who is 3 days postoperative is experiencing incisional pain rated a 6 on a scale of 1 to 10.
4. A client admitted for congestive heart failure has a blood pressure of 146/84.

9 The quality improvement nurse reads several nurses' notes from different records that refer to clients' moods. Examples are that the client "is in good spirits today," "feels depressed today," and "is withdrawn today." Based on these pieces of documentation, which of the following actions would be best for the quality improvement nurse to take?

1. Communicate findings to nursing administration.
2. Report findings to Joint Commission on Accreditation of Healthcare Organizations.
3. Communicate findings to the agency's Nursing Staff Development Department.
4. Do nothing, as this is acceptable documentation practice.

10 Before going off duty, a nurse reviews the notes written for a client and discovers that there has been an omission of important assessment findings. Which nursing action is most appropriate at this time?

1. Insert omitted data in the appropriate area.
2. Recopy the entire section, include missing data, and throw the original away.
3. Record the time of the entry, time of the assessment, and missing data and label as "late entry."
4. Verbally relay the assessment finding during intershift report and leave the record unchanged.

➤ *See pages 82–83 for Answers & Rationales.*

I. OVERVIEW OF COMMUNICATION

A. Effective *communication* occurs when there is an exchange of information, ideas, attitudes, and emotions; therefore, successful communication occurs when the message intended is the message received

B. Effective communication is a basic skill in providing health care to clients; nurses communicate with other healthcare providers and healthcare consumers (clients) and their support systems (family, significant others)

C. The nurse needs to understand the basic elements of communication that tend to promote accurate dissemination of information as well as elements that may inhibit successful communication so that the client receives effective health care

D. A therapeutic helping relationship is enhanced by the nurse's ability to care for and comfort clients with an empathetic understanding and other strategies

E. Phases of the therapeutic relationship

1. Pre-interaction phase

a. Occurs prior to initial contact with a client and is similar to the planning stage before an interview

b. Any information that the nurse has related to the client is organized and analyzed prior to contact with the client; during this phase the nurse prepares for initial contact

2. Orientation phase

a. May also be called the introductory phase or prehelping phase

b. During this phase the nurse and client get to know one another and develop a degree of trust

c. The three processes that occur during this phase are opening the relationship, clarifying the problem, and structuring and formulating the contract

3. Working phase

a. Includes exploring and understanding thoughts and feelings, along with facilitating and taking action

b. Skills required during this phase are empathetic listening and understanding, respect, genuineness, concreteness, and confrontation

c. At the completion of this phase the client makes decisions and takes action, while the nurse provides information, collaborates, and is supportive of the client

4. Termination phase

a. During this phase, the nurse and client have reached their goals and conclude their communication

b. This phase may be difficult for both the nurse and client; to reduce feelings of loss and ambivalence, the nurse summarizes the relationship and may make follow-up phone calls to help the client transition to independence

c. The nurse should prepare the client for the termination phase early in the communication process

F. Elements of communication

1. Sender

   a. Sometimes referred to as the *encoder;* is the person or group who initiates the communication in order to convey information, thoughts, ideas, or feelings to another

   b. The sender encodes the information by selecting the signs and symbols used in the communication (language, word selection, voice intonations, gestures, etc.)

2. Message

   a. Is the information to be communicated and includes the codings (vocabulary, tone of voice, body language, and way the message is transmitted)

   b. Effective communication occurs when the message intended is the message received

3. Channel

   a. The *channel* or *medium* or is the vehicle used to convey the message and can target any of the five senses; e.g., written documentation (sight), oral communication (hearing), and therapeutic touch

   b. It is important that the nurse use the correct medium to send the message; for example, it may be necessary to write the message for a client who is hearing impaired to ensure the message intended is the message received

4. Receiver

   a. Is the person or group that the message is intended for, also referred to as the *decoder* of the message

   b. The decoder or receiver perceives or interprets the message

5. Environment

   a. Is the set of physical, cultural, and social conditions in which the information is transmitted

   b. This is sometimes referred to as the *context* of the communication

6. **Feedback** (sometimes referred to as *response*)

   a. Requires that the receiver respond to the message communicated by the sender; the response may be verbal or nonverbal

   b. The nature of the response helps to determine whether communication was effective or ineffective

G. Levels of communication

1. Intrapersonal: *intra-* is a prefix meaning "within"; this level of communication refers to communication that occurs within oneself and happens constantly; it involves thinking about a message before it is sent, interpreting the message, and evaluating the message (self-talk)

2. Interpersonal: *inter-* is a prefix meaning "between"; this level of communication refers to communication occurring between people and involves the sending and receiving of a message and feedback

3. Public communication: involves sending a message to a group of people for the dissemination of information; it generally does not require feedback

H. Forms of communication

1. Communication occurs both verbally and nonverbally in a therapeutic relationship; purposeful communication between nurse and client is often termed *therapeutic communication*

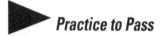

Practice to Pass

An unconscious client with a closed head injury has been admitted to the intensive care unit following a motor vehicle accident. How should the nurse respond to this client to promote effective communication?

2. The nurse needs to be aware of the form of communication chosen to ensure the message sent is the message received

   a. For instance, if the nurse's body language indicates the verbal information given is not important, then the client will also view it as unimportant

   b. Using a different example, if the nurse invades the client's territorial space, then the client may not be able to focus on the message sent

3. **Verbal communication:** involves the use of words that are either spoken or written

   a. *Therapeutic rapport:* verbal communication can be facilitated by a trusting relationship between the nurse and the client, in which the client believes that the nurse cares about the client's well-being and want to assist the client in meeting health-related goals

   b. *Pacing:* the rhythm and speed with which the verbal message is sent can have an impact on the way that the words of the message are received; the pace may indicate interest, disinterest, or anxiety, among others

   c. *Intonation:* the pattern of pauses and accents or stresses when sending a message can also impact on how it is received; it can reflect an underlying mood of the sender, such as anger, boredom, excitement, etc.

   d. *Clarity/brevity:* clear and brief messages are more likely to be interpreted correctly by the receiver than, vague and lengthy messages; the clarity of a message is influenced by congruence between the content of the message and the nurse's body language (nonverbal behavior)

   e. *Timing/relevance:* messages need to be delivered at a time when the client is interested in receiving them and the content of the message needs to be of interest to the client at the time the communication is taking place; for example, a client newly diagnosed with diabetes may not be interested in listening to information about a diabetic diet if relatives from out of state have just arrived for a visit

4. **Nonverbal communication:** communication that occurs without the use of words; is often referred to as body language

   a. Facial expressions: can either convey or mask emotions; cautiously interpret eye and facial movements and validate these impressions with further assessment before drawing final conclusions; some expressions are more universal, such as a smile for happiness and a frown for displeasure

   b. Eye contact: can be influenced by cultural norms; avoiding eye contact may be culturally appropriate or can indicate other feelings, such as embarrassment or lack of interest in communicating

   c. Gestures: can convey the urgency of a client's message or can be a coping response when an urgent message cannot be expressed quickly enough using words; some gestures (such as a wave) have almost universal meanings while others are culture specific; gestures can also be used as signals when a client cannot communicate with words

   d. Posture/gait: can indicate a client's physical well-being, self-concept, and mood

      1) An erect posture and a steady purposeful gait generally indicate a sense of well-being

      2) Slouching or a shuffling slow gait may indicate depressed mood or being physically tired or uncomfortable

      3) A client who guards the abdomen or who is lying down with knees drawn up to the chest is most likely experiencing pain

    4) Be sure to validate with the client any impressions gained from observing his or her posture and gait

  e. Territoriality and space

    1) All people, clients and nurses alike, have a physical zone around the body that is considered an extension of self and that should not be entered by others, often referred to as *personal space*

    2) The size of the space can vary considerably from culture to culture and even person to person

    3) Often other forms of body language are used as signals to indicate when someone has violated personal space (such as taking a step back or holding up a hand in front of the person)

  f. Personal appearance

    1) Can be a general indicator of self-esteem, social status, emotional status, culture or other group association

    2) Selection of clothing is often highly personal

    3) Hygiene may be influenced by physical ability, emotional status, mental illness, energy level, and time

    4) Be careful not to judge clients on the basis of personal appearance

I. Effective communication techniques

  1. *Using silence:* allows for quiet time without conversation for several seconds or minutes to allow for reflection about a discussion that just occurred, to reduce tension, or to gather thoughts about how to proceed

  2. *Offering self:* offers the nurse's presence without attaching any expectations or conditions about the client's behavior during that time

  3. *Restating or paraphrasing:* ensures the nurse understands the message sent; consists of verbalizing the main thought of the message sent

  4. *Clarifying:* asks for additional information to ensure understanding of the message sent; a statement like "Would you tell me more about what you have just said?" indicates that understanding the client's message is important to the nurse

  5. *Focusing:* draws the client's attention to pertinent information and helps the client expand on that information; this technique directs the client toward information that is important

  6. *Acknowledging:* gives nonjudgmental recognition to a client for a certain behavior or contribution, or indicates attention to and care of the client

  7. *Reflecting:* redirects the content of a client's message back to the client for further thought or consideration

  8. *Giving information:* provides specific information to a client either with or without the client's request

  9. *Summarizing:* may be used at the end of an interaction to identify material discussed; it helps to sort out relevant information from irrelevant

J. Communication techniques to avoid

  1. *Self-disclosure*

    a. Involves relating to a client by communicating a personal experience to the client that focuses the relationship on the nurse

    b. For instance, if a client is having difficulty adjusting to an altered body image related to an amputation, it is not helpful for the nurse to communicate how he or she would feel if faced with a similar problem

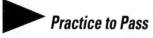

Practice to Pass

A client who has chest pain has been brought to the Emergency Department. The client is acutely intoxicated, angry, and belligerent. How should the nurse proceed?

  c. The therapeutic helping relationship should be client-centered and goal-directed

 2. *Inattentive listening*

  a. Inattentive listening blocks communication by indicating that the client's needs are not important

  b. A nurse who is thinking about another client when providing care to an individual will seem distracted and uncaring

 3. *Overuse of medical jargon*

  a. Overuse of medical jargon confuses clients and indicates the nurse is not interested in ensuring healthcare information is understood

  b. For instance, if the nurse asks the client how many times he/she has voided and the client does not understand the word *void,* the client may not know what the appropriate response should be

 4. *Giving personal opinions*

  a. Expressing one's opinion may give the impression that a person is closed to new ideas; in a helping relationship, clients need to manage their own lives and problems and should be assisted to formulate their own ideas and plans

  b. Giving advice needs to be avoided

 5. *Prying*

  a. Prying or probing techniques only provide information to satisfy the nurse's curiosity

  b. If a client states that a problem was not discussed with the healthcare provider and the nurse asks, "Why not?" it may place the client in a defensive position

  c. Asking for information not pertinent to the client's health status actually violates the client's right to privacy

 6. *Changing the subject*

  a. Changing the subject blocks therapeutic communication by indicating that the client should not continue to talk about the previous topic; this leads the conversation to only those areas that the nurse wants to discuss

  b. For instance, if a female client asks if her breast will be removed because of a tumor, and the nurse asks if she has had a bowel movement since admission, this implies the nurse's unwillingness to discuss the client's concern

K. Communicating with clients who have special needs

 1. Difficulty hearing

  a. To ensure that effective communication occurs with a client who is hearing-impaired, stand or sit near to the client and speak clearly and slowly using a low-pitched voice

  b. The environment should have adequate lighting and be quiet and free from distractions

  c. Use therapeutic communication techniques to ensure that the message sent is the message received

  d. It may also be necessary to use writing to enhance communication with a client who is hearing impaired

  e. Avoid using a loud voice when speaking to a client who is hearing impaired; instead, speak directly into the ear that has better hearing

2. Difficulty seeing

a. When communicating with a visually impaired client, ensure the environment has adequate light

b. Ensure that the quality of the spoken word matches the message communicated

c. Remember that the visually impaired client may not have the ability to use nonverbal cues to help interpret the message

3. Mute/unable to speak clearly

a. When communicating with a client who is unable to speak clearly, has an artificial airway, or is mute, encourage the client to write a response or utilize word boards or pictures to ensure effective communication

b. Utilize the therapeutic technique of clarification or paraphrasing as needed to assist in communication

4. Cognitively impaired

a. When communicating with a client who is cognitively impaired, use language that is simple and concise, and speak words slowly and calmly

b. Verbalize only one thought or question at a time to allow the client to focus on the message

c. Allow adequate time for the client to process the information

d. Use environmental cues when possible to convey the message to the client; for instance, holding a toothbrush for the client to see while asking if he/she would like to brush the teeth helps the client understand the message

5. Unresponsive

a. When communicating with an unresponsive person, use touch along with the spoken word and try to elicit a response from the client

b. Asking a closed question such as, "Can you hear me?" and observing for nonverbal cues that may indicate the client has received the message is one way to elicit a response

c. Speak to the client in a manner that assumes the client can hear every word that is spoken; avoid having conversations about the client's status or that are irrelevant to the client at the bedside

6. Non–English speaking

a. Seek an interpreter fluent in the client's primary language if the client does not speak English; until an interpreter is available, communicate through nonverbal means

b. Use pictures, environmental cues, and body language to communicate with a client who speaks a different language

c. For procedures requiring informed consent, follow agency policy to obtain an approved interpreter before explaining procedure and obtaining client signature

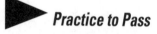

Practice to Pass

A nurse needs to complete an admission assessment on a hearing-impaired client. How should the nurse proceed?

II. DOCUMENTING AND REPORTING

A. Documentation

1. The act of making an entry in the client's medical record is referred to as **documentation** or charting

2. Communicating healthcare information is an important aspect of providing nursing care

3. The client record (medical record) provides a description of the nursing and medical care received by the client

4. The information should be written clearly, concisely, and accurately; it should be factual and free of personal opinions or judgments

5. The record is a written or computer-based legal documentation of the client's health status that includes the client's healthcare problems, treatment, and responses

B. **Purpose of records**

1. Communication tool for healthcare team

   a. The record serves as a means of communication between nursing personnel and other care providers to plan a client's health care

   b. Communication among healthcare professionals is essential in providing care to clients and prevents fragmentation, repetition, and delays in client care

2. Legal document

   a. The record is a legal document that provides verification of the quality of care that a client receives

   b. All information in the client record is confidential and access to the record is restricted to only those health professionals involved in the client's care

3. Financial billing

   a. Documentation of health care received by the client is also a means for reimbursement for services provided

   b. Before the client's record can be released to insurance companies, the client must authorize in writing what portions of the record to release

4. Education

   a. Healthcare students may also use documentation for educational purposes by comparing actual cases to textbook cases

   b. Educators may use client records as a source for teaching students

   c. A review of the medical records may indicate a need for continuing education for the nursing staff or other healthcare providers

   d. It is important that records used for educational purposes protect clients' privacy at all times

5. Assessment: health records help an agency identify services utilized by clients in order to plan for staffing, educational, and fiscal needs

6. Research: the record may also provide vital statistics and data for research purposes to improve treatment protocols, identify frequency of diseases, and causes of death; client identifying information must be removed

7. Auditing and monitoring

   a. Medical records serve as a source by which to evaluate health care received by clients to ensure quality care

   b. *Quality improvement* refers to evaluation of the level of care provided in a healthcare agency and can be done internally or externally

   c. These auditing procedures are completed to ensure continuity of care and that healthcare standards are being met by the institution; the Joint Commission on the Accreditation of Healthcare Organizations (JCAHO) is an example of an accrediting agency; **standards of care** are detailed guidelines that describe minimal nursing care needed to ensure high-quality care in a defined situation

C. Common forms used in written or electronic documentation

1. Admission nursing assessment: a comprehensive form that is organized according to a specific scheme, such as body systems, functional abilities, health problems, a nursing model, or type of unit (labor and delivery versus surgical); it may also be called an admission database or nursing history

2. Client care plans (nursing or interdisciplinary): individualized care plans or standardized care plans (plans that address the usual needs of a client with an identified health problem)

3. **Kardex** or clinical worksheet: lists demographic data, including allergies, medications ordered, IV fluids ordered, currently ordered treatments and procedures, scheduled diagnostic or laboratory tests, and orders or data for meeting basic needs (diet, self-feeding ability, activity, safety, hygiene, and elimination), and possibly a problem list; a Kardex may or may not be part of the permanent client record

4. Flowsheets: forms that cluster specific data in one place for easy reference, to assess trends in data, or to document care; these include vital signs, blood glucose, intake and output, medication record, or daily nursing care; some agencies combine many of these onto one large flowsheet that is used for a 24-hour period

5. Progress notes: provide information about client progress in meeting health goals; are more fully described in a section to follow

6. Nursing discharge or referral summaries: include a concise summary of the course of hospitalization or treatment, resolved and unresolved health problems, current treatments and medications (including time of last dose), functional abilities for activities of daily living, activity restrictions, comfort level, client education completed, referrals to other healthcare providers, and discharge destination (home, rehabilitation facility, long-term care facility) and mode of transport (ambulatory, wheelchair, stretcher/ambulance)

D. Guidelines for legal documentation

1. Documentation is a form of verbal communication because words are used for the exchange of information

2. Use words that are clear, easy to read, and complete

3. Be aware that documentation will stand alone without the benefit of nonverbal communication; avoid words with unclear meanings

4. The client's chart documents the client's healthcare problems, needs, and services; it truly provides the total picture of the client's health care

5. Follow these guidelines when making notations in the client's healthcare record:

   a. Accurate: documentation should include facts and observations rather than the nurse's opinions, judgments, or interpretation of the client's behavior

   b. Complete: documentation should include all relevant aspects of care, including assessments, interventions, client comments, client response to care (including nursing care, diagnostic tests, and therapeutic procedures), progress toward goal achievement, care that was omitted with reasons why and who was notified, and the substance of any communication with other disciplines

   c. Current: documentation should be done as soon as care is provided whenever possible and should reflect the client's present condition; late entries must be so noted

    d. Organized: documentation should have a logical flow of ideas; pieces of information that relate to each other should be grouped together; this includes proper sequencing of information and events

    e. Appropriateness: documentation should only include information that relates to the client's current healthcare status and care being delivered; inclusion of irrelevant personal information about the client can be considered an invasion of privacy (at the least) or to be libelous (at worst)

    f. Agency policies: documentation should be consistent with all agency policies, which often includes that each note contain date and time of charting; be legible; use permanent ink, correct spelling, approved style of documentation (see section to follow on methods of recording), and proper terminology; contain a signature

6. Pitfalls of documentation

    a. Writing illegibly: interpreting notes that are written illegibly may be difficult or impossible to do either in present time or at a later date; it is important to write carefully so everyone understands the contents of the note

    b. Leaving blank lines: provides an opportunity for someone to insert information at a later date; is generally inconsistent with healthcare agency policies on documentation; use a pen to draw a line through blank lines of a page and draw on "X" through blank portions of a page for the same reason

    c. Altering someone else's notes: the record is a legal document and entries must not be altered once recorded; a separate entry can be made to record own observations or care if needed

    d. Back-dating records: do not back-date late entries; instead include the date and time of the actual charting as well as the date and time of the original observations or care being recorded; for example, if an event that happened at 10:30 was going to be charted at 11:15 and a notation was already made at 11:00, then the entry should be made for 11:15 with the words *Addendum 10:30* at the beginning of the note

    e. Correcting errors incorrectly: agency policy dictates how to correct a mistaken entry; this usually includes drawing a single line through the error and writing *error* or *void* above it with the nurse's initials; the purpose of the single line is to maintain the legibility of the words under the line

    f. Inserting information between lines: should be avoided; new or omitted information should be added as an addendum note

    g. Documenting for someone else: should not be done; each nurse should document own observations and care and be legally accountable for own entries

    h. Expressing opinions: is not advisable; documentation should contain facts and observations; opinions that could be interpreted as negative or prejudicial could be libelous

    i. Using unmeasurable terms: tends to make documentation vague; notes should reflect clarity and brevity (use as few words as possible)

    j. Failing to document communication with other healthcare members regarding client care: all aspects of care (including communications) that have an impact on the client's health status must be documented; the familiar saying "If it wasn't documented, it wasn't done" applies to this situation as well as many others in nursing practice

Practice to Pass

The nurse documents a note for one client in another client's medical record. What action should the nurse take to correct the error?

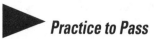

Practice to Pass

What principles of documentation should the nurse follow every time an entry is made in the client's record?

E. Methods of recording

1. Narrative charting

   a. Is considered a source-oriented record whereby each department has a separate section in the record

   b. Provides documentation of the total health status of the client, including nursing interventions received, treatments performed on the client, and the client's reaction to the care received

   c. Is generally written in chronological order; this format is time-consuming because a complete head-to toe-assessment is usually documented every shift

   d. Makes it sometimes difficult to focus on the client's pertinent problem(s) because all routine care and normal assessment findings are integrated with the documentation about problems

2. Problem-oriented medical record (POMR)

   a. Data is arranged according to the problems a client has rather than the source of information

   b. Each health professional involved in the client's care contributes to a given list of client problems

   c. The POMR has four basic components, including the database, problem list, plan of care, and **progress notes** (a written narrative of client progress, treatments, and other important information)

   d. Notes may be written using SOAP (subjective, objective, assessment, plan), APIE (assessment, problem, intervention, evaluation), or PIE (problem, intervention, evaluation) format

3. Charting by exception

   a. Charting by exception is a form of documentation whereby only the exceptions to the rule are documented; notes may follow PIE format

   b. The information may be documented in narrative form, but often several standardized flow sheets are used to simplify documentation of the client's health status

   c. The PIE system eliminates the traditional care plan and incorporates an ongoing care plan into the progress notes

   d. Standards of care may be preselected or preprinted and included in the client's medical record; these may also be individualized as needed to provide quality nursing care

4. Focus charting

   a. This method focuses on client needs that deviate from the normal

   b. The intent of this format is to make the client's needs and strengths the focus of care that results in a holistic approach for nursing

   c. The progress notes are organized into data (D), action (A), and response (R) categories

5. Critical pathways

   a. Critical pathways (clinical pathways, care maps) are a set of documentation forms that identify outcome criteria that certain groups are expected to achieve on each day of care

   b. This format is based on cost-effective care delivered within an established length of stay

      c. An example of an outcome criterion is that a client having a laparoscopic cholecystectomy is afebrile for the first 24 hours after surgery; if this client develops a fever, this would be a **variance** or a goal not met and would be recorded as such

  6. Computerized charting

      a. Computer systems are becoming more popular in healthcare facilities for maintaining client records, which often includes nursing documentation

      b. Nurses use computers to store clients' databases, add new data, create and revise care plans, document medication administration, and document overall client progress

      c. Computerization of the client's medical record in some healthcare institutions has made the transfer of the client from one setting to another relatively easy

      d. Benefits of computer-driven records include legibility of records and more efficient use of nurses' time

F. Reporting: refers to the transfer of information from nurses to nurses, or from nurses to other members of the healthcare team; can be written or oral in form

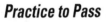

  1. Oral change-of-shift (intershift) report

      a. An oral report is given to all nurses on the next shift for the purpose of ensuring continuity of care; may take place in a designated private area or utilize a walking rounds format

      b. The report should be organized, concise, and efficient

      c. The report should include:

         1) Demographics: client's name, age, hospital day, room number, and physician

         2) Medical diagnosis

         3) General physical and psychological condition as well as any changes in condition

         4) New physician orders

         5) Scheduled diagnostic test or therapies

         6) Dietary modifications and fluid requirements

         7) Activities permitted

         8) Client teaching needs

         9) Nursing diagnoses

         10) Safety needs

         11) Other information pertinent to the client's healthcare needs

  2. Tape-recorded intershift report

      a. Some agencies utilize a tape recorder to provide nurses with an intershift report

      b. The elements of a taped report are the same as for an oral report

      c. It is important for nurses who utilize this method to recognize that the verbal communication must be accurate and detailed because the oncoming nurses may not be able to ask questions, and there is minimal opportunity for feedback

      d. Procedures for maintaining confidentiality of material recorded on the tape and for destroying or erasing information on the tape must be followed; concerns about confidentiality are making this a less popular method in several healthcare agencies

▶ Practice to Pass

A nurse is preparing to give a report to staff members coming on duty. What information needs to be reported to ensure the continuity of care?

3. Written intershift report

   a. Some agencies have implemented written reports in lieu of oral or taped reports

   b. The information conveyed is the same as for other types of report

   c. Agency-specific or unit-specific forms are developed and utilized

   d. A benefit is that the nurse has immediate access to all previous written reports from the time of the client's admission for easy retrieval of information in an efficient manner

   e. A new report is written at the end of each shift and all forms are passed on to the oncoming nurse

   f. Upon discharge or transfer, shift reports are disposed of or shredded according to agency policy

III. TEACHING AND LEARNING

A. Standards for client education (see Box 3-1)

B. Purposes of client teaching

1. Maintenance and promotion of health and illness prevention

   a. Examples include prenatal classes, immunization requirements, nutrition, exercise, and parenting

   b. Generally these programs are aimed towards groups of people with a health-care need and designed to disseminate information and skills needed for clients to develop positive **health practices** (personal habits or behaviors that promote health)

2. Restoration of health

   a. These programs are intended for clients with an active health problem and focus on the cause, condition, and/or treatment

   b. An example of this type of client teaching would be insulin administration for a client that has new onset type 1 (formerly insulin-dependent) diabetes

3. Coping with impaired functioning

   a. This type of client teaching centers around providing instruction to an individual who has not made or cannot make a complete recovery

   b. An example is a client who modifies activities of daily living because of a lower limb amputation

C. Domains of learning

1. Cognitive learning involves acquiring and using knowledge; for instance, when teaching a parenting class, the nurse provides information on the developmental stages of children; applying that knowledge to toilet training the child, the parent is learning in the **cognitive domain**

2. Affective learning occurs when a client changes unhealthy attitudes or feelings and values; a parent who accepts and understands that children have specific developmental stages and may not become toilet trained until after the age of 2 is learning in the **affective domain**

3. Psychomotor: learning to complete a physical act is learning in the **psychomotor domain;** a client learning to self-administer injections is an example of learning in this domain

Box 3-1	➤ The client's learning needs, abilities, preferences, and readiness to learn are assessed.

Joint Commission for the Accreditation of Healthcare Organizations (JCAHO) Client and Family Education Standards

➤ The client's learning needs, abilities, preferences, and readiness to learn are assessed.

➤ The assessment considers cultural and religious practices, emotional barriers, desire and motivation to learn, physical and cognitive limitations, language barriers, and the financial implications of care choices.

➤ When called for by the age of the client and the length of stay, the hospital assesses and provides for client's academic and educational needs.

➤ Clients are educated about the safe and effective use of medication according to law and their needs.

➤ Clients are educated about potential drug-food interactions and are provided counseling on nutrition and modified diets.

➤ Clients are educated about rehabilitation techniques to help them adapt or function more independently in their environment.

➤ Clients are informed about access to additional resources in the community.

➤ Clients are informed about when and how to obtain any further treatment they may need.

Modified from Joint Commission on Accreditation of Healthcare Organizations: Accreditation manual of hospitals, Chicago, 1997, The Commission.

D. Factors that influence client learning

1. Motivation

   a. Motivation is the desire to learn; important to learning is that the client recognizes the need to learn a new behavior

   b. Nurses can assist a client in solving problems and identifying needs that may increase his or her desire to learn

2. Health beliefs

   a. A client's health beliefs may or may not be congruent with the information being taught

   b. The nurse may assist a client in this way by showing a cause and effect type of relationship between negative health practices and poor health outcomes; for example, if the cardiac client believes that smoking will worsen his/her cardiac status, the individual may be more likely to stop smoking

   c. Nurses need to assess a client's healthcare beliefs in order to develop beneficial teaching plans

   d. Nurses need to be aware that a client's healthcare beliefs may not change, despite concentrated efforts, because of multiple psychological, cultural, and environmental factors

3. Psychosocial adaptation to illness

   a. Psychosocial adaptation to illness describes the transition from a healthy independent state to an illness state

   b. Successful adaptation depends on the client's emotional makeup

   c. It is important for the nurse to understand that a client is unlikely to learn new health-related behaviors when he/she is not ready or motivated to learn, or experiencing problems unrelated to his or her health

   d. The nurse should assess how a client is adapting on a regular basis

4. Active participation

    a. Active participation by the client in the teaching/learning process makes learning more meaningful

    b. The nurse needs to assess a client's learning needs and to involve the client in the learning process to make this happen

5. Literacy level/educational level: ability of the client to read materials provided and understand the spoken word

6. Developmental level

7. Individual learning style: learning is enhanced when the nurse uses instructional methods that match the client's preferred learning style (such as visual, auditory, kinesthetic)

E. Basic teaching principles

1. *Set priorities:* the client and nurse rank the client's learning needs according to importance; it is imperative the nurse involve the client in ranking needs because learning is more likely to occur when the needs perceived by the client are met

2. *Use appropriate timing:* plan the period of time between when the client receives information and actively uses that information; for example, a client with diabetes is more likely to successfully administer insulin immediately after watching a video, rather than waiting until the next morning

3. *Organize materials:* learning occurs from simple to complex; it is important that the material be organized in this manner to allow the learner to assimilate information more readily

4. *Promote/maintain learner attention and participation:* learning is enhanced if the environment is comfortable and free from distractions, and if there is opportunity for client feedback; involve the client actively in the learning process to facilitate assimilation of information; ensure the client is physically comfortable to help maintain client attention; ensure that the information is personally relevant to the client

5. *Build on existing knowledge:* assess the client's knowledge of the material to be presented before beginning client teaching; when the nurse builds on the client's existing knowledge, the material becomes more personal to the client, learning is enhanced and the learner's confidence is increased

6. *Select appropriate teaching methods*

    a. Discussion: one-on-one formal or informal instruction allows the client to set the pace of learning and engage in verbal exchange with the nurse; promotes customized learning for the client

    b. Question and answer: meets the needs of clients for specific pieces of information as requested by the client; often beneficial as a follow-up to other teaching methods

    c. Role-play, discovery: a creative strategy that allows the client to simulate real-life situations and apply new knowledge or skills in an artificial or "safe" setting; helps to build the client's confidence in newly acquired knowledge and skills once feelings of being shy, embarrassed, or awkward are worked through

    d. Computerized instruction: can include CAI (computer-assisted instruction) or interactive computer programs (using touch-screen technology) to more actively engage the client in the process; allows the client to regulate the pace of

► Practice to Pass

A 16-year-old client is to check the blood glucose level every 8 hours after discharge from the hospital. What does the nurse have to consider when designing a teaching plan for this client?

the instruction and may allow the client to direct the nature of the material that is presented next (interactive programs)

7. *Use appropriate teaching aids:* these are useful supplements to instruction if they are well-selected in terms of the content and the client's learning style; may include visual aids (drawings, charts, models, printed materials), audiotapes, films or videotapes, programmed instruction, games, and others

8. *Provide teaching related to developmental level*

a. Infant

1) Guidelines for health promotion teaching for this age group include immunizations, infant safety, nutrition, rest/sleep patterns, and sensory stimulation

2) It is important for the nurse to assess the parents' learning needs and provide instruction accordingly

3) Choose to complete client teaching when the infant is calm and happy to minimize the parents' distraction

b. Toddler

1) Guidelines for health promotion teaching for this age group include accident prevention, toilet training, dental hygiene, and appropriate play activities

2) Toddlers fear pain and separation from parents

3) Parent teaching for a hospitalized toddler includes participation in the care the child receives, purpose of care plans, and developmental regression that can occur as a result of hospitalization

c. Preschooler

1) Health promotion teaching for a preschooler includes accident prevention, dental health, nutrition, cognitive stimulation, and sleep patterns

2) The nurse can assist the hospitalized preschooler by using visual, tactile, and auditory images to decrease a toddler's fear of procedures

3) Use of therapeutic play is also important to this age group; using dolls or puppets to demonstrate procedures prior to their being done is also helpful to the child

d. School-age

1) Health promotion teaching for the school-age child includes dental hygiene, safety measures, promotion of physical fitness, and hygiene measures to prevent the spread of infection

2) Nurses can assist the hospitalized school-age child by providing concrete examples and explanations of procedures to help the child understand health care

3) Encourage the child to identify his/her own learning needs; forms of play may assist the child to learn as well

e. Adolescent

1) Health promotion teaching for this age group includes information about the effects of drugs and alcohol, sexually transmitted infections, reducing risk of injury (e.g., motor vehicle accidents, sports), nutrition, and reducing exposure to sun

2) Actively involve the adolescent in learning to help him or her assimilate the information provided

3) Client contracting and peer education also promote learning

     f. Young/middle-aged adult

       1) Health promotion teaching for this age group may include importance of routine health tests and screening, sun protection measures, importance of nutrition (especially adequate protein and calcium intake), and exercise to maintain health

       2) It is important that the nurse evaluate the client's learning needs and determine learning needs that the client believes are important to maintain his or her health

     g. Older adult

       1) Health promotion teaching for this age group includes importance of exercise in maintaining joint mobility, nutritional information (including caloric and fluid requirements), and fall prevention information

       2) The nurse should ensure there is adequate lighting and should use large print if necessary for the client who is visually impaired

       3) If the client is hearing impaired, the nurse should use written teaching materials, and it may be necessary to utilize visual aids

Case Study

An 80-year-old man is being discharged from the hospital with the medical diagnosis of neurogenic bladder. His physician has ordered self-catheterization three times a day. He lives with his daughter but is very independent. He is also very religious and went to church daily prior to becoming ill. The daughter reported that in addition to going to church he used to volunteer at the local school, mentoring high school students for 2 hours each day. She added that since he developed the bladder problem, he hasn't left the house and has talked more about dying.

1. Devise a teaching plan for this client and describe how to document the client teaching provided.

2. What information is necessary to assess prior to presenting the teaching plan?

3. How might the nurse approach the client to discuss end-of-life issues and possible increasing dependency issues?

For suggested responses, see pages 335–336.

4. From the information provided identify possible nursing diagnoses for this client and specify the supporting case study information.

5. Identify criteria that can be used to evaluate client outcomes based on the nursing diagnoses identified.

POSTTEST

1 A nurse observes a client pacing the halls, and it appears as if the client has been crying. What is the most appropriate action by the nurse?

1. Consider the behavior as a normal reaction to illness.

2. Validate perceptions with the client.

3. Discuss the client's actions with another nurse for verification.

4. Discuss the morning schedule with the client to decrease apprehension.

2 What would be the best approach for the nurse to use when a client conveys anxiety immediately prior to surgery? Select all that apply.

1. Reassure the client of the surgeon's competency.
2. Provide teaching about the surgical procedure.
3. Explore the client's feelings with him or her.
4. Relate the nurse's personal experience of having a similar surgery.
5. Check on the client frequently until the client is transported to the operating room.

3 A nurse is preparing to complete an admission assessment on a client who is partially hearing impaired. What would be the best approach for the nurse to use?

1. Request that a family member be present.
2. Prepare written questions that cover the assessment criteria.
3. Speak slowly in a low-pitched voice while facing the client.
4. Perform only the physical assessment at this time.

4 A client states, "I am so sick, I know I am going to die." The best way for the nurse to document this data would be to write:

1. Client is depressed today.
2. Client thinks he is going to die.
3. Client is frustrated with being sick.
4. Client states, "I am so sick, I know I am going to die."

5 A 68-year-old female client needs to learn how to take her pulse before taking prescribed heart medication. Before beginning the client teaching, the nurse should evaluate which of the following about the client?

1. Cardiac status
2. Reading ability
3. Psychomotor abilities
4. Motivation to attain optimal wellness

6 A nurse can best evaluate a client's ability to self-administer insulin by using which of the following methods?

1. Have the client write the procedure.
2. Demonstrate the techniques on a mannequin.
3. Have the client tell the nurse the steps to take when administering the insulin.
4. Observe the client self-administering an insulin dose.

7 Which of the following behaviors by a client indicates to the nurse that learning in the cognitive domain has taken place?

1. Explaining the rationale for taking a new medication
2. Actively demonstrating the new skill
3. Telling the nurse he has accepted the illness and its effects on lifestyle
4. Physically demonstrating insulin injections

8 Which of the following options would be typical outcome criteria likely to appear on a critical pathway for a postoperative appendectomy client?

1. Morphine sulfate 6 mg IM Q 4 hours prn for pain
2. Limit visitors at the bedside to immediate family.
3. Client will be afebrile within 24 hours after surgery.
4. Encourage ambulation and self-care after breakfast.

9 In order to provide care to clients, the nurse would give high priority to which information received in intershift report?

1. Physical assessment data and client response to care
2. Client's list of active and resolved problems and associated medical treatments
3. Physician visits and new orders
4. Intake/output data and vital signs

10 Charting by exception is used by a hospital for documentation. Using this format, how would the nurse document routine morning care in the narrative notes?

1. Morning care completed
2. Morning care completed, client tolerated well
3. Morning care completed by client
4. Not necessary to document morning care if uneventful

➤ *See pages 84–85 for Answers & Rationales.*

POSTTEST

ANSWERS & RATIONALES

Pretest

1 **Answer: 4** Asking the client to describe feelings seeks additional information and indicates to the client that the nurse is attentive. Asking for the reason (option 1) may force the client to defend himself or herself because the client may or may not know the reason for these feelings. Stating that the client looks nervous may be interpreted as unsupportive. Providing a backrub does not allow the client to express feelings.
Cognitive Level: Application **Client Need:** Psychosocial Integrity **Integrated Process:** Communication and Documentation **Content Area:** Fundamentals **Strategy:** The critical words in the question are *the nurse's best reply.* Recall that the best way to obtain information related to the client's health is to have the client elaborate or clarify a statement the client made. **Reference:** Kozier, B., Erb, G., Berman, A., & Snyder, S. J. (2004). *Fundamentals of nursing: Concepts, process and practice* (7th ed.). Upper Saddle River, NJ: Pearson Education, pp. 430–431.

2 **Answer: 4** Therapeutic communication involves assessing the client's coping strengths and encouraging the client to problem solve. Asking what the client has done before focuses him or her on solving his or her own problems and helps the nurse assess the client's coping mechanisms. This is the best first step. From there, the nurse can assist the client in problem solving. Option 2 is empathetic but does not seek further information, while option 1 rushes to a solution. Option 3 places the client's issue on hold and assumes the client would like to speak to a chaplain. Each of the incorrect options could block the communication process if made early in the conversation.
Cognitive Level: Application **Client Need:** Psychosocial Integrity **Integrated Process:** Communication and Documentation **Strategy:** The critical words are *best initial response.* Use knowledge of communication techniques and the process of elimination to choose the option that gathers more information by assessing the client's ability to cope with this situation. **Reference:** Kozier, B., Erb, G., Berman, A., & Snyder, S. J. (2004). *Fundamentals of nursing: Concepts, process and practice* (7th ed.). Upper Saddle River, NJ: Pearson Education, pp. 430–431.

3 **Answer: 3** Comatose clients may retain cognition and hearing even when they are unable to respond. They should be spoken to and cared for just as an alert, hearing client would be. Using touch along with the spoken word is appropriate for unresponsive clients. Discus-

sions of the client's condition (option 4) should be avoided at the bedside.
Cognitive Level: Application **Client Need:** Psychosocial Integrity **Integrated Processes:** Caring **Content Area:** Fundamentals **Strategy:** Use knowledge of basic communication techniques to answer the question. To choose the correct option, recall the critical concept that clients in comatose states may still hear what is said. **Reference:** Kozier, B., Erb, G., Berman, A., & Snyder, S. J. (2004). *Fundamentals of nursing: Concepts, process and practice* (7th ed.). Upper Saddle River, NJ: Pearson Education, pp. 949–950.

4 **Answer: 3** Clients are more likely to successfully complete a new procedure if they can actively demonstrate the procedure immediately after instructions have been given with the nurse present the first several times. Written literature and a video do not allow for active participation; however, they can be used as supplementary learning aids.
Cognitive Level: Application **Client Need:** Health Promotion and Maintenance **Integrated Process:** Teaching/Learning **Content Area:** Fundamentals **Strategy:** Recall that learning is measured by a change in client behavior. Recall that a return demonstration would evaluate psychomotor skill needed to perform wound care. **Reference:** Kozier, B., Erb, G., Berman, A., & Snyder, S. J. (2004). *Fundamentals of nursing: Concepts, process and practice* (7th ed.). Upper Saddle River, NJ: Pearson Education, p. 460.

5 **Answer: 4** Learning is more likely to take place when the client's perceived needs are met. The nursing assessment identifies areas for client teaching and the client's ability to learn. The amount of time needed to implement a teaching plan (option 3) is not associated with establishing priorities. The physician's orders often do not address client teaching (option 1). A thorough nursing assessment will gather much data, but teaching needs are assessed in a focused manner (option 2).
Cognitive Level: Application **Client Need:** Health Promotion and Maintenance **Integrated Process:** Teaching/Learning **Content Area:** Fundamentals **Strategy:** The critical words are *most effective* and *learning needs of a client.* Recall factors that influence client learning and use the process of elimination to identify the best areas for client teaching. **Reference:** Kozier, B., Erb, G., Berman, A., & Snyder, S. J. (2004). *Fundamentals of nursing: Concepts, process and practice* (7th ed.). Upper Saddle River, NJ: Pearson Education, p. 452.

ANSWERS & RATIONALES

6 **Answer: 2** A description of the client's self-care abilities provides data to the referral nurse about information needed to continue the client's care at home. Vital sign information is only one parameter and does not provide enough information about the client's overall status. Last dose of medications is important data but does not identify all of the medications the client is currently taking, which is helpful in developing a comprehensive plan of care. The surgical report does not have direct relevance to the client's home care needs.

Cognitive Level: Application **Client Need:** Health Promotion and Maintenance **Integrated Process:** Communication and Documentation **Content Area:** Fundamentals **Strategy:** Use the process of elimination and knowledge of discharge planning principles to systematically eliminate options that do not provide comprehensive or crucial information to other healthcare agencies/providers. **Reference:** Kozier, B., Erb, G., Berman, A., & Snyder, S. J. (2004). *Fundamentals of nursing: Concepts, process and practice* (7th ed.). Upper Saddle River, NJ: Pearson Education, p. 340.

7 **Answer: 1, 3, 4** A change-of-shift report is given to ensure continuity of care. It should be concise and efficient. Client learning needs (option 1), dietary modifications (option 4), and permitted activities (option 3) are all essential information so the next nurse can provide appropriate care. Family visitation and modes of transportation for diagnostic tests (options 2 and 5) are not considered necessary information.

Cognitive Level: Application **Client Need:** Safe, Effective Care Environment: Management of Care **Integrated Process:** Communication and Documentation **Content Area:** Fundamentals **Strategy:** The core issue of the question is knowledge of important information to include in an intershift report. Use knowledge of reporting guidelines and the process of elimination in selecting key information to report to the oncoming shift. **Reference:** Kozier, B., Erb, G., Berman, A., & Snyder, S. J. (2004). *Fundamentals of nursing: Concepts, process and practice* (7th ed.). Upper Saddle River, NJ: Pearson Education, p. 345.

8 **Answer: 1** A client who has not urinated following catheter removal would require immediate nursing intervention, specifically assessing the client's abdominal distention, reviewing intake and output records, and possibly calling the physician for an order to do a straight catheterization. The second priority would be the client who has incisional pain (option 3); however, since the client is 3 days postoperative, this is not as urgent a problem as option 1. The third priority would be to compare the blood pressure of the client in option 4 with baseline blood pressure. The client in option 2 is not a priority since the normal orientation status indicates no threat to the health status of the client.

Cognitive Level: Analysis **Client Need:** Physiological Integrity: Basic Care and Comfort **Integrated Process:** Communication and Documentation **Content Area:** Fundamentals **Strategy:** The critical phrases are *most useful information* and *priority setting.* Analyze each client in the various options and choose the one that has the most critical need. **Reference:** Kozier, B., Erb, G., Berman, A., & Snyder, S. J. (2004). *Fundamentals of nursing: Concepts, process and practice* (7th ed.). Upper Saddle River, NJ: Pearson Education, p. 345.

9 **Answer: 3** The quality improvement nurse's best action is to report the findings to the Nursing Staff Development Department to improve the standards of nursing documentation in the facility. The documentation of mood reviewed by the nurse reflects that the wording of the documentation does not describe the client behavior or quote the client's original words; rather it reflects the nurse's opinion or judgment about the client status. For this reason, alerting the department that could provide corrective action is the most important action of the quality improvement nurse.

Cognitive Level: Application **Client Need:** Safe, Effective Care Environment: Management of Care **Integrated Process:** Communication and Documentation **Content Area:** Fundamentals **Strategy:** The critical words are *best action.* This implies that more than one option is a realistic possibility but that one option will be more effective. Use knowledge of the purpose of quality improvement to make a selection. **Reference:** Kozier, B., Erb, G., Berman, A., & Snyder, S. J. (2004). *Fundamentals of nursing: Concepts, process and practice* (7th ed.). Upper Saddle River, NJ: Pearson Education, pp. 322–323.

10 **Answer: 3** Recording the time of the entry, the time of the assessment, and the missing data is an acceptable documentation practice. Inserting information in the client record is not an appropriate documentation action. Clients' records should not be recopied. Verbally reporting the omission solely is not acceptable.

Cognitive Level: Application **Client Need:** Safe, Effective Care Environment: Management of Care **Integrated Process:** Communication and Documentation **Content Area:** Fundamentals **Strategy:** The critical phrase is *at this time.* Recall that client records must reflect accuracy to determine that missing data must be provided as an addendum. Recall guidelines for legal documentation to aid in making a selection. **Reference:** Kozier, B., Erb, G., Berman, A., & Snyder, S. J. (2004). *Fundamentals of nursing: Concepts, process and practice* (7th ed.). Upper Saddle River, NJ: Pearson Education, p. 341.

ANSWERS & RATIONALES

Posttest

1 **Answer: 2** The nurse should validate his or her perceptions with the client to ensure the correct interpretation of the client's nonverbal behavior. The nurse does not need to verify this observation with another nurse (option 3). The nurse should not make false assumptions (option 1) and should not ignore the client's behavior (option 4).
Cognitive Level: Application **Client Need:** Psychosocial Integrity **Integrated Process:** Communication and Documentation **Content Area:** Fundamentals **Strategy:** The critical phrase is most appropriate. Recall that client behavior, feelings, and concerns must be validated and explored by the nurse. **Reference:** Kozier, B., Erb, G., Berman, A., & Snyder, S. J. (2004). *Fundamentals of nursing: Concepts, process and practice* (7th ed.). Upper Saddle River, NJ: Pearson Education, p. 274.

2 **Answer: 3, 5** Exploring the client's feelings indicates that the client's feelings are important to the nurse. Checking on the client frequently conveys that the nurse is concerned with the client's status. Providing reassurance about surgeon competency (option 1) may dismiss the client's feelings as unimportant. Providing teaching to a client at this time (option 2) is inappropriate because it may not be assimilated because of anxiety. Relating a personal experience focuses the attention on the nurse, rather than the client (option 4).
Cognitive Level: Application **Client Need:** Psychosocial Integrity **Integrated Processes:** Caring **Content Area:** Fundamentals **Strategy:** The critical words in the question are *best approach*. Recall that client behavior, feelings, and concerns must be validated and explored. Use this principle and knowledge of effective communication techniques to make a selection. **Reference:** Kozier, B., Erb, G., Berman, A., & Snyder, S. J. (2004). *Fundamentals of nursing: Concepts, process and practice* (7th ed.). Upper Saddle River, NJ: Pearson Education, p. 431.

3 **Answer: 3** For a client who is hearing impaired, speaking slowly in a low-pitched voice and facing the client will promote understanding of the message sent. Option 4 will not provide enough information to effectively care for the client. Options 1 and 2 may be appropriate if the client cannot hear at all.
Cognitive Level: Application **Client Need:** Health Promotion and Maintenance **Integrated Process:** Communication and Documentation **Content Area:** Fundamentals **Strategy:** The core issue of the question is knowledge of appropriate communication techniques to use with clients who are hearing impaired. Recall that one should always face the hearing-impaired client so the client can see the facial expression of the examiner and may be able to read

lips. **Reference:** Kozier, B., Erb, G., Berman, A., & Snyder, S. J. (2004). *Fundamentals of nursing: Concepts, process and practice* (7th ed.). Upper Saddle River, NJ: Pearson Education, p. 559.

4 **Answer: 4** Documentation needs to be accurate and complete and should not express the opinions or judgment of the nurse. The incorrect options are unclear, judgmental, and/or represent the nurse's interpretation of data.
Cognitive Level: Application **Client Need:** Psychosocial Integrity **Integrated Process:** Communication and Documentation **Content Area:** Fundamentals **Strategy:** The core issue of the question is knowledge of principles of documentation. Recall that documentation must be factual and accurate and that the nurse should not interpret the statement made by the client. **Reference:** Kozier, B., Erb, G., Berman, A., & Snyder, S. J. (2004). *Fundamentals of nursing: Concepts, process and practice* (7th ed.). Upper Saddle River, NJ: Pearson Education, p. 264.

5 **Answer: 3** A prerequisite to learning a new psychomotor skill is that the client is able to physically perform the skill. In this case if the client doesn't have the dexterity to palpate a pulse or ability to see a clock's second hand, the client will need assistance with the skill. Options 1 and 2 are unnecessary for the nurse to assess prior to implementing the teaching plan. Motivation to attain better health is also important, but the nurse must first evaluate the client's ability to perform the skill.
Cognitive Level: Application **Client Need:** Health Promotion and Maintenance **Integrated Process:** Teaching/Learning **Content Area:** Fundamentals **Strategy:** Recall information about the three domains of learning (cognitive, affective, and psychomotor) and that the nurse needs to ensure that the client has the mental and physical ability to carry out the intervention. **Reference:** Kozier, B., Erb, G., Berman, A., & Snyder, S. J. (2004). *Fundamentals of nursing: Concepts, process and practice* (7th ed.). Upper Saddle River, NJ: Pearson Education, p. 451.

6 **Answer: 4** Having the client actively demonstrate the procedure is the best way for the nurse to evaluate the client's level of skill. The other options are less effective ways for the nurse to evaluate the client's learning of the new skill.
Cognitive Level: Application **Client Need:** Health Promotion and Maintenance **Integrated Processes:** Teaching/Learning **Content Area:** Fundamentals **Strategy:** The critical phrase is *best evaluate a client's ability*. To choose the correct option, recall that the nurse needs to ensure that the client has the mental and physical ability to carry out the action. **Reference:** Kozier, B., Erb, G., Berman, A., & Snyder, S. J. (2004). *Fundamentals of nursing: Concepts, process*

and practice (7th ed.). Upper Saddle River, NJ: Pearson Education, p. 462.

7 **Answer: 1** Learning in the cognitive domain involves the acquisition and use of knowledge mentally or intellectually. Option 3 involves learning in the affective domain, which involves changing feelings and values toward a positive health behavior. Options 2 and 4 involve learning in the psychomotor domain.
Cognitive Level: Application **Client Need:** Health Promotion and Maintenance **Integrated Process:** Teaching/Learning **Content Area:** Fundamentals **Strategy:** Knowledge of the three domains of learning (cognitive, affective, and psychomotor) will allow you to accurately asses client education needs and select appropriate teaching strategies. Recall that the cognitive domain is thinking, the affective domain is the feeling or emotional response, and the psychomotor domain involves acquiring a new skill. **Reference:** Kozier, B., Erb, G., Berman, A., & Snyder, S. J. (2004). *Fundamentals of nursing: Concepts, process and practice* (7th ed.). Upper Saddle River, NJ: Pearson Education, p. 458.

8 **Answer: 3** Critical pathways are documents that identify outcome criteria that a group of patients are expected to achieve on each day of hospitalization. Only option 3 would be an outcome criterion. Option 1 is a medical order. Option 2 is a nursing intervention (and not necessarily an appropriate one), and option 4 is also a nursing intervention.
Cognitive Level: Application **Client Need:** Safe, Effective Care Environment: Management of Care **Integrated Process:** Communication and Documentation **Content Area:** Fundamentals **Strategy:** The critical terms are *outcome criterion* and *critical pathway.* Recall that critical pathways contain outcome criteria that require documentation of variances whenever the outcomes are not met. Then recall the differences between goals or outcomes and orders/interventions to make a final selection. **Reference:** Kozier, B., Erb, G., Berman, A., & Snyder,

S. J. (2004). *Fundamentals of nursing: Concepts, process and practice* (7th ed.). Upper Saddle River, NJ: Pearson Education, p. 336.

9 **Answer: 1** Physical assessment data and client response to care are pieces of information that are most important in ensuring that client's healthcare needs are being met. The other options are useful to a nurse assuming care of a client but are more limited in the scope of information they provide (options 3 and 4) or are not as relevant to the client's status in real time (option 2).
Cognitive Level: Analysis **Client Need:** Safe, Effective Care Environment: Management of Care **Integrated Process:** Communication and Documentation **Content Area:** Fundamentals **Strategy:** Knowledge of reporting guidelines would assist you to be concise and still relay necessary information. Recall that a summary of care, physical status, needs, and response to treatment should be given high priority during report. **Reference:** Kozier, B., Erb, G., Berman, A., & Snyder, S. J. (2004). *Fundamentals of nursing: Concepts, process and practice* (7th ed.). Upper Saddle River, NJ: Pearson Education, p. 345.

10 **Answer: 4** Charting by exception is a form of documentation in which notations are made if there was an exception to the standard of care or the client's response to care. All other options are normal and are therefore not necessary to include in documentation using this format.
Cognitive Level: Application **Client Need:** Safe, Effective Care Environment: Management of Care **Integrated Process:** Communication and Documentation **Strategy:** The core issue of the question is knowledge of the method of charting by exception. Recall that care is documented on a flowsheet unless there is a problem or potential problem. **Reference:** Kozier, B., Erb, G., Berman, A., & Snyder, S. J. (2004). *Fundamentals of nursing: Concepts, process and practice* (7th ed.). Upper Saddle River, NJ: Pearson Education, p. 335.

References

Bastable, S. (2003). *Nurse educator: Principles of teaching and learning for nursing practice* (2nd ed.). Sudbury, MA: Jones & Bartlett.

Berman, A., Snyder, S., Kozier, B., & Erb, G. (2008). *Fundamentals of nursing: Concepts, process, and practice* (8th ed.). Upper Saddle River, NJ: Prentice Hall, pp. 245–267, 486–510.

Craven, R. & Hirnle, C. (2006). *Fundamentals of nursing: Human health and function* (5th ed.). Philadelphia: Lippincott Williams & Wilkins, pp. 248–263, 428–457.

Harkreader, H., Hogan, M. & Thobaben, M. (2004). *Fundamentals of nursing: Caring and clinical judgment* (3rd ed.). St. Louis, MO: Elsevier Science, pp. 230–255, 274–290.

Joint Commission on Accreditation of Healthcare Organizations (2006). *Accreditation manual of hospitals.* Chicago: The Commission.

Potter, P. & Perry, A. (2005). *Fundamentals of nursing* (6th ed.). St. Louis, MO: Mosby, Inc., pp. 423–499.

Riley, J. (2004). *Communication in nursing* (5th ed.). St. Louis, MO: Mosby, pp. 14–236.

Taylor, C., Lillis C., & LeMone, P. (2005). *Fundamentals of nursing: The art and science of nursing care* (5th ed.). Philadelphia: Lippincott Williams & Wilkins, pp. 195–228, 335–365, 441–472.

ANSWERS & RATIONALES

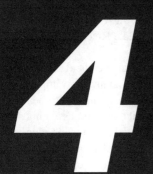

Overview of Professional Standards

Chapter Outline _____

Overview of Nursing Leadership and Management

Overview of Delegation

Ethics, Morals, and Values

Legal Concepts of Nursing Practice

The Roles of the Professional Nurse

 NCLEX-RN® Test Prep

Use the CD-ROM enclosed with this book to access additional practice opportunities.

Objectives _____

➤ Compare the concepts of leadership and management in relation to nursing.

➤ Identify common management functions.

➤ Contrast the various models for delivery of nursing care.

➤ Identify the components of effective delegation.

➤ Discuss the relationship of ethics, morals, and values in professional nursing practice.

➤ Discuss legal concepts and issues as they pertain to the healthcare environment.

➤ Describe the four primary roles of the professional nurse.

Review at a Glance

accountability acceptance of ownership for the results or lack of results of client care

ANA Code of Ethics for Nurses a statement of values developed by the American Nurses Association to provide guidance to the nurse and protection for the client and family

case manager an individual who oversees all aspects of nursing and health care; one who supervises the client's services and care rendered through communication, brokering of services, and procurement of available resources

decision making ability to sort through issues and data and develop a reasonable and prudent plan of action

that will lead to the resolution of an actual or potential issue or problem

delegation a process of assigning staff to complete a task or assignment; the goal of delegation is to maintain seamless client care, improve the skills of novice nurses, and spread tasks to appropriate personnel; complex tasks requiring specialized knowledge should not be delegated

ethics a code on which a person bases his or her actions and decisions; the process of determining right from wrong or good from bad

leadership use of a person's interpersonal skills to guide followers to achieve personal and/or organizational goals

malpractice professional failure to carry out or perform duties that results in the injury of another

management ability to deploy resources in the achievement of the organization's goals

negligence an unintentional act or failure to act as a reasonably prudent person would act in the same or similar situation that results in injury to another; negligence can be an act of omission or commission

Nurse Practice Act determines the scope of professional nursing practice in a state and establishes guidelines whereby the nurse can perform skills or services

PRETEST

1 The client is to undergo an invasive procedure. While providing information about the procedure, the nurse provides legal protection of a client's right to autonomy with which of the following?

1. Informed consent
2. Beneficence
3. Good Samaritan law
4. Advance directives

2 The unit manager is meeting with the director of nursing for the unit manager's yearly performance review. The director of nursing states that the unit manager needs to improve in leadership skills. In differentiating leadership from management, the nurse manager recognizes that which of the following will demonstrate an improvement in leadership skills?

1. Manager attends a workshop on budgeting unit resources
2. Manager applies for a higher position within the institution
3. Unit demonstrates a decreased number of staff sick calls per month
4. Manager uses interpersonal skills to motivate and encourage staff to achieve unit and institutional goals

3 Which of the following would be an example of a nurse using "expert power" to influence fellow staff members?

1. Using a sense of humor and good interpersonal skills to convince other nurses that change is needed
2. Offering a day off with pay to staff members who comply with requested change
3. Giving staff members who are reluctant to accept the change less desirable assignments and longer scheduled night rotations
4. Using valid and current data to speak positively to staff about advantages of the change over the current system

4 The nurse observes that which of the following nurse colleagues is maintaining client confidentiality?

1. Nurse who reads the records of clients not assigned to become more familiar with their disease processes
2. Nurse who shares information about an interesting client with nurses from another unit who may eventually care for the client
3. Nurse who allows the client's family to review the medical record to provide answers to questions
4. Nurse who shares information about the client with those involved in care for the purpose of planning nursing care

5 The unit manager formulates rules and insists that everyone follow them. At unit meetings, the manager reads the rules to staff members with no discussion allowed. The nurse interpret that the staff is working under which type of leadership?

1. Autocratic
2. Democratic
3. Laissez-faire
4. Situational

6 A client is admitted for a medical procedure that is contrary to the nurse's personal views. Despite personal objections to the procedure, the nurse provides a high level of care to the client. In making the decision to provide care based on what is right and wrong, or good and bad, related to the client, the nurse's decision was generated from which of the following?

1. Laws
2. Ethics
3. The state Nurse Practice Act
4. State statutes

7 The client tells the nurse not to inform family members about the medical diagnosis or to share other details of the medical record. In meeting this request, the nurse would be upholding which of the following?

1. Informed consent
2. Confidentiality
3. Living will
4. Justice

8 Four nursing students are discussing the American Nurses Association (ANA) Code of Ethics for Nurses. The student who correctly understands the purpose of the statement is the one who concludes that the purpose of the code is to do which of the following?

1. Assure the public that nurses will display ethical behaviors when providing client care.
2. Compare expected behavior of nurses with other healthcare providers such as physicians.
3. Provide guidelines regarding care of individuals, and for accountability to the profession and society.
4. Prevent certain individuals from practicing nursing by enforcing regulations that prohibit attainment of licensure.

9 The nursing unit is considering changing the mode of nursing care delivery to one that holds a nurse responsible and accountable over a 24-hour period for the care and treatment of a caseload. The nursing staff practicing this delivery system is using:

1. Primary nursing
2. Functional nursing
3. Total client care nursing practice
4. Team nursing

10 A nurse sees a motor vehicle accident and stops to provide first aid, knowing that this action is protected by the Good Samaritan law. The nurse should provide assistance after recalling which of the following about this law?

1. It was created specifically for RNs and LPNs.
2. It differs from state to state.
3. It allows nurses to be paid for rendering emergency aid.
4. It prohibits licensed nurses from providing help during an accident.

➤ *See pages 100–102 for Answers & Rationales.*

I. OVERVIEW OF NURSING LEADERSHIP AND MANAGEMENT

A. Leadership

1. Definition: a person's use of interpersonal skills to guide others to achieve personal goals and goals of the organization; a good leader will utilize managerial skills to encourage, motivate, and create change

2. Essential leadership skills include delegation, problem-solving skills, good communication skills, decision-making, confrontation and conflict resolution, time management, team building and leading, negotiation, motivation, and supervision

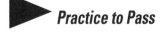

Practice to Pass

Discuss the classic leadership style that is most useful when working with a professional staff.

3. Leadership styles: should be modified to meet the needs of the situation; leader should have a flexible style to maximize success; leadership styles include:

   a. Classic leadership styles

   1) Autocratic: no participation from others; the person in charge makes all of the decisions; there is no other input

   2) Democratic: the person in charge asks for input from group members; the group makes the decisions; the leader facilitates discussion

   3) Laissez-faire: no one makes decisions; chaos can result; no goals are achieved; no direction is offered

   4) Situational: the leader changes leadership style to meet the needs of the situation; if it is an emergent situation, the leader is more autocratic; other situations call for the group to make the decision

   b. Contemporary leadership styles

   1) Charismatic: characterized by an emotional relationship between staff followers and leader in which the leader evokes strong feelings of commitment to leader's cause and beliefs (rare)

   2) Transactional: characterized by the leader's engaging in a relationship or transaction with the staff/followers in exchange for a resource valued by the follower (i.e., working overtime on one shift for a holiday off)

   3) Transformational: characterized by the leader's ability to foster creativity, commitment, and collaboration by empowering staff/followers to share in the organization's vision and achieve goals

   4) Shared: characterized by organizational belief that many staff members are leaders and leadership emerges in response to the challenges confronting a work group (i.e., shared governance)

B. Management

1. Definition: the ability to deploy resources to achieve the organization's goals; includes being accountable and responsible for accomplishing goals, coordinating and integrating resources, and using the management process (plan, staff, direct, organize, and control)

   a. A manager's power is vested within the position; a manager is not necessarily a leader

   b. Management skills can be learned

   c. A manager must effectively utilize resources, communicate effectively, and develop employees' skills to increase productivity and effectiveness

   d. Staff accomplishes work through mandates and protocols

   e. A manager has formal position and authority; it is an assigned role

2. Common management processes

   a. Planning: schedules, job description, client care, staffing mixes, assignments, established goals, prognostication skills, strategic planning, contingency planning

   b. Staffing: hiring, firing, staff development, performance appraisals

   c. Organizing: daily activities, coordinate staff and work to be done, division of labor, chain of command in bureaucracy, delivery system, generating the skill mix of staff and staffing patterns

   d. Directing: leading, problem solving, decision making, work completion, meeting goals, use of communication skills

   e. Controlling: establish performance standards; determine means of measuring performance, evaluating performance, and giving feedback

   f. **Decision making:** the ability to sort through issues and data and develop a reasonable and prudent plan of action that will lead to the resolution of an actual or potential issue or problem

      1) Multiple models

         a) Vroom–Yetton Expectancy Model: leader determines the amount of participation in making a decision; depends on quality and acceptance of decision; assists in determining the decision style

         b) Decision tree: the problem is depicted with outlining of alternatives coupled with their potential consequences

         c) Program evaluation and review technique (PERT): is a network systems model; outlines and prioritizes activities and flow of events toward goal attainment within a set time frame

         d) Critical path method (CPM): depicts the order in which tasks are to be completed

      2) Types of power

         a) Reward: power comes with the notion that the manager/coordinator can offer a reward that the nurse wants; reward can include assignment, schedule, transfer, and promotion

         b) Coercive: power is derived from the fear of repercussion

         c) Legitimate: power is vested in the position and sanctioned by the bureaucracy

         d) Expert: power comes from knowledge and skill; staff looks to gain knowledge from the expert

         e) Referent: power is based upon admiration and respect; followers are compliant because they like the person

         f) Information: power is derived from information or data that the follower desires

         g) Connection: power is generated by the leader's networking skills and links to influential people

         h) Position: power is vested within the actual job description, duties, responsibilities, authority, decision making, and the withholding and releasing of resources and money

3. Quality management

   a. Refers to purposeful processes that are instituted to assure and improve quality of client care

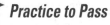

Practice to Pass

How does the management process assist in the attainment of organizational goals?

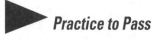

Practice to Pass

What types of power does a new graduate in nursing have?

      b. Involves input by staff nurses, managers, and administration for most optimal program outcomes

      c. Quality improvement teams may be unit-based

      d. Quality programs may focus on one or more specific procedures or types of care delivery

C. Nursing care delivery models

    1. Total patient care: nurse is responsible for carrying out all aspects of client care; case method; nurse gives care for entire shift; usually seen in critical care and postanesthesia care units

    2. Functional: task-based nursing; clients' needs are divided into tasks and assigned to nurse and other staff, such as unlicensed assistants

    3. Team nursing: nurse is either the team leader or a member of a delivery team; the team leader delegates tasks and responsibilities; the leader is the designated authority but should use democratic or participative style with team members; communication is essential for success

    4. Primary: total responsibility for client care; the nurse facilitates care for client from admission to discharge; has 24-hour accountability and responsibility; plans, coordinates, and evaluates care for caseload of clients

    5. Case management: nurse assigned as case manager ensures that needed services continue to be provided when client is discharged from hospital to home or other healthcare facility; it includes making arrangements for the transfer as well

II. OVERVIEW OF DELEGATION

A. Delegation

    1. The process of assigning staff to complete a task or assignment

    2. The goal of delegation is to maintain quality client care, improve the skills of novice nurses, and spread tasks to appropriate personnel

    3. Complex tasks requiring specialized knowledge should not be delegated

B. Process for delegation

    1. Determine complexity of client needs or nature of work to be delegated

    2. Identify staff member to whom tasks are to be delegated

    3. Determine that work is consistent with staff member's job description, level of competency, and normal duties

    4. Clearly communicate expectations and results using measurable terms; convey trust and reasonable authority

    5. Secure staff member's voluntary acceptance of work request

    6. Keep communication lines open

    7. Compare actual results with expectations giving feedback and praise

    8. Evaluate achievement of goals or outcomes

C. Obstacles to delegation

    1. Nonsupportive environment: the environment must be conducive to developing all personnel and achieving goals

    2. Limited resources: financial issues may prevent the ability to delegate; these may relate to either finances, number of qualified personnel, or necessary equipment

3. Inexperience: a staff member's inexperience can be a hindrance to delegation; an institution can minimize this through competency-based orientation and testing; the nurse delegating the task sometimes must teach the novice the necessary skills to complete the task; with proper guidance, delegating can improve the novice's skills

4. Fear of liability: the nurse must have the skill and knowledge to perform the task or oversee the completion of the request; it should only be done with thorough knowledge of what needs to be done as well as appropriate supervision

5. Fear of burdening co-workers: requesting assistance or delegating a task should be done after assessing the workload of other nurses; the assignment should not overwhelm the nurse thereby causing omissions/mistakes to occur

6. Unwillingness of workers to accept delegated tasks: the staff should not refuse a request unless it will compromise the care of their clients

7. Fear of failure: this can serve to motivate the nurse to learn more about the task or work toward developing the necessary skills to successfully complete the task; if the nurse is afraid of failure, these concerns must be articulated to the supervisor and assistance requested; the task or assignment should not be delegated to an unprepared nurse

D. Inappropriate delegation

1. Underdelegation: can occur if delegator does not think that a staff member can perform an assignment and completes the assignment without delegating
   a. It is crucial to develop staff that can provide comprehensive client care
   b. If unable to perform tasks, staff development should occur to improve skills
   c. Delegation should be done with caution until staff are prepared to complete assigned skills
   d. Nurses who need assistance should ask for it

2. Reverse delegation: staff requests that manager or leader completes the task because of their inability or unwillingness to do so; this can be minimized with the use of competency-based orientation programs and in-services

3. Overdelegation: the tasks are delegated inappropriately; the nurse cannot successfully achieve goals if overwhelmed by numerous requests; each nurse must scrutinize the ability to take the assigned request; a good leader will balance requests after assessing the needs of the unit and clients; unlicensed assistive personnel (UAPs) and new graduate nurses should not be assigned tasks for which they are not prepared or that are beyond their scope of practice

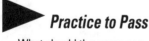

Practice to Pass

What should the nurse consider when delegating tasks to unlicensed assistive personnel?

III. ETHICS, MORALS, AND VALUES

A. Ethics

1. A code upon which a person bases actions and decisions
2. The process of determining right from wrong, good and bad
3. Decisions are guided by beliefs and values
4. Governs relationships with family and society
5. Are moral truths that guide thought process and actions
6. Represent the practical application of a moral philosophy

Box 4-1

Ethical Principles

> Autonomy: consists of freedom to make decisions that will impact welfare and take action for self; is self-governing; includes four basic elements:
>> Respect for others
>> Ability to determine personal goals
>> Complete understanding of choice
>> Freedom to implement plan/choice

> Beneficence: to act in the best interest of others; to contribute to the well-being of others; includes client advocacy; has three major components:
>> To promote good
>> To prevent harm or evil
>> To remove harm or evil

> Paternalism: acting in a fatherly or motherly manner, usually restricts client's autonomy and coerces decision making, restricts autonomy

> Justice: fair, equitable, and appropriate treatment; resources are distributed equally to all

> Fidelity: remaining faithful to ethical principles and the ANA Code of Ethics for Nurses (see section below); keeping commitments and promises

> Virtues: compassion, discernment, trustworthiness, and integrity; virtue ethics emphasize the character of the moral agent

> Confidentiality: to maintain the privacy of the client of family; nondisclosure of data or personal information; is a component of ANA Code of Ethics for Nurses (see text)

B. **Ethical theories:** values and behaviors are explained based on a particular viewpoint

   1. Duty-oriented: the intention of the act makes it right or wrong (Kantism)

   2. Rights-oriented: based on principles of justice/fairness; human rights are moral rights of a very important kind; shared equally by all persons

   3. Goal-oriented: goals are defined, medical intervention is weighed against whether it will promote a desired goal

   4. Intuitionist: looks inward; makes sense out of imagination; possesses insight

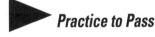

Practice to Pass

How does the ANA Code of Ethics for Nurses guide nursing practice?

C. **Ethical principles:** guide practice and decision making (see Box 4-1)

D. **Code of Ethics**

   1. The **ANA Code of Ethics for Nurses** was developed by American Nurses Association to provide guidance to the nurse and protection for the client and family; see Box 4-2

   2. The guidelines delineate values and standards for professional practice

E. **Morals:** a personal philosophy based on what is right or wrong, or good or bad; ethics is practical way of putting morals into practice; leads to decision making and problem solving; ethical considerations define morals essential to practice

F. **Values:** are personally and professionally developed and are based on philosophy and principles; values shape actions and reactions to issues and problems; provide guidance in determining actions; socialization and experiences help mold the value system

> **Box 4-2**
>
> **American Nurses Association Code of Ethics**
>
> 1. The nurse, in all professional relationships, practices with compassion and respect for the inherent dignity, worth and uniqueness of every individual, unrestricted by considerations of social or economic status, personal attributes, or the nature of health problems.
>
> 2. The nurse's primary commitment is to the patient, whether an individual, family, group, or community.
>
> 3. The nurse promotes, advocates for, and strives to protect the health, safety, and rights of the patient.
>
> 4. The nurse is responsible and accountable for individual nursing practice and determines the appropriate delegation of tasks consistent with the nurse's obligation to provide optimum patient care.
>
> 5. The nurse owes the same duties to self as to others, including the responsibility to preserve integrity and safety, to maintain competence, and to continue personal and professional growth.
>
> 6. The nurse participates in establishing, maintaining, and improving healthcare environments and conditions of employment conducive to the provision of quality health care and consistent with the values of the profession through individual and collective action.
>
> 7. The nurse participates in the advancement of the profession through contributions to practice, education, administration, and knowledge development.
>
> 8. The nurse collaborates with other health professionals and the public in promoting community, national, and international efforts to meet health needs.
>
> 9. The profession of nursing, as represented by associations and their members, is responsible for articulating nursing values, for maintaining the integrity of the profession and its practice, and for shaping social policy.

Reprinted with permission from American Nurses, Code of Ethics for Nurses, © 2001 American Nurses Publishing, American Nurses Foundation/American Nurses Association.

IV. LEGAL CONCEPTS OF NURSING PRACTICE

A. **The practice of nursing** must be done within the confines of the law; it is mandatory that nurses know the law and parameters of the nursing license

B. **Legal limits of nursing:** dictated by each state's board of nursing as well as state and federal laws and guidelines

   1. Constitution: the law of the land; defines structure, power and limits of government, guarantees fundamental rights and liberty; other laws may not infringe on the rights granted by the Constitution

   2. Statutory laws: laws enacted by the legislative branch of government; includes licensing laws, guardianship codes, statutes of limitation, informed consent, living will legislation, protective and reporting laws; regulatory agencies are established through statutes

   3. Common laws: judge-made law, derived from court decisions that establish a precedent by which other cases are judged

   4. Administrative laws: laws made by administrative agencies, such as a state board of nursing

C. **Accountability:** accepting the ownership for results or the lack of results; there is responsibility to provide professional nursing practice for all; efforts are made to provide quality care

D. **Responsibility:** obligates a person to accomplish a task; with delegation, the responsibility must transfer also to the one assigned to complete the assignment; accountability is shared

E. **Good Samaritan laws:** designed to protect those who aid victims in emergencies

1. Statutes vary from state to state

2. It is important for each nursing professional to review that state's law

3. Situation must be an emergency; care rendered must be free of charge; provided care must be in good faith; cannot willingly or intentionally harm the victim

4. Will not protect the nurse if nurse is grossly negligent

5. Once aid is offered, must stay with victim until the victim is stable or another provider with equal or greater training can take over

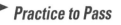

Practice to Pass

How does the Good Samaritan law protect nurses?

F. **Licensure:** a credential determined by state boards of nursing; requires completion of a nursing curriculum that leads to the successful passage of a licensing examination; licensure qualifies individual to perform designated skills and services

1. **Nurse Practice Act:** determines the scope of the professional nurse in a specific state

a. Establishes guidelines whereby the nurse can perform skills or services

b. The Nurse Practice Act is a set of state statutes (rules and regulations) that provide guidance to professional nurses

c. Establishes educational, examination, and behavioral standards for nurses that protect the public

d. To enforce these requirements, each state has a board of registration in nursing in the role of overseer

2. Liability: nurses are responsible and accountable for actions or inactions

G. **Negligence:** unintentional failure to act or not perform an act that a reasonable person in the same role would or would not do and results in injury to another; the failure to act as a reasonable person; elements include:

1. Duty: the nurse has a responsibility to care for and watch over the person as a component of employment; duty indicates a legal relationship between the client and the nurse

2. Breech of duty: the nurse failed to complete this duty; this can include acts of commission (activities the nurse did) or omission (activities the nurse failed to do)

3. Cause: there is a reasonably close causal connection between the nurse's conduct and a resulting injury

4. Injury occurred: the client has suffered physical, emotional, or financial injury; there is an actual loss or damage resulting from conduct

H. **Malpractice**

1. Negligence by a professional; professional failure to carry out or perform duties that result in the injury of another; scope of practice should be delineated in order to operate within it

2. The boundaries of malpractice are defined by statute, rules, and educational requirement

3. Malpractice is usually filed as a civil tort; a court finding of guilty usually results in restitution

4. The nurse may carry personal malpractice insurance to provide for restitution if malpractice occurs

5. Rarely are malpractice charges filed as criminal charges (under a finding in which a guilty verdict results in punishment, either jail or capital punishment)

6. Nursing activities to reduce risk of liability in lawsuits

   a. Practice within the provisions of the state's Nurse Practice Act

   b. Follow the ANA Code of Ethics for Nurses and standards of professional practice

   c. Treat every client with kindness and respect

   d. Maintain skills and knowledge base by completing continuing education programs

   e. Recognize personal strengths and weaknesses; seek help when facing new experiences and job requirements

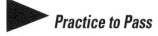

Practice to Pass

How can the nurse avoid accusations of malpractice?

I. Issues in nursing practice

1. Physician orders

   a. Determine the prescriptive course of action; guide the course of action for the client and family

   b. Includes prescriptive orders for:

   1) Medications

   2) Diet

   3) Activity level

   4) Length of stay

   5) Tests: diagnostic, blood, x-rays, procedures

   c. Nurses' actions are led by the physician's orders

   d. If orders are inappropriate, the nurse should question and clarify the orders; the nurse should ensure the prescribed amount of medication is a proper dose; the nurse is responsible for knowing pharmacological principles, drug interactions, and proper dosages

   1) If an order does not seem correct, the nurse should act on the client's behalf

   2) A nurse should never give a medication that is ordered as a toxic dose

   e. Explain ordered procedures to client and ask for feedback

   f. Physician's orders should be scrutinized for legibility and accuracy; when in doubt, clarify them with the physician

2. **Informed consent:** a legal protection of a client's rights; the client has the right to choose the type of care desired and make own decisions

   a. Informed consent is required before providing care except in an emergency situation, when the assumption exists that the client would consent if able (implied consent)

   b. The client can refuse treatment

   c. Informed consent must meet three requirements

   1) The individual has capacity to consent

   2) It is voluntarily done

   3) The individual understands the treatment and information presented

   d. Informed consent involves two steps

   1) Provision of information to the client that includes what is being done, why it is being done, the risks of the procedure, and possible alternatives to the procedure (with sufficient detail to allow the client to decide whether to proceed with treatment or not

2) Actually obtaining the consent (the person performing the procedure is required to obtain the consent)

3. Organ/tissue donation: an end-of-life issue; the client must be legally dead to donate organs; the decision can be made in advance when client is alive and competent or may be made at time of death by the family

a. The transplant team harvests the organs after consent is obtained

b. The bereaved family must be approached with compassion in requesting a discussion on organ donation

c. The goal is to assist those in need of transplant with the organ necessary to prolong life

d. Clinical death is defined as having no brain waves, no spontaneous breathing, and no superficial or deep reflexes

4. **Advance directives:** a document the individual completes when competent outlining the care desired to receive in the future; advance directives are followed if decision-making powers are altered and provides guidance to the healthcare team

5. Incident reports: each agency develops a protocol for reporting unusual or adverse events involving clients; incident reports are communication tools designed to provide information to risk managers, administration, and may be used in legal cases; incident reports are used to identify problems and develop solutions to prevent the same incident from happening again

6. Risk management: the goal of risk management is to protect the client and the nurse from harm, and protect the organization from liability related to harm

a. Risk management includes:

1) Organizational commitment to employee health and safety

2) Comprehensive worksite risk analysis

3) Employee participation

4) Hazard prevention and control including waste management

b. Guidelines are consistent with those of the Occupational Safety and Health Administration (OSHA)

7. The Joint Commission on Accreditation of Healthcare Organizations (JCAHO) establishes guidelines for accreditation of the institution or agency; the healthcare institutions abide by standards or lose accreditation; accreditation demonstrates an acceptable level of performance

V. THE ROLES OF THE PROFESSIONAL NURSE

A. Direct care provider

1. The nurse provides total care for the client

2. The nurse uses the nursing process to develop an appropriate plan of care, carry it out and evaluate its effectiveness

3. The nurse utilizes the skills of assessment, planning, intervention, and evaluation to meet the needs of the client

4. Documentation methodically records all data acquired through interaction with the client and other healthcare workers

5. The direct care provider may delegate some responsibilities to professional and nonprofessional personnel

B. Client advocate

1. In this role, the nurse becomes an activist speaking up for the client who cannot or will not speak for self
2. The client advocate seeks what is best for the client
3. The client advocate:
   a. Respects and upholds client's rights
   b. Ensures that client needs are met
   c. Can act as a mediator among client, family, and health care provider
   d. Provides support to the client
4. Client advocacy requires good communication skills and assertiveness on the part of the nurse
5. State Nurse Practice Acts may include nurse advocacy roles in the definition of nursing

C. Case manager

1. A case manager oversees all aspects of care
2. This individual attempts to procure medications and equipment, consults other disciplines, holds conferences about clients, prepares clients for discharge, and makes appropriate referrals
3. In doing these things, the case manager:
   a. Facilitates delivery of cost-efficient care
   b. Individualizes care
   c. Coordinates care
   d. Applies tools, skills, and techniques toward the desired outcome
   e. Collaborates with other healthcare professionals to coordinate care
   f. Monitors and evaluates options and services to meet individual and family needs

D. Client/family educator

1. Involves instruction regarding medications, health promotion, disease prevention, and discharge
2. Includes referring client and family to appropriate resources, literature, and Web sites
3. Incorporates good communication among client, family, and healthcare team members

Case Study

While driving home from the hospital on a rainy evening, a registered nurse (RN) witnesses a minivan slide off the road into a tree. The nurse stops the car and runs to the mangled minivan. As the nurse looks inside the driver's window, two semiconscious teenagers are observed in seatbelts and are moaning for help.

1. As an RN, does the nurse have a legal obligation to stop?

2. Are Good Samaritan laws uniform from state to state?

3. If the driver and passenger are slightly injured, is the nurse bound by law to assist them?

4. If the nurse intentionally injures the victim, does the Good Samaritan law cover the nurse from liability?

5. When can the nurse leave the scene of this accident?

For suggested responses, see page 336.

POSTTEST

1 Because a nurse caring for a surgical client fails to monitor the client adequately during the postoperative period according to the standard of care, the client experiences surgical complications. The nurse concludes that this action is consistent with which of the following?

1. Practicing medicine without a license
2. Negligence
3. A misdemeanor
4. Failure to follow the Good Samaritan law

2 A nurse accidentally administers a drug to the wrong client and the client reacts adversely to that drug. The nurse anticipates that this event could lead to which of the following charges?

1. A tort
2. Malpractice
3. Fraud
4. Assault

3 A 45-year-old male Hispanic client who speaks very little English is scheduled for surgery tomorrow. The nurse is concerned that the informed consent signed by the client on admission may not be valid for which of the following reasons?

1. The surgical consent form was not notarized.
2. It was witnessed by unlicensed personnel.
3. The client may not understand the document he signed, which outlines treatment and associated risks.
4. The client may be an undocumented immigrant.

4 The new graduate nurse asks the nursing unit manager to share strategies aimed at risk management. The manager correctly recommends which of the following? Select all that apply.

1. Treat every client with kindness and respect.
2. Seek help when facing new situations if unsure about which course of action is best.
3. Observe and report suspicious behavior of colleagues.
4. Be aware of the provisions of the state's Nurse Practice Act and function within those provisions.
5. Refuse to assist in the care of clients assigned to other nurses.

POSTTEST

POSTTEST

5 The clinic managers want nurses working in the unit to administer moderate sedation. To legally include this procedure in their practice, the staff nurses determine first that it is acceptable under which of the following?

1. The agency's policy and procedure book
2. The nurse's liability insurance
3. Good Samaritan law
4. The state's Nurse Practice Act

6 A client diagnosed with Alzheimer's disease is currently competent to make healthcare decisions regarding future needs. The nurse counsels the client to contact a lawyer about which of the following?

1. Advance directives
2. Temporary power of attorney
3. Self-determination
4. Informed consent

7 The nurse is aware that no physician has visited a hospitalized client for three consecutive days. The nurse reports this event to the nursing supervisor after determining that it is a priority to execute which nursing role?

1. Direct care provider role
2. Case manager role
3. Client educator role
4. Client advocate role

8 The nurse has assigned ancillary personnel to take vital signs (VS) of all the clients on the unit. After noting one set of VS that is questionable, the nurse retakes the VS after considering which of the following principles?

1. Supervision
2. Obligation
3. The highest level of empowerment
4. Accountability

9 A nurse who is enrolled in a continuing education leadership course considers that which of the following would be an example of overdelegation in the workplace?

1. A registered nurse with three months of experience recently finished orientation to a hospital unit. The nurse manager assigns the new nurse to be charge nurse for the evening shift because the regular nurse has called in sick.
2. The evening staff expects the charge nurse to give report on all clients to the night shift so they can leave the unit on time.
3. A staff nurse is reluctant to ask a nursing assistant to take vital signs on her clients, so the nurse takes all vital signs without assistance.
4. An experienced staff nurse is assigned to orient a new graduate to the unit after the new nurse completes general orientation to the hospital.

10 A new staff nurse is assigned responsibility for the care of an assigned client from admission to discharge. When the staff nurse is not on duty, others provide care based on instructions left by the staff nurse. The nurse understands that which care delivery system is being utilized on this unit?

1. Primary nursing
2. Team nursing
3. Case management
4. Functional nursing

See pages 102–104 for Answers & Rationales.

ANSWERS & RATIONALES

ANSWERS & RATIONALES

Pretest

1 **Answer: 1** Informed consent provides legal protection of a client's right to personal autonomy and to choose medical treatment. Advanced directives determine the actions of the healthcare team when the client is unable to make a decision. *Beneficence* is an ethical term that means that a person will act for the benefit of others.

The Good Samaritan law protects healthcare professionals who come to the aid of others during an emergency. **Cognitive Level:** Application **Client Need:** Safe, Effective Care Environment: Management of Care **Integrated Process:** Communication and Documentation **Content Area:** Fundamentals **Strategy:** The critical words are *right to autonomy*. Use knowledge of ethical principles to guide nursing practice and assist in making correct practice decisions. **Reference:** Kozier, B., Erb, G., Berman, A., & Snyder, S. J. (2004). *Fundamentals of nursing: Concepts, process and practice* (7th ed.). Upper Saddle River, NJ: Pearson Education, p. 70.

2 **Answer: 4** A good leader can incorporate managerial theories into practice, whereas a manager does not necessarily utilize leadership techniques. Use of interpersonal skills to motivate others to achieve goals is a hallmark of leadership. All other options would be related to managerial skills alone.
Cognitive Level: Application **Client Need:** Safe, Effective Care Environment: Management of Care **Integrated Process:** Nursing Process: Implementation **Content Area:** Leadership/Management **Strategy:** The critical phrase is *improvement in leadership skills.* Recall basic principles of nursing leadership and management to determine which skill needs to be developed for improved performance. **Reference:** Kozier, B., Erb, G., Berman, A., & Snyder, S. J. (2004). *Fundamentals of nursing: Concepts, process and practice* (7th ed.). Upper Saddle River, NJ: Pearson Education, pp. 475–476.

3 **Answer: 4** Expert power relies on the expert skills of the practitioner to gain the admiration and confidence of the group. Referent power relies on interpersonal skills, whereas coercive skills use the fear of threats. Use of rewards is positive feedback or reinforcement, but it is not expert power.
Cognitive Level: Application **Client Need:** Safe, Effective Care Environment: Management of Care **Integrated Process:** Nursing Process: Implementation **Content Area:** Fundamentals **Strategy:** The critical phrase is *expert power.* Recall the types of power and their appropriate uses to make a selection. **Reference:** Kozier, B., Erb, G., Berman, A., & Snyder, S. J. (2004). *Fundamentals of nursing: Concepts, process and practice* (7th ed.). Upper Saddle River, NJ: Pearson Education, p. 475.

4 **Answer: 4** The client has a right to confidentiality. Unless a nurse is assigned currently to care for an individual, the nurse should not seek or share known details about a client's status. Family members would need approval from the client and the physician prior to reviewing a medical record.
Cognitive Level: Application **Client Need:** Safe, Effective Care Environment: Management of Care **Integrated Process:** Communication and Documentation **Content Area:** Fundamentals **Strategy:** The core issue of the question is knowledge about how to maintain client confidentiality. Recall that the ANA Code of Ethics guides you to protect client rights and that all client information is confidential. **Reference:** Kozier, B., Erb, G., Berman, A., & Snyder, S. J. (2004). *Fundamentals of*

nursing: Concepts, process and practice (7th ed.). Upper Saddle River, NJ: Pearson Education, p. 28.

5 **Answer: 1** The unit manager allows no input from anyone else, and all decisions are made by this individual. This is consistent with autocratic leadership. Democratic leadership gives voice to those affected; laissez-faire leadership is characterized by lack of decision making. In situational leadership, the individual adapts his or her style according to the needs at the time.
Cognitive Level: Application **Client Need:** Safe, Effective Care Environment: Management of Care **Integrated Process:** Communication and Documentation **Content Area:** Fundamentals **Strategy:** The core issue of the question is knowledge of various leadership styles. Use knowledge of the definitions of styles of leading to choose the option that best matches the behavior of the manager in the question. **Reference:** Kozier, B., Erb, G., Berman, A., & Snyder, S. J. (2004). *Fundamentals of nursing: Concepts, process and practice* (7th ed.). Upper Saddle River, NJ: Pearson Education, p. 476.

6 **Answer: 2** Ethics is a science that deals with rights and wrongs, the "good and bad" of human decision making and behavior. Laws are considered rules of society and would include statutes and practice acts.
Cognitive Level: Application **Client Need:** Safe, Effective Care Environment: Management of Care **Integrated Process:** Caring **Content Area:** Fundamentals **Strategy:** The core issue of the question is knowledge of when a client situation has a bearing on ethics. Use knowledge of how to discriminate legal from ethical matters to make an appropriate selection. **Reference:** Kozier, B., Erb, G., Berman, A., & Snyder, S. J. (2004). *Fundamentals of nursing: Concepts, process and practice* (7th ed.). Upper Saddle River, NJ: Pearson Education, p. 73.

7 **Answer: 2** Confidentiality protects the privacy of clients and their records. Informed consent is necessary prior to the treatment of the client. A living will is a document that is developed in which the client chooses end-of-life procedures. Justice demands that fair and equitable treatment is given to all and resources are distributed equally.
Cognitive Level: Application **Client Need:** Safe, Effective Care Environment: Management of Care **Integrated Process:** Nursing Process: Implementation **Content Area:** Fundamentals **Strategy:** Recall the definitions of the various terms in the options and determine the one that protects client rights as outlined in this question. **Reference:** Kozier, B., Erb, G., Berman, A., & Snyder, S. J. (2004). *Fundamentals of nursing: Concepts, process and practice* (7th ed.). Upper Saddle River, NJ: Pearson Education, p. 28.

ANSWERS & RATIONALES

8 **Answer: 3** Option 3 is the stated purpose of the ANA Code of Ethics; others contain incorrect information. **Cognitive Level:** Application **Client Need:** Safe, Effective Care Environment: Management of Care **Integrated Process:** Communication and Documentation **Content Area:** Fundamentals **Strategy:** The critical phrase in the question is *the purpose of the statement.* Recall that the ANA Code of Ethics delineates the values and standards for professional nursing practice. **Reference:** Kozier, B., Erb, G., Berman, A., & Snyder, S. J. (2004). *Fundamentals of nursing: Concepts, process and practice* (7th ed.). Upper Saddle River, NJ: Pearson Education, p. 75.

9 **Answer: 1** Primary nursing holds the nurse accountable for the care of a caseload of clients over a 24-hour period. Functional nursing is task-central nursing; total patient care is also known as the case method; and team nursing is a group of personnel that provide care to clients. **Cognitive Level:** Comprehension **Client Need:** Safe, Effective Care Environment: Management of Care **Integrated Process:** Nursing Process: Implementation **Content Area:** Fundamentals **Strategy:** The critical phrase is *accountable over a 24-hour period.* Recall that the hallmark of primary nursing is total accountability and responsibility for the care a client receives 24 hours a day until discharge. **Reference:** Kozier, B., Erb, G., Berman, A., & Snyder, S. J. (2004). *Fundamentals of nursing: Concepts, process and practice* (7th ed.). Upper Saddle River, NJ: Pearson Education, p. 100.

10 **Answer: 2** Good Samaritan laws are designed to protect healthcare professionals who offer assistance during an emergency and may apply to various licensed personnel. The laws vary from state to state and should be reviewed by the practicing RN. Care must be rendered free of charge and provided in good faith. **Cognitive Level:** Comprehension **Client Need:** Safe, Effective Care Environment: Management of Care **Integrated Process:** Caring **Content Area:** Fundamentals **Strategy:** The critical term is *Good Samaritan law.* Knowledge of this law will provide guidance for the nurse seeking to render aid in an emergency. **Reference:** Kozier, B., Erb, G., Berman, A., & Snyder, S. J. (2004). *Fundamentals of nursing: Concepts, process and practice* (7th ed.). Upper Saddle River, NJ: Pearson Education, p. 61.

Posttest

1 **Answer: 2** *Negligence* is defined as the failure to act as a reasonably prudent person would act in the same or similar situation, or doing something that a reasonably prudent person would not do. Giving a medication without an order is an example of option 1. Option 3 is incorrect because it relates to criminal statues that may not have been violated in this case. Option 4 does not relate to hospital-based care. **Cognitive Level:** Application **Client Need:** Safe, Effective Care Environment: Management of Care **Integrated Process:** Nursing Process: Implementation **Content Area:** Fundamentals **Strategy:** Recall legal concepts of nursing practice to recognize which principle is related to the current situation. Recalling that the nurse's actions are in essence an act of omission may help to determine that the correct answer is negligence. **Reference:** Kozier, B., Erb, G., Berman, A., & Snyder, S. J. (2004). *Fundamentals of nursing: Concepts, process and practice* (7th ed.). Upper Saddle River, NJ: Pearson Education, p. 57.

2 **Answer: 2** Malpractice occurs when any form of negligence causes injury to the client. It is the failure to act as a reasonably prudent person with the same knowledge and experience would act in the same or similar situation. A tort is a wrong or injury that a person has suffered from another's actions. Fraud is deliberate deception, and assault is an injury inflicted on one person by another. **Cognitive Level:** Application **Client Need:** Safe, Effective Care Environment: Management of Care **Integrated Process:** Nursing Process: Analysis **Content Area:** Fundamentals **Strategy:** Recall the definitions of the various terms used in the options and use the process of elimination to make a selection. **Reference:** Kozier, B., Erb, G., Berman, A., & Snyder, S. J. (2004). *Fundamentals of nursing: Concepts, process and practice* (7th ed.). Upper Saddle River, NJ: Pearson Education, p. 57.

3 **Answer: 3** Informed consent must always meet three requirements; it must be voluntary, the individual must have the capacity to consent, and the individual must understand the treatment and associated information in the consent document. Because of the language barrier, the client might not understand what he was consenting to, and if so, the document is not valid. It is not necessary for witnesses to be licensed personnel, and the document is not required to be notarized. The client's immigration status is unrelated to consent. **Cognitive Level:** Analysis **Client Need:** Safe, Effective Care Environment: Management of Care **Integrated Process:** Communication and Documentation **Content Area:** Fundamentals **Strategy:** Consider the necessary requirements to have an informed consent, and use the process of elimination to make a selection. **Reference:** Kozier, B., Erb, G., Berman, A., & Snyder, S. J. (2004). *Fundamentals of nursing: Concepts, process and practice* (7th ed.). Upper Saddle River, NJ: Pearson Education, p. 53.

4 **Answers: 1, 2, 4** Practice within the provisions of the Nurse Practice Act is essential to legal nursing practice. Treating all clients with kindness and respect and seek-

ing assistance when confronted with new situations will reduce the nurse's risk of liability in lawsuits. Seeking help when unsure in new situations also helps reduce risk of error by providing more expert opinions. Observing and reporting suspicious behavior (option 3) is vague and does not relate directly to risk management. Refusing to help other nurses (option 5) is unprofessional and at times could increase the risk of harm to clients if the unit were understaffed.
Cognitive Level: Application **Client Need:** Safe, Effective Care Environment: Management of Care **Integrated Process:** Nursing Process: Implementation **Content Area:** Fundamentals **Strategy:** The core concept in the question is risk management. Recall that common strategies for reducing the nurse's risk of liability in lawsuits such as the ones in the correct options may help prevent unnecessary involvement in legal proceedings. **Reference:** Kozier, B., Erb, G., Berman, A., & Snyder, S. J. (2004). *Fundamentals of nursing: Concepts, process and practice* (7th ed.). Upper Saddle River, NJ: Pearson Education, p. 476.

5 **Answer: 4** Each state has its own Nurse Practice Act that provides parameters in which nurses practice. Each state has a different interpretation of the individual acts; the Nurse Practice Act delineates the scope of practice. The agency's policy and procedures would be modified if new nursing responsibilities are assigned; however, agency policy must be consistent with the state Nurse Practice Act. Liability insurance coverage determines under what conditions the insurance company will pay a claim. The Good Samaritan law covers emergency aid rendered outside employment.
Cognitive Level: Application **Client Need:** Safe, Effective Care Environment: Management of Care **Integrated Process:** Communication and Documentation **Content Area:** Fundamentals **Strategy:** The critical word in the question is *first*. Nurse Practice Acts determine the scope of practice for registered nurses within each state. Recall that knowledge of this Act is key to legal nursing practice in any state. **Reference:** Kozier, B., Erb, G., Berman, A., & Snyder, S. J. (2004). *Fundamentals of nursing: Concepts, process and practice* (7th ed.). Upper Saddle River, NJ: Pearson Education, p. 54.

6 **Answer: 1** Advance directives offer guidance to the healthcare team when the client cannot make a decision regarding treatment. Advance directives are written while the client is competent. A durable (not temporary) power of attorney allows a competent person the power to act on behalf of the client in the event that the client loses decision-making capacity. The Self-Determination Act mandates that healthcare staff must offer the client information regarding healthcare deci-

sions. Informed consent is a crucial component of health care and seeks to alert the client to all avenues of care and treatment.
Cognitive Level: Application **Client Need:** Safe, Effective Care Environment: Management of Care **Integrated Process:** Teaching/Learning **Content Area:** Fundamentals **Strategy:** The critical phrase is *currently competent to make decisions regarding future needs.* Recall advanced directives give healthcare providers guidance to the desired course of treatment a client may wish when he or she becomes incapacitated. **Reference:** Kozier, B., Erb, G., Berman, A., & Snyder, S. J. (2004). *Fundamentals of nursing: Concepts, process and practice* (7th ed.). Upper Saddle River, NJ: Pearson Education, pp. 1043–1044.

7 **Answer: 4** A client advocate is one who expresses and defends the cause of the client. It is the nurse's responsibility to ensure the client has access to healthcare services that meet health needs. A direct care provider administers nursing care. A case manager provides for continuity of care, and a client educator provides instruction.
Cognitive Level: Application **Client Need:** Safe, Effective Care Environment: Management of Care **Integrated Process:** Nursing Process: Implementation **Content Area:** Fundamentals **Strategy:** Recall that advocacy is protecting the rights of others, which in this case indicates ensuring that clients have their healthcare needs met. **Reference:** Kozier, B., Erb, G., Berman, A., & Snyder, S. (2004). *Fundamentals of nursing; concepts, process, and practice* (7th ed.). Upper Saddle River, NJ: Pearson Education, p. 81.

8 **Answer: 4** Delegation is the transference of responsibility for the performance of an activity from one person to the next. The delegator, however, retains accountability for the outcome of the activity that has been delegated. An obligation to complete a task is responsibility. Empowerment is conferring power in a situation to another. Supervision involves directly or indirectly observing the care provided.
Cognitive Level: Analysis **Client Need:** Safe, Effective Care Environment: Management of Care **Integrated Process:** Communication and Documentation **Content Area:** Fundamentals **Strategy:** The core issue of the question is the role of the nurse in delegation. Recall that the nurse retains accountability for the care of the client and for the results of activities delegated to make a selection. **Reference:** Kozier, B., Erb, G., Berman, A., & Snyder, S. J. (2004). *Fundamentals of nursing: Concepts, process and practice* (7th ed.). Upper Saddle River, NJ: Pearson Education, p. 470.

9 **Answer: 1** Overdelegation occurs when too much authority or accountability is transferred to the delegate.

ANSWERS & RATIONALES

Reverse delegation occurs when authority is transferred to an individual of higher rank (option 2). Option 3 is an example of failure to delegate, and option 4 is an example of appropriate delegation. **Cognitive Level:** Comprehension **Client Need:** Safe, Effective Care Environment: Management of Care **Integrated Process:** Nursing Process: Implementation **Content Area:** Fundamentals **Strategy:** The core concept being tested is overdelegation. Use knowledge of the concept of overdelegation to select the option in which too much responsibility is conferred to another. **Reference:** Kozier, B., Erb, G., Berman, A., & Snyder, S. J. (2004). *Fundamentals of nursing: Concepts, process and practice* (7th ed.). Upper Saddle River, NJ: Pearson Education, p. 471.

10 **Answer: 1** In primary nursing, one nurse is responsible for total care of a number of clients 24 hours a day, 7 days a week. Team nursing provides individualized nursing care to clients by a nursing team led by a profes-

sional nurse. The case manager may not provide direct client care but coordinates health care among numerous healthcare workers. Functional nursing is task-based and assigns different team members to complete various nursing activities, such as taking vital signs, changing dressings, or administering medications. **Cognitive Level:** Analysis **Client Need:** Safe, Effective Care Environment: Management of Care **Integrated Process:** Nursing Process: Implementation **Content Area:** Fundamentals **Strategy:** The critical phrase is *responsible for the care of a client from admission to discharge.* Use knowledge of nursing care delivery models and the process of elimination to make a selection. **Reference:** Kozier, B., Erb, G., Berman, A., & Snyder, S. J. (2004). *Fundamentals of nursing: Concepts, process and practice* (7th ed.). Upper Saddle River, NJ: Pearson Education, p. 100.

References

American Nurses Association (2001). *Code for nurses with interpretative statements.* Kansas City, MO.

Finkelman, A. (2006). *Leadership and management in nursing.* Upper Saddle River, NJ: Pearson Education.

Guido, G. (2006). *Legal and ethical issues in nursing* (4th ed.). Upper Saddle River, NJ: Pearson Education.

Harkreader, H. & Hogan, M. (2007). *Fundamentals of nursing: Caring and clinical judgment* (3rd ed.). St. Louis, MO: Elsevier Science, pp. 16–43, 291–305.

Huber, D. (2006). *Leadership and nursing care management.* (3rd ed.). St. Louis, MO: Saunders.

Katz, J., Carter, C., Bishop, J., & Kravitz, S. L. (2004). *Keys to nursing success.* (2nd ed.). Upper Saddle River, NJ: Pearson Education.

Berman, A.J., Snyder, S., Kozier, B. & Erb, G. (2008). *Fundamentals of nursing: Concepts, process, and practice* (8th ed.). Upper Saddle River, NJ: Pearson Education, pp. 52–96, 511–595.

Sullivan, E. (2005). *Effective leadership and management in nursing* (6th ed.). Upper Saddle River, NJ: Pearson Education.

Tappen, R., Weiss, S., & Whitehead, K. (2006). *Essentials of nursing leadership and management* (4th ed.). Philadelphia: F. A. Davis.

Health Promotion Throughout the Lifespan

5

Chapter Outline

Health Promotion
Self-Concept
Sexual Development
Growth and Development
Culture and Health Promotion
Overview of the Family
Spirituality
Loss and Grief

Objectives

➤ Review how body image, self-esteem, roles, and identity affect an individual's self-concept.

➤ Discuss both the concept of sexuality and health promotion activities to foster a client's sexual health.

➤ Explore growth and development changes as they occur from infancy through late adulthood.

➤ Describe how an individual's culture affects all aspects of life including health.

➤ Describe the various family units, theoretical frameworks, and how illness can affect family dynamics.

➤ Distinguish spirituality from religion and the relationship to health promotion.

➤ Identify elements of the grieving process, usual grief symptoms, and methods for health promotion related to loss and grief.

NCLEX-RN® Test Prep

Use the CD-ROM enclosed with this book to access additional practice opportunities.

Review at a Glance

body image the perception of size, appearance, and function of one's body

child abuse any abuse whether physical, sexual, emotional, or neglect inflicted upon a child

colic crying that lasts 10 to 12 hours per day characterized by acute abdominal pain caused by intestinal contractions

ethnicity a demonstration of the characteristics shared by a group of people belonging to the same race or national origin

ethnocentrism the belief of superiority of one's race

failure to thrive a condition that may result from an inadequate parent-child relationship characterized by feeding difficulties, irritability, and inhibited weight gain; metabolic abnormalities and malabsorption syndrome are physiologic causes of failure to thrive

faith absolute belief in a set of ideologies though not demonstrated logically, nor visibly apparent

health a dynamic state of being that exists on a continuum, with high-level wellness of one end, a neutral state of neither wellness nor illness in the middle, and illness and death at the other end

health promotion an effort to advance health that engages a person in activities to enhance wellness

health protection modification of behavior to alter or reduce the effects of illness and disease

health restoration process of bringing the client back to a state of homeostasis

hope the thought process used by an individual in goal setting and successful attainment of these goals

identification to perceive oneself like another and mimic behavior of that person

infertility inability to conceive despite a period of unprotected intercourse for 12 months

introjection claiming attributes of others as one's own

loss absence of an object, person, body part, emotion, idea, or function, that was valued

maturity a state of maximal development of the physical, psychosocial, and cognitive being, enabling a person to function efficiently in the environment

race a group of individuals characterized by shared biological traits inherited from a common ancestor

regressive behavior temporary return to behaviors identified with previous stages of development

religion the organized expression of one's spirituality, faith, and hope

repression inhibition of experiences, thoughts, and impulses from conscious thought

self-concept complex integration of conscious and unconscious feelings, attitudes and perception, which affects behaviors and relationships with others

self-esteem emotional evaluation of self-worth

separation anxiety fear and frustration expressed by a child when absent from parents

sexual abuse sexual behavior forced upon another person

sexual orientation feelings of erotic potential directed toward members of opposite gender or one's own gender

sexual response cycle physiological changes that occur in response to sexual arousal; four phases are excitement, plateau, orgasm, and resolution

spirituality belief or faith in and establishment of a relationship with a higher being; this belief includes unknown aspects of life

sudden infant death syndrome the unexplained death of an infant under 1 year of age

PRETEST

1 A new mother informs the nurse that a neighbor just lost a baby to Sudden Infant Death Syndrome (SIDS). She is requesting information on ways she can prevent her baby from dying of SIDS. Which response by the nurse would be best?

1. "We do not know what causes SIDS and there really is not anything you can do to prevent it."
2. "Always be sure to put your baby to sleep on her back."
3. "Breastfeeding an infant for the first 6 months of life is the best start a mother can give her baby."
4. "Always make sure your baby is on her abdomen after feeding so she will not choke if she vomits."

2 An elderly, terminally ill client is being cared for by her only daughter. The daughter expresses a fear of not knowing how to care for her mother appropriately. Which nursing diagnosis is most appropriate?

1. Social isolation
2. Powerlessness
3. Situational low self-esteem
4. Ineffective role performance

3 The nurse is evaluating clients in a mental health clinic. One assessment the nurse makes is determining whether the clients are working on the appropriate psychosocial tasks as described by Erikson. Which statement(s) by the 45-year-old client indicate to the nurse that the client is working on meeting the appropriate developmental task? Select all that apply.

1. "I have a new girlfriend."
2. "My doctor says I shouldn't be driving a car, but if I don't drive, I will have to depend on others to bring me to clinic."
3. "I am now coaching a tee-ball team for our local baseball league."
4. "I was thinking of changing my hairstyle, what do you think?"
5. "I am helping my daughter plan her wedding."

4 A client states that his wife is going through a midlife crisis. The nurse would validate the husband's statement if the wife states she has been:

1. Buying a new wardrobe.
2. Writing a novel.
3. Wallpapering her mother's bedroom.
4. Baking bread for neighbor.

5 A family has a new pool and the mother asks the pediatric nurse how to protect her 2-year-old from drowning. Which of the following statements would be the best response?

1. Provide swimming lessons given by a certified instructor.
2. Place a fence around the pool.
3. Provide adult supervision at all times.
4. Purchase an approved flotation device.

6 When learning of the diagnosis of deep vein thrombosis, a client states, "If it is God's will, I will get better." Which of the following would be the highest priority intervention by the nurse to provide culturally competent care?

1. Notify the health care provider immediately.
2. Convey respect for the client's belief.
3. Further assess the client's knowledge of the disease.
4. State name and request to interview the client.

7 In order to provide culturally competent care, the nurse would plan to provide a Chinese American client with which of the following as the highest priority?

1. Visit from a rabbi
2. Choice of diet
3. Written discharge instructions rather than oral
4. Teaching video instead of oral and written instructions

8 A Jewish client shares with the nurse that he fears he will never walk again following back surgery. He feels his lack of health stems from punishment for past sin. The nurse concludes that what goal is of high priority for this client?

1. Restore spiritual well-being.
2. Enhance relationships with support people.
3. Walk within 3 days of surgery to facilitate coping.
4. Pray the rosary for forgiveness.

9 Since the client was diagnosed with terminal liver cancer, the nurse observes that the client's family assists with all of the activities of daily living. The nurse should communicate which rationale for self-care to the family?

1. Strengthening muscles may encourage healing of the cancer.
2. The client needs time alone to reason through her diagnosis.
3. Sense of loss can be lessened by retaining control in certain areas of life.
4. Increased mental activity required for self-care will enhance mood.

10 The nurse has been assigned to care for a client with a medical diagnosis of end stage renal disease; the client has recently begun hemodialysis. The client's care plan includes a diagnosis of spiritual distress. Which of the following comments by the client would validate that diagnosis? Select all that apply.

1. "I can't see much point in going on like this."
2. "I really hate this place. I'll be glad to get out of here and back to my own bed."
3. "Can you find a priest to come and talk to me sometime?"
4. "What kind of a God would let this happen to me?"
5. "Being in the hospital is really depressing."

➤ *See pages 128–129 for Answers & Rationales.*

I. HEALTH PROMOTION

A. Healthy People 2010

1. Is a document that serves as a guide to the nation's goal to improve health across the lifespan
2. Includes strategies to promote health, and to prevent disease, disability, and death
3. Overarching goals are to increase quality and years of healthy life, and eliminate health disparities
4. Identifies leading health indicators of concern in the United States
   a. Physical activity
   b. Overweight and obesity
   c. Tobacco use
   d. Substance abuse
   e. Responsible sexual behavior
   f. Mental health
   g. Injury and violence
   h. Environmental quality
   i. Immunizations
   j. Access to health care

B. Definitions related to health

1. **Health:** a dynamic state of being that exists on a continuum, with high-level wellness at one end, a neutral state of neither wellness nor illness in the middle, and illness and death at the other end
2. **Health promotion:** an effort to advance health that engages a person in activities to enhance wellness
3. **Health restoration:** the process of bringing the client back to homeostasis
4. **Health protection:** modification of behavior to alter or reduce the effects of illness and disease

C. Levels of prevention

1. Primary: consists of general health promotion activities and measures to protect against illness or infection (such as immunizations)
2. Secondary: consists of activities designed to identify health problems early and to decrease risk of exposure to disease, so as to limit future impairment
3. Tertiary: consists of measures aimed at returning a person to an optimum level of functioning through health restoration and rehabilitation

II. SELF-CONCEPT

A. Self-concept: complex integration of conscious and unconscious feelings, attitudes and perception, which affects behaviors and relationships with others

B. Development

1. Erikson defined eight psychosocial stages, also called developmental crises, which must be completed successfully in order to develop a healthy self-concept
2. Each stage or developmental crisis builds on the tasks of the previous stage
3. Erikson's psychosocial stages outline the age-associated developmental tasks assigned by Erikson (see Table 5-1)

Table 5-1	Physical, Psychosocial, and Cognitive Development from Birth to Adolescence		
Age	**Physical Development**	**Psychosocial Development (Erikson)**	**Cognitive Development (Piaget)**
Infancy (Birth to 1 year)	Weight: Average weight at birth is 7 to 8 pounds; should triple birth-weight by 1 year of age Height: 20 inches Head circumference: 33 to 35 cm Chest circumference: 30 to 33 cm Head circumference is greater than chest circumference until after 7 months of age	Trust versus Mistrust: The child learns to identify his or her physical self as separate and different from the environment; the development of trust is essential to the self-esteem of the child and is achieved through consistently having needs met	Sensorimotor period: At beginning of period (birth), child responds in a reflexive manner; by the end of this period (2 years), child has the ability to communicate and is mobile; at this point, the child's cognitive development involves goal distinction and attainment
Toddler (1 to 3 years)	Motor skills progress from walking to running to riding a tricycle Toilet training will be accomlished Physiologic anorexia will result because metabolism slows as growth rate slows	Autonomy versus Shame and Doubt: The child learns to internalize the attitudes of others towards self Toddler asserts autonomy by saying "no" frequently Separation anxiety occurs when parents are absent from child; regressive behaviors may occur when child reverts to less mature behavior by trying to return to a "safer period of time"	Sensorimotor period continues until age 2; then child begins the preoperational period Logic is not well developed; child often doesn't understand the cause-and-effect relationship Child often utilizes "magical thinking" as a way to explain the world around him or her
Preschool (3 to 5 years)	The child's body build changes from short, chubby toddler to slender, long-legged preschooler Physical skills continue to develop, focusing primarily on large motor skills The child learns to climb, ride a bicycle, use utensils, and dress him or herself	Initiative versus Guilt: The child continues learning self-esteem Failure to successfully achieve goals in this period will lead the child to have feelings of guilt and poor self-esteem	Continues in the preoperational period; thought process is continuing to mature but still has difficulty with causality; the child begins to develop intuitive thought; the development of conscience is an important component of this age period
School-age (6 to 12 years)	Boys and girls remain close in size and body proportions Beginning around age 6, the child loses the deciduous teeth; with the eruption of the permanent teeth, the facial proportions change	Industry versus Inferiority: The child takes pride in accomplishments Activities of this age should focus on developing a sense of competence and perseverance Self-concept develops as the school-age child internalizes the standards of society School-age children learn cooperation and become less self-centered	Preoperational cognitive development gives way to concrete operational thinking; during this period, the child's thought process continues to mature; in learning new information, the child benefits from concrete applications, which will give way to abstraction
Adolescent (13 to 18 years)	Between the ages of 10 and 18, males grow an average of 16 inches and gain 72 pounds Girls grow an average of 9 inches and gain 55 pounds Primary and secondary sexual characteristics develop as a result of increased hormone production In the male, ejaculation first occurs around age 14; menarche in females may occur between ages 8 and 16	Identity versus Role Confusion: The child establishes an identity; confidence and self-concept increases and the need for independence leads the adolescent to prefer spending time with the peer group rather than parents	Formal operational thought process begins at 11 years and progresses through adulthood; the child develops the ability to think abstractly

Table 5-1	(continued)		
Age	**Physical Development**	**Psychosocial Development (Erikson)**	**Cognitive Development (Piaget)**
Early adulthood (18 to 40 years)	Growth is complete, body systems function at peak efficiency Musculoskeletal system well-developed	Intimacy versus Isolation: The individual is developing intimate relationships with another individual or a cause, institution, or creative effort This relationship allows the individual to share components of the personality with another and allows adjusting of behavior to the behavior of another	
Middle-age (40 to 65 years)	Body changes include decreasing hormonal production Menopause (cessation of menstruation) occurs in women	Generativity versus Stagnation: The individual is concerned with providing for others When successful, the individual will have feelings of being needed, and being vital to establishing and nurturing the next generation	
Older adult (65 years to death)	Skin becomes drier, hair loses color Subcutaneous fat and muscle tissue is lost Decrease in physical strength, senses are less efficient All body organs are affected	Acceptance of self-worth, uniqueness, and death; this period is described as the coming together of all previous phases of the life cycle When ego has been achieved, the individual will remain creative	

   C. **Components of self-concept**

      1. **Self-esteem:** emotional evaluation of self-worth; heavily influenced by love and approval received as an infant

      2. **Body image:** the perception of size, appearance, and function of one's body

      3. Life role: a set of behaviors identified and expected by one's self, culture, and society

      4. Identity: a sense of individuality and uniqueness often affected by sex, race, occupation, marital status, education, talents, beliefs, personality, etc.

   D. **Stressors affecting self-concept:** real or imagined factors can threaten body image, self-esteem, role, or identity

      1. Stressors affecting body image include amputation, incontinence, and acne

      2. Self-esteem stressors include physical and emotional abuse, demotion in the workplace, and lack of success in an educational setting

      3. Role stressors include death of loved one, divorce, and unrealized life goals

      4. Stressors affecting identity include physical changes experienced in aging, lack of sexual performance, and pressures exerted by peers that are inconsistent with family values

   E. **Assessment:** the nurse should seek to identify behaviors suggestive of altered self-concept (see Box 5-1)

Box 5-1	1. Overly apologetic	7. Unusually dependent
Behaviors Suggestive of Altered Self-Concept	2. No eye contact	8. Has difficulty expressing opinions
	3. Hesitant speech	9. Lack of interest in daily activities
	4. Excessive, inappropriate anger	10. Passive
	5. Frequent crying	11. Difficulty making decisions
	6. Demeans self	12. Haphazard appearance

F. Nursing diagnoses: Impaired adjustment; Anxiety; Disturbed body image; Ineffective coping; Fear; Parental role conflict; Powerlessness; Ineffective role performance; Situational low self-esteem; Spiritual distress

G. Planning

1. The nurse develops a plan of care based on assessment data gathered, including information on state of health, anxiety level, support structure, culture, and religion

2. Goals and outcome criteria are developed with client's participation; goals would include a realistic perception of body, increased sense of self-worth, and adequate performance of roles

H. Implementation

1. To encourage an increased sense of self-concept, interventions should assist the client in identifying strengths and to maintain a sense of self

2. Examples of interventions for nursing diagnosis *Anxiety*

   a. Help client define level of anxiety

   b. Explore coping skills used in past and teach new ones as needed

   c. Encourage verbalization of concerns

   d. Decrease new stressors

   e. Alleviate pain before it progresses

   f. Teach relaxation techniques

I. Evaluation

1. Client demonstrates improved self-concept; evidence may be nonverbal cues such as resumed eye contact

2. The nurse should provide review of situation to the client and reinforce change

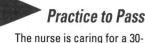

Practice to Pass

The nurse is caring for a 30-year-old female client who is postoperative following a mastectomy. Following assessment, the nurse has chosen the nursing diagnosis "Situational low self-esteem related to loss of body part." What client outcomes are appropriate for this diagnosis?

III. SEXUAL DEVELOPMENT

A. Phases of sexual development (see Table 5-2)

B. Sexual orientation: feelings of erotic potential directed toward members of opposite gender or one's own gender

C. Sexual response cycle: physiological changes that occur in response to sexual arousal; four phases are excitement, plateau, orgasm, and resolution

1. Excitement is the phase of increasing sexual arousal that can last from minutes to hours

Table 5-2	Phases	Age	Characteristics
Sexual Development	Infancy	Birth–18 months	Gender is assigned; genitals sensitive; males may have erections; females have vaginal lubrication
	Preschool	1–5 years	Identifies gender; labels body parts correctly; parent of opposite sex is focus of love
	Childhood	6–12 years	Becomes curious about sex roles and reproduction; friends are usually of same sex
	Adolescence	12–18 years	Sex characteristics develop; friendships may include the opposite sex; may engage in masturbation and sexual activity
	Adulthood	18–65 years	Establishes family, to include sexual activity, values, and family roles; between 40 and 65, hormone production decreases leading to climacteric in both sexes
	Older adulthood	65 years–death	Frequency of sexual activity decreases; men and women experience altered sexual functioning

2. Plateau is the phase that lasts from 30 seconds to 3 minutes and is a period of increasing sexual tension; it is manifested by elevated heart and respiratory rate and increased blood pressure

3. The orgasmic phase is the climax of sexual tension which lasts only a few seconds; during this phase, the male ejaculates

4. Resolution is the phase when the body returns to the unaroused state; is often accompanied by sleepiness and a feeling of relaxation

D. **Alterations in sexual health**

1. **Infertility:** inability to conceive despite a period of unprotected intercourse for 12 months

   a. Primary infertility refers to the couple who have never conceived

   b. Secondary infertility refers to the couple who have conceived before but are unable to do so at this time

2. **Sexual abuse:** sexual behavior forced upon another person; the behavior varies from inappropriate touching to rape; the abuser can be of either gender although male perpetrators are more common; the abused can be an adult or a child but often is a person with less power than the abuser; the impact of sexual abuse can be long-lasting

3. Sexual dysfunction: change in sexual functioning altering the normal sexual pattern; males may have erectile dysfunction; females may have orgasmic dysfunction or dyspareunia; sexual dysfunction can arise from many factors, including prescribed medications, drug categories that may contribute to dysfunction and the problems that they may cause include:

   a. Antihypertensives: may decrease sexual desire and cause erectile dysfunction

   b. Antidepressants: may decrease sexual desire or cause erectile or orgasmic dysfunction

   c. Antihistamines: may cause decreased vaginal lubrication and sexual desire

   d. Anticholinergics: may decrease sexual response

   e. Sedatives/tranquilizers: in large doses may decrease sexual desire or cause orgasmic dysfunction and impotence

   f. Ethyl alcohol: in moderate amounts increases sexual functioning, while chronic use may cause decreased sexual desire, female orgasmic dysfunction, and impotence

g. Barbiturates: increase sexual pleasure in low dose, while chronic use decreases desire and causes sexual dysfunction

h. Diuretics: decrease vaginal lubrication and sexual desire and cause erectile dysfunction

i. Opioid analgesics and other narcotics: inhibit sexual desire and response

E. Common nursing diagnoses related to change in sexuality: Disturbed body image; Decisional conflict; Deficient knowledge: STD prevention; Rape-trauma syndrome; Disturbed self-esteem; Sexual dysfunction; Ineffective sexuality patterns

F. Health promotion for sexual functioning

1. Client teaching is important to prevent sexual difficulties and to assist in behavior change needed to restore sexual health

a. Subject matter for client teaching is chosen according to client age; for instance, women over 50 need teaching regarding comfort measures for symptoms of menopause while priority teaching for women 20 years of age would be contraception and prevention of sexually transmitted diseases (STDs)

b. Sexual matters usually involve intimate content therefore the nurse provides client privacy to facilitate a proper learning environment

2. Sexual health promotion in acute care includes early disease detection; prompt intervention; prevention of complications and disabilities, such as teaching self-examination of breasts and testicles, STD prevention, contraceptive use

3. Sexual health promotion in restorative care assists the client in rehabilitation to optimum level of functioning; most likely includes both partners; specific teaching includes dealing with impotence, orgasmic dysfunction, and infertility

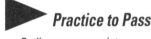

Practice to Pass

Outline an appropriate teaching plan for a 20-year-old male who has significant risk factors for testicular cancer.

IV. GROWTH AND DEVELOPMENT

A. General information relative to growth and development (refer back to Table 5-1)

1. Growth refers to an increase in size of the body

2. Development describes an increase in function and capability of the body; principles of development include:

a. Cephalocaudal development refers to head to tail maturation; the child will learn control over the head before learning control of the legs

b. Proximodistal development describes the development of the trunk prior to development in the extremities

3. The cognitive development of the child is described by Piaget's theory; unlike Erikson's theory which goes throughout life, Piaget's theory describes development from birth to the end of adolescence

B. Infancy (birth to 1 year)

1. Physical development: significant physical change occurs in weight, length, head circumference, refinement of sight, hearing, smell, taste and touch, reflexes, and motor skills; develop from turning head side-to-side to walking alone and feeding self

2. Psychosocial development: trust versus mistrust (refer again to Table 5-1)

3. Cognitive/intellectual development: Piaget outlines cognitive development as progressing from reflexive action to goal distinction and attainment

4. Health promotion: major health concerns

   a. Failure to thrive is a condition that may result from an inadequate parent-child relationship and is characterized by feeding difficulties, irritability and inhibited weight gain; this impaired parent-infant relationship must be differentiated from physiologic causes of failure to thrive, which include inadequate feeding and malabsorption syndromes

   b. Colic is acute abdominal pain lasting 10 to 12 hours per day caused by intestinal contractions; it typically occurs in the first 3 months of life; the cause is unknown, but the result is an infant who cries for long periods; the crying upsets the caregiver whose distress may contribute to the infant's emotional distress

   1) Possible causes include allergy to infant formula, rapid feeding, and swallowing air

   2) Treatment to reduce colic may include changing formula, changing nipples, and increased burping; cuddling and swaddling may be of benefit; the caregivers need to be reassured that the colic will end at approximately 3 months of age

   c. Sudden infant death syndrome (SIDS) is the unexplained death of an infant under 1 year of age; although an autopsy is performed, no reason for the death can be found

   1) SIDS occurs more frequently in males, preterm infants, and those with family history of SIDS

   2) Parents need to know that there was nothing they could have done to predict the infant's death

   3) Studies have shown that putting the infant to sleep on his or her back reduces the risk of SIDS

   d. Child abuse can include any abuse whether it is physical, sexual, emotional, or neglectful in nature

   1) Symptoms will depend upon the type of abuse

   a) Physical abuse can be manifested by bruises, burns, and fractures; the history of the injury does not match the physical findings; for instance, the history states the child fell off a porch, but the fracture is a spiral fracture, which occurs with twisting of a limb

   b) Sexual abuse may be discovered when the child is found to have a sexually transmitted disease

   c) Neglect may be noted when the child is severely undernourished without physical cause

   d) Emotional abuse is harder to identify but may be observed if abuser is verbally abusing the child; at other times it may be quite difficult to detect

   2) Take the history without comment; make no accusations to the parents; note that the child is improperly dressed for the weather; teachers may report a sudden change in behavior or school performance

   3) Nurses have a responsibility to report suspected abuse to the authorities; failure to report suspected abuse can lead to the nurse's liability; possible abuse reported in good faith will not lead to legal repercussions

5. Screening and assessment

   a. Healthcare examinations should be done at 2 weeks and at 2, 4, 6, and 12 months

   b. Immunizations are high priority (see Table 5-3)

Table 5-3	Vaccine	Recommended Age
Immunization Schedule for Ages 0 to 11 Years, 2007	Hepatitis B (Hep B)	First dose at birth to 2 months Second dose at 1–4 months Third dose at 6–18 months
	Rotavirus (Rota)	First dose at 2 months Second dose at 4 months Third dose at 6 months
	Diphtheria, tetanus, pertussis (DTaP)	First dose at 2 months Second dose at 4 months Third dose at 6 months Fourth dose at 15–18 months Fifth dose at 4–6 years Tetanus booster at 11–15 years Every 5–10 years thereafter
	H. influenza type B (Hib)	First dose at 2 months Second dose at 4 months Third dose at 6 months Fourth dose at 12–18 months
	Inactivated polio (IPV)	First dose at 2 months Second dose at 4 months Third dose at 6–18 months Fourth dose at 4–6 years
	Pneumococcal conjugate (PCV)	First dose at 2 months Second dose at 4 months Third dose at 6 months Fourth dose at 12–18 months
	Measles, mumps, rubella (MMR)	First dose 12–18 months Second dose 4–6 years
	Varicella	First dose 12–15 months Second dose 4–6 years
	Hepatitis A (HepA)	In selected areas 2–18 years
	Human papillomavirus (HPV)	First dose females age 11–12 years Second and third doses 2 and 6 months later
	Influenza	Yearly for children age 6–59 months
	Meningococcal (MCV4 or MPSV4)	Age 11 years (MCV4) and age 2 or older (MPSV4) if high risk

    c. Assess for safety issues such as risks for falls, burns, motor vehicle accidents, drowning, poisoning, choking, suffocation, and strangulation

    d. Assess feeding method techniques and schedule

    e. Developmental assessment includes physical, psychosocial, and cognitive areas

C. Early childhood: toddlers (1 to 3 years) and preschool children (4 to 5 years)

    1. Physical development

        a. Motor skills in the toddler progress from walking to running to riding a tricycle; the preschool child runs well, jumps, balances on toes, and dresses himself or herself

        b. Toilet training may begin after the child can walk well, pull clothing up and down, recognize the urge for elimination and control that urge until in the proper setting

      c. The toddler often experiences physiologic anorexia caused by a slowing of metabolism to accommodate the moderate growth rate

      d. Growth in the preschool child is greater in height than weight

2. Psychosocial development

      a. Toddler: autonomy versus shame and doubt (refer again to Table 5-1)

       b. **Separation anxiety** occurs when the parents are absent from the child and is expressed by fear and frustration

          1) It is also called toddler hospitalization reaction and consists of three stages

             a) Protest: the child is angry, screams and hollers; may bite or kick when healthcare personnel try to console the child; some children remain in this phase throughout hospitalization, while others quickly move into the next phase

             b) Despair: the child mourns the loss of the parent or caregiver; may continue to refuse to eat and have difficulty sleeping; may draw up into a fetal position and avoid contact with healthcare personnel; often cries softly

             c) Denial: in the third phase, the child is often thought to have recovered or adapted to the separation; this is incorrect, and the child may have severe difficulty resulting from the separation; in this phase, the child appears happy and plays, eats, and sleeps without difficulty; when the parents visit, the child may ignore them

          2) Support both the child and the parents or caregivers when separation occurs; nursing activities include the following:

             a) Provide physical comfort to the child

             b) Remind the child that the parents or caregivers love him or her and will return

             c) Encourage parents or caregivers to visit or stay with the child as appropriate

             d) Encourage the parents or caregivers to leave an article of clothing or a possession with the child

       c. **Regressive behavior** such as bed wetting or baby talk may occur when the child feels threatened; during these periods, the child attempts to return to a safer period of development; regression is common during and after a hospitalization; provide emotional support and allow the child to exhibit the regressive behavior

      d. Preschool children: initiative versus guilt (refer to Table 5-1); the preschooler learns **identification,** the ability to perceive oneself like another and mimic behavior of that person; he or she also has **introjection** (claiming attributes of others as one's own); imagination is an important part of the child's play life; **repression,** inhibition of experiences, thoughts, and impulses from conscious thought, is also expected at this stage

3. Cognitive/intellectual development: at the age of two, the child enters the preoperational period; logic is not well-developed; the child often doesn't understand cause-and-effect relationships; the child often utilizes "magical thinking" as a way to explain the world

4. Health promotion: major health concerns for the toddler and preschooler include:

   a. Accidents, including car accidents, drowning, burns, poisoning and falls; these are the leading cause of mortality in toddlers and are common in preschoolers as well

   b. Respiratory tract and ear infections are common to toddlers and preschoolers

5. Screening and assessment

   a. Healthcare examinations for the toddler should be scheduled at 15 and 18 months of age and then as needed; toddlers should visit the dentist by age 3; preschoolers should have exams every 1 to 2 years

   b. Immunizations (see Table 5-3)

   c. Discuss safety issues and methods to use to avoid accidents

   d. Developmental assessment includes physical, psychosocial, and cognitive areas; the Denver Developmental Screening Tool (Denver II) can be used by the nurse to evaluate development

D. School age (6 to 12 years)

1. Physical development

   a. Deciduous teeth are lost and permanent teeth begin to erupt; this occurrence changes the physical appearance of the child's face

   b. Weight gain occurs rapidly and is usually related to preadolescent growth spurts; females growth spurt in height begins some years prior to males

   c. Preadolescence begins about age 10 for females and age 12 for males; endocrine functions increase leading to increased perspiration and active sebaceous glands

2. Psychosocial development

   a. Industry versus inferiority: self-concept develops as the school-age child internalizes the standards of society (refer to Table 5-1)

   b. School-age children learn cooperation and to become less self-centered through peer interaction; parental relationships contribute more to self-esteem than peer groups

3. Cognitive/intellectual development: the child develops an understanding of logical reasoning, money, time, and day of the week; self-motivation develops

4. Health promotion

   a. Major health concerns: communicable diseases, parasitic infestations, homicide, and violence

   b. Screening and assessment

      1) Annual health care examinations

      2) Immunizations (refer to Table 5-3)

      3) Teach sports safety, emphasizing personal responsibility

      4) Developmental assessment includes physical, psychosocial, and cognitive areas

E. Adolescence (12 to 18 years)

1. Physical development: between the ages of 10 and 18, males grow an average of 16 inches and gain 72 pounds; during this same period, females grow an average of 9 inches and gain 55 pounds

2. Psychosocial development: the adolescent seeks to establish identity; appearance and perception of others is important; when valued, loved, and

accepted by family and peers, confidence and self-concept increases; the need for independence leads the adolescent to prefer spending time with the peer group rather than parents

3. Psychosexual development: increased hormone production leads to the development of primary (maturation of reproductive organs) and secondary sexual characteristics (pubic hair growth, breast development, voice changes); in males, ejaculation first occurs around age 14; in females, menarche may occur between ages 8 and 16; intimacy with a partner lays the foundation for commitment necessary for adult relationships; sexual experimentation may occur

4. Health promotion

   a. Major health concerns: alcohol and/or drug abuse, motor vehicle and other types of accidents, suicide, homicide, heart disease, depression

   b. Screening and assessment

      1) Health care examination as necessary

      2) Immunizations (refer to Table 5-3)

      3) Offer education concerning contraception, STDs, and emotional issues

      4) Offer safety assessment and teaching concerning motor vehicles, sports, and substance abuse

      5) Assess for nutritional alterations such as anorexia nervosa, bulimia, or obesity

      6) Developmental assessment includes physical and psychosocial areas

F. Early adult (20 to 40 years)

1. Physical development: the body systems function at peak efficiency; weight changes occur from influences of diet and exercise

2. Psychosocial development: in early adulthood **maturity** develops; maturity is the state of maximal development of the physical, psychosocial, and cognitive being, enabling a person to function efficiently in the environment; important lifestyle decisions are made such as education, occupation, marriage, children, and social responsibility

3. Psychosexual development: sexual activity increases; lifestyle choices are established based on adopted values

4. Health promotion

   a. Major health concerns: accidents, suicide, hypertension, substance abuse, STDs, domestic abuse, and malignancies

   b. Screening and assessment

      1) Healthcare examination should be done every 1 to 3 years for females; every 5 years for males

      2) Dental checkups are recommended every 6 months; vision and hearing assessments should be done as needed

      3) Females should have a Papanicolaou (Pap) smear yearly, breast self-examination (BSE) should be done monthly, clinical breast exam should be done every 1 to 3 years

      4) Males should perform testicular self-examination (TSE) monthly

      5) Screening for cardiac disease should be done as needed

      6) Teach motor vehicle safety, sun protection, and occupational safety

G. Middle adulthood (40 to 65 years)

   1. Physical development: the hair thins and grays, skin turgor declines, fat is redistributed to the abdominal area, loss of height caused by thinning of intervertebral discs occurs, blood vessels thicken and lose elasticity, visual acuity decreases, males are more prone to decline in auditory acuity, metabolism slows, constipation is common caused by a decrease in intestinal tone

   2. Psychosocial development: the middle adult is concerned with guiding the next generation through acts of service such as church, social, or political work; value of intellectual abilities surpasses physical attractiveness; individuals with difficulty in psychosocial development often demonstrate self-centeredness

   3. Psychosexual development: a decrease in hormone production produces menopause in females 40 to 55 years and the climacteric in males; couples may focus more on the quality of sexual encounters rather than the quantity

   4. Health promotion

   a. Major health concerns: accidents, cancer, cardiac disease, obesity, alcoholism, mental health changes

   b. Screening and assessment

   1) Healthcare examinations for females should be done yearly; for males they should be scheduled every 2 to 3 years

   2) Regular dental examinations should continue

   3) Continue BSE and TSE monthly

   4) Screen for cardiac disease and for colorectal, breast, cervical, uterine, and prostate cancers

   5) Discuss safety hazards in the home, the workplace, and in a motor vehicle

H. Late adulthood (over 65 years)

   1. Physical development

   a. Integumentary changes include dryness, pallor, wrinkling, age spots, decreased perspiration, and thinning of hair

   b. Neuromuscular changes include loss of height, osteoporosis, joint stiffness, and impaired balance

   c. Sensory changes include loss of visual and auditory acuity, decreased sense of taste and smell, and increased sensitivity to pain, touch, and temperature

   d. Pulmonary changes include decreased lung expansion and possible dyspnea

   e. Cardiovascular changes include increased blood pressure and decreased cardiac output

   f. Gastrointestinal changes include delayed swallowing, increased indigestion, and constipation

   g. Urinary changes include urgency and frequency, and impaired renal function

   h. Genital changes include male prostate enlargement and atrophy of reproductive organs in the female

   2. Psychosocial development: issues may include retirement, economic change, relocation, maintaining independence, and experiences of grief

   3. Psychosexual development: lessening sexual activity

   4. Health promotion

   a. Major health concerns: accidents, arthritis, cardiac disease, pulmonary disease, pharmaceutical misuse, alcoholism, dementia, and abuse

    b. Screening and assessment

        1) Health examinations should continue as they did during middle adulthood

        2) Explore safety issues such as fall prevention

        3) Encourage older adults to have lower intake of calories including adequate roughage and to maintain moderate exercise as able

        4) Assess for cognitive impairment and abuse

V. CULTURE AND HEALTH PROMOTION

A. Four basic characteristics of culture

    1. Learned from birth by family and peers through language (both nonverbal and verbal) and socialization

    2. Values, beliefs, patterns of behavior, language, food, dress, and other factors are shared by members of the same cultural group

    3. Common cultural aspects are influenced by specific conditions such as environment, technology, and resources

    4. Culture is dynamic and ever-changing as the members' needs change

B. Culturally based characteristics

    1. Space and distance: culture defines the relationship of the body to objects and other individuals; e.g., the Chinese may view being in close proximity to others as impolite

    2. Eye contact: a form of nonverbal communication with specific meaning for the culture; e.g., Americans view eye contact as a demonstration of self-confidence and interest, while the Navajo Indian considers eye contact a sign of disrespect

    3. Time: the past, the present and the future are defined and emphasized by a culture; e.g., Irish Americans value their heritage and tend to be past-oriented, whereas Native Americans are more often present-oriented, viewing time casually and accomplishing work as the need arises; Americans tend to be future-oriented, planning tasks to accomplish goals

    4. Touch: may be interpreted as casual or intimate; Hispanics value close relationships that include physical touching; in the Hmong culture, the head is never touched by anyone other than an elder

    5. Observance of holidays: these are specific to the culture and are valued differently; the significant winter holiday for many Christians is Christmas, while Hanukkah is the valued holiday for the Jewish culture

    6. Diet: culture dictates staple foods, food preparation, presentation of food, behaviors related to diet, and foods used as cures for illnesses; rice is a staple food for Asians, and pasta is plentiful in the Italian diet

C. Cultural assessment: systematic examination of individuals, groups, or communities in terms of cultural beliefs values or practices; to evaluate culture, ask questions such as the following:

    1. Where were you born? Your mother? Your father? Your grandparents?

    2. What is necessary to maintain health? Certain foods? Certain behaviors? Certain religious practices?

    3. Where do you think illness originates? What aspects of illness concern you?

    4. What difficulties arise when you are ill? For your family? Related to your employment?

    5. Describe how you seek to restore your health when ill.

Practice to Pass

In order to communicate with a Russian client, an interpreter is necessary. List characteristics of an ideal interpreter. Discuss key points in working with an interpreter.

6. Who do you seek assistance from when ill?

7. Are there remedies used for illness? Describe these.

8. What role do women have in health practices? During illness?

9. What role do men have in health practices? During illness?

10. Please list any other practices important to your culture that are important to you.

D. Ethnicity

1. A demonstration of the characteristics shared by a group of people belonging to the same race or national origin

2. **Race:** a group of individuals characterized by shared biological traits inherited from a common ancestor

   a. Races may be discriminated against as a result of **ethnocentrism:** the belief of superiority of one's race; federal, state, and local laws govern discrimination based on race

   b. Economic status may be related to race and also be a result of discrimination and lack of opportunities

   c. Political campaigns and practices may target specific racial issues

VI. OVERVIEW OF THE FAMILY

A. Family diversity: definitions of the family as the basic unit of society have broadened to include varying forms of the family

1. Nuclear family: consists of parents and children includes first marriage families, blended or stepparent families, and adoptive families

2. Binuclear family: a postdivorced family in which children are part of two nuclear families with varying amounts of time spent in each family

3. Intergenerational family: includes more than one generation of a family living together, such as older parents (grandparents)

4. Extended family: consists of parents, children, grandparents, aunts, and uncles

5. Single-parent family: consists of one male or female parent and children

B. Frameworks used for understanding the family

1. General systems theory: the family is a dynamic system with identifiable parts that interact; this system is composed of matter (people), energy, and communication (interactions with members and with those outside the family); the family is an open system continually interacting with and influenced by the community

2. Structural-functional theory: this theory defines two aspects of the family, structure and function; structure is the constantly evolving members and their relationships; functions of the family include assigning purpose, providing affiliation, socialization of members, and providing care

3. Developmental theory: families (like individuals) progress through stages of development; families must create an environment that encourages progression through the developmental stages

4. Nursing theories can be adapted to assist in health promotion activities provided by the nurse

   a. In Betty Neuman's systems model, the client or the family would be considered an open system surrounded by three levels of boundaries, which, when activated, protect the entity; health promotion would focus on strengthening these boundaries

    b. Sr. Callista Roy defines an adaptive system in which the client/family inter-
acts with the environment to meet needs; these needs can by physiologic, self-
concept, role function, or interdependence; the nurse can facilitate
interactions that promote health

    c. Imogene King developed a nursing theory that assists in defining the social
system in which a family functions; goal attainment occurs through transactions; transactions may include bargaining, negotiating, and common frames
of references; the nurse can facilitate a family's transactions and therefore
goal attainment

C. Illness impacts the family in a variety of ways

    1. Anxiety, stress, and/or depression may occur as members consider the outcome
of the illness; the degree of anxiety, stress, and/or depression experienced is
related to coping skills utilized

    2. Careers of family members may be affected as increased time demands interfere
with work schedules; anxiety, stress and/or depression may also interfere with
job performance; financial strain may occur with extended absences from work

    3. Roles may change within the family during illness particularly if a matriarch or
patriarch is the ill member and children must become caregivers

    4. Caregiver strain occurs as an illness becomes lengthy and additional
responsibilities are assumed

D. Common nursing diagnoses: Ineffective family processes; Disabled family coping;
Compromised family coping; Readiness for enhanced family coping

VII. SPIRITUALITY

A. Spirituality is belief or faith in and establishment of a relationship with a higher being; this
belief includes unknown aspects of life; these beliefs bring meaning, purpose, and hope;
faith provides inner strength

    1. Faith: absolute belief in a set of ideologies though they are not demonstrated
logically or visibly apparent; strength and trust are derived from faith

    2. Hope: the thought process used by an individual in goal setting and successful
attainment of these goals; hope is enhanced through inner strength,
relationships, and faith in God; the absence of hope leads to despair

    3. Religion: the organized expression of one's spirituality, faith, and hope

B. Promotion of spiritual health

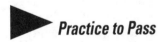

Practice to Pass

How can the nurse assess
spiritual development of the
preschooler?

    1. Definition: spiritual health is a state of wellness encompassing personal
fulfillment as well as fulfillment in life and with others; characterized by
expression of peace, love, and joy; a defined life purpose; and existence within a
set of values as outlined by the community and oneself

    2. Nursing interventions

        a. Encourage hope by: assisting the client in recalling past experiences where
hope was used while in crisis; goal revision to emphasize small steps of
progress; defining important, future events such as trips or family celebra-
tions that the client can anticipate; providing reading material or companionship to encourage the client; and support of religious practices

        b. Encourage evaluating the crisis with clarity; give factual information about
the client's state of health; refer the client as necessary to members of the
healthcare team; encourage a trusting relationship where emotions and fears
can be expressed

Table 5-4	Religion	Belief about Health
Religious Beliefs about Health	Christianity	Prayer for healing is appropriate; rosary may be used Catholic and Eastern Orthodox Christians may request a priest to administer sacrament of communion, reconciliation, or annointing (sacrament of the sick) Pictures of saints and angels may provide comfort
	Judaism	Dietary restrictions: milk and meat are not mixed; non-kosher products include predatory fowl, shellfish, and pork Prayer for healing is appropriate Artificial insemination, autopsy, use of birth control, use of blood and blood products, medications, and surgery are permitted Euthanasia is prohibited
	Hinduism	Characterized by the belief that for every action there is a corresponding reaction, therefore illness is caused by previous actions, even those in another life Eating meat is prohibited Medications, surgery, organ donation, and use of blood or blood products are acceptable
	Jehovah's Witness	Abortion, artificial insemination, use of blood or blood products, and organ donations are forbidden Healing prayer may be requested Reading of Scripture may provide comfort

   c. Assist with suffering by encouraging the client to interpret suffering; listen and be available; assist the client in discovering the positive aspects of suffering

C. Spiritual distress

   1. May occur in acute illness, chronic illness, terminal illness, or near-death experience
   2. Characteristics of spiritual distress
      a. Questioning of belief of life, death, and suffering
      b. Losing hope and developing feelings of discouragement or despair
      c. Doubting or abandoning religious practices
      d. Requesting spiritual assistance

D. Religious beliefs about health (see Table 5-4)

E. Religious rituals related to birth and death (see Table 5-5)

VIII. LOSS AND GRIEF

A. Loss

   1. Absence of an object, person, body part, emotion, idea, or function that was valued
   2. Actual versus perceived loss: actual losses are identified and verified by others while a perceived loss cannot be verified by others; for example, loss of a home caused by fire is an actual loss while loss of companionship following a move to a distance city is a perceived loss
   3. Maturational versus situational loss: maturational losses occur in normal development while situational losses occur without expectation; for example, parental sorrow produced from a child going away to college is a maturational loss while the death of the same child would be a situational loss
   4. Death, the ultimate loss: death results in a loss for the dying person as well as for those left behind; can be viewed as a time of growth for all who experience it (see Table 5-6 for an overview of the concept of death by age)

Table 5-5	Religion	Birth Rituals	Death Rituals
Religious Rituals Related to Birth and Death	Judaism	Males are circumcised on the eighth day following birth Females are named in the synagogue on the Sabbath following birth	When death is likely, no new heroic measures are taken Euthanasia is prohibited
	Islam	After birth, a prayer is recited in the child's ear Child is named on seventh day following birth Tuft of hair is shaved from head on seventh day following birth	Request that following death head be turned to Mecca Ritual bath following death
	Christianity	Baptism is done after birth to document that the child was born into a Christian family Baptism is done at birth of a seriously ill child; family or nurse may perform baptism	Speaking of afterlife is comforting as client is dying

Table 5-6	Age	Beliefs/Attitudes
Development of the Concept of Death	Infancy to 5 years	Does not understand concept of death Infant's sense of separation forms basis for later understanding of loss and death Believes death is reversible, a temporary departure, or sleep Emphasizes immobility and inactivity as attributes of death
	5 to 9 years	Understands that death is final Believes own death can be avoided Associates death with aggression or violence Believes wishes or unrelated actions can be responsible for death
	9 to 12 years	Understands death as the inevitable end of life Begins to understand own mortality, expressed as interest in afterlife or as fear of death
	12 to 18 years	Fears a lingering death May fantasize that death can be defied, acting out defiance through reckless behaviors (e.g., dangerous driving, substance abuse) Seldom thinks about death, but views it in religious and philosophic terms May seem to reach "adult" perception of death but be emotionally unable to accept it May still hold concepts from previous developmental stages
	18 to 45 years	Has attitude toward death influenced by religious and cultural beliefs
	45 to 65 years	Accepts own mortality Encounters death of parents and some peers Experiences peaks of death anxiety Death anxiety diminishes with emotional well-being
	65 + years	Fears prolonged illness Encounters death of family members and peers Sees death as having multiple meanings (e.g., freedom from pain, reunion with already deceased family members)

Table 5-7		
Theories of Grief, Dying, and Mourning	**Bowlby's Three Phases of Grief**	*Protest:* lack of acceptance concerning the loss; characterized by anger, ambivalence, and crying *Despair:* denial and acceptance occur simultaneously causing disorganized behavior; characterized by crying and sadness *Detachment:* loss is realized; characterized by hopefulness, accurately defining the relationship with the lost individual, and energy to move forward in life
	Kübler-Ross's Five Stages of Grieving	*Denial:* characterized by shock and disbelief; serves as a buffer to mobilized defense mechanisms *Anger:* resistance of the loss occurs; anger is typically directed toward others *Bargaining:* deals are sought with God or other higher power in an effort to postpone the loss *Depression:* loss is realized; may talk openly or withdraw *Acceptance:* recognition of the loss occurs; disinterest may occur; future thinking may occur
	Worden's Four Tasks of Mourning	1. Accept the reality of the loss; the loss is accepted 2. Experience the pain of grief; healthy behaviors are accomplished to assist in the grieving process 3. Adjust to the environment without the deceased; tasks are accomplished to reorient the environment, i.e., removing the clothes of the deceased from the closet 4. Emotionally relocate the deceased and move forward with life; correctly align the past, the present, and look toward the future

B. Grieving process (see Table 5-7)

C. Anticipatory grief: expression of the symptoms of grief prior to the actual loss; grief period following the loss may be shortened and the intensity lessened because of the previous expression of grief; for example, a child told that a family move is expected may grieve about losing friends prior to actually leaving

D. Complications of bereavement

1. Chronic grief: symptoms of grief occur beyond the expected time frame and the severity of symptoms is greater; depression may result

2. Delayed grief: when symptoms of grief are not expressed and are suppressed, a delayed grief reaction occurs; the nurse should discuss the normal process of grieving with the client and give permission to express these symptoms

E. Symptoms of normal grief

1. Feelings include sadness, exhaustion, numbness, helplessness, loneliness, disorganization, preoccupation with the lost object or person, anxiety, depression

2. Thought patterns include fear, guilt, denial, ambivalence, anger

3. Physical sensations include nausea, vomiting, anorexia, weight loss or gain, constipation or diarrhea; diminished hearing or sight; chest pain; shortness of breath; tachycardia

4. Behaviors include crying, difficulty carrying out activities of daily living, and insomnia

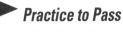

Practice to Pass

A parent is caring for her terminally ill child at home. She asks the nurse, "How will I know when death is near?" What should the nurse's response be?

! ▸ **F. Nursing health promotion to facilitate mourning (Worden, 1991)**

1. Help client accept that the loss is real by providing sensitive, factual information concerning the loss

2. Encourage the expression of feelings to support people; this builds relationships and enhances the grief process

3. Support efforts to live without the deceased person or in the face of disability; this promotes a client's sense of control as well as a healthy vision of the future

4. Encourage establishment of new relationships to facilitate healing

5. Allow time to grieve; the work of grief may take longer for some; observe for a healthy progression of symptoms

6. Interpret "normal" behavior by teaching thoughts, feelings, and behaviors that can be expected in the grief process

7. Provide continuing support in the form of a presence for therapeutic communication and resource information

8. Be alert for signs of ineffective coping such as inability to carry out activities of daily living, signs of depression, or lack of expression of grief

Case Study

A client is an 82-year-old Polish female who states that her religion is Catholic. She has congestive heart failure and receives weekly visits from a home health nurse. The client states that she is a burden to everyone and wishes it wasn't against her religious beliefs to commit suicide.

1. What spiritual assessment data should the nurse obtain?

2. What spiritual nursing diagnosis might be appropriate?

3. State the expected outcomes for this nursing diagnosis.

4. What interventions are appropriate to help this client?

5. How would the nurse evaluate the stated outcomes?

For suggested responses, see pages 336.

POSTTEST

1 The nurse is caring for a male client who has recently had his left leg amputated. To assess body image, the nurse should gather subjective data such as the:

1. Client's feelings regarding surgery.
2. Strength of femoral pulses bilaterally.
3. Client's description of his personality.
4. Status of wound healing.

2 A nurse is admitting a client who became ill while visiting in this country. The nurse is unfamiliar with the cultural practices and health beliefs of the client's home country. Which of the following questions would be appropriate to ask in the admission assessment? Select all that apply.

1. Are there remedies you have used for this illness before coming to the hospital?
2. Who do you usually see for help or care when you are ill?
3. What do you believe is causing your current illness?
4. Why do you dress in that type of clothing?
5. Can you tell me about your usual diet?

3 A client reports a decrease in sexual desire. The nurse should examine the client's medication list for which of the following medications? Select all that apply.

1. Azithromycin (Zithromax)
2. Propranolol (Inderal)
3. Ascorbic acid (vitamin C)
4. Warfarin (Coumadin)
5. Sertraline (Zoloft)

4 The nurse is interviewing an adolescent client. The nurse can best facilitate communication with the adolescent client by making which statement?

1. "If you read the pamphlet you'll know all you need to know."
2. "We can talk about this with your mother."
3. "Other teenage girls also feel depressed."
4. "Tell me about the last time you had sexual intercourse."

5 Several parents have asked the pediatric nurse to assess whether their toddlers are ready for toilet training. The nurse concludes that which of the following toddlers demonstrates readiness for toilet training?

1. One who can dress and undress self and walks well
2. One who pulls to a standing position and says "pee" when urinating
3. One who walks and needs assistance with removing clothes
4. One who crawls well and cries loudly after urination

6 A 4-year-old Mexican American child has recently been diagnosed with leukemia. When considering the client's culture, the nurse would employ which of the following as the most appropriate intervention?

1. Limit all visitors, including extended family.
2. Encourage visits from extended as well as immediate family.
3. Ban all visits from alternative healers.
4. Make diet selections for the child and family.

7 Before acting upon the perceived nonverbal behavior of a client from Italy, the nurse should do which of the following?

1. Validate his or her perception.
2. Use a translator.
3. Get another nurse to assess the client.
4. Form a nursing diagnosis.

8 An elderly client expresses difficulty sleeping because her spirit is disturbed due to sin in her life. The nurse should select which of the following as the priority intervention?

1. Call the chaplain and schedule a visit.
2. Ascertain what religious practice is appropriate to the client.
3. Pray immediately with the client.
4. Administer sleep medications as ordered.

9 A client who is in the final stage of cancer is depressed and distant. The client asks the nurse, "Why is God punishing me?" Which of the following would be the most appropriate action for the nurse to take?

1. Be available to the client.
2. Share personal religious belief with the client.
3. Tell the client to pray for answers.
4. Call the physician for antianxiety medication orders.

10 A nurse finds multiple bruises in various stages of healing and signs of old injuries on an infant during an assessment. The nurse suspects the child may be the victim of abuse. Which of the following would be most important for the nurse to do?

1. Investigate the mother's feelings toward the infant.
2. Refer the child to a center for abused children.
3. Document objective findings and report suspected abuse as outlined in agency policy.
4. Make a note on the chart so the child will be assessed carefully on future visits.

➤ *See pages 129–131 for Answers & Rationales.*

POSTTEST

ANSWERS & RATIONALES

Pretest

1 **Answer: 2** Studies have shown that infants who are put to sleep on their backs have a much lower incidence of SIDS than infants who are placed on the abdomen. Breastfeeding has many health benefits for the newborn but is unrelated to risk of SIDS.
Cognitive Level: Application **Client Need:** Health Promotion and Maintenance **Integrated Process:** Teaching/Learning **Content Area:** Fundamentals **Strategy:** The critical words are *prevent SIDS.* Use knowledge of major health concerns of infants to select the response that represents sound parent teaching. **Reference:** Kozier, B., Erb, G., Berman, A., & Snyder, S. J. (2004). *Fundamentals of nursing: Concepts, process, and practice* (7th ed.). Upper Saddle River, NJ: Pearson Education, p. 374.

2 **Answer: 4** There has been a change in the daughter's responsibilities; therefore, her role has changed, making the appropriate nursing diagnosis *Ineffective role performance.* There is insufficient data to support the other nursing diagnoses listed.
Cognitive Level: Analysis **Client Need:** Health Promotion and Maintenance **Integrated Process:** Nursing Process: Analysis **Content Area:** Fundamentals **Strategy:** The core issue of the question is knowledge of various psychosocial nursing diagnoses. Use this information and the process of elimination to make a selection. **Reference:** Kozier, B., Erb, G., Berman, A., & Snyder, S. J. (2004). *Fundamentals of nursing: Concepts, process, and practice* (7th ed.). Upper Saddle River, NJ: Pearson Education, p. 148.

3 **Answer: 3, 5** Option 3 indicates an interest in guiding the next generation, which is an appropriate task for the client's age. Option 5 represents a similar example. Option 1 deals with relationships and is most frequently seen in late adolescence/early adulthood. The concern for loss of independence is seen in the older adult, and the adolescent is more likely to be concerned with personal appearance because it affects body image.
Cognitive Level: Analysis **Integrated Process:** Nursing Process: Evaluation **Client Need:** Health Promotion and Maintenance **Content Area:** Fundamentals **Strategy:** Recall that the psychosocial tasks of the middle adult include establishing a steady income, developing leisure, assisting/teenage children to become adults, and enjoying spouse and caring for aged parents. **Reference:** Kozier, B., Erb, G., Berman, A., & Snyder, S. J. (2004). *Fundamentals of nursing: Concepts, process, and practice*

(7th ed.). Upper Saddle River, NJ: Pearson Education, pp. 398–399.

4 **Answer: 1** Erikson's stage of development for middle-aged adulthood is Generativity versus Stagnation. Behaviors indicating lack of progression would be self-centered (option 1) and demonstrate lack of commitment. Successful progression would be demonstrated by creativity and concern for others (options 2, 3, and 4).
Cognitive Level: Analysis **Client Need:** Psychosocial Integrity **Integrated Process:** Nursing Process: Analysis **Content Area:** Fundamentals **Strategy:** Use knowledge of Erikson's stages of psychosocial development to guide you in assessing client status. **Reference:** Kozier, B., Erb, G., Berman, A., & Snyder, S. J. (2004). *Fundamentals of nursing: Concepts, process, and practice* (7th ed.). Upper Saddle River, NJ: Pearson Education, p. 357.

5 **Answer: 3** A toddler may still drown even though swimming lessons, fences, and flotation devices are present. Only adult supervision can ensure the safety of a toddler when water is present.
Cognitive Level: Application **Client Need:** Safe, Effective Care Environment: Safety and Infection Control **Integrated Process:** Teaching/Learning **Content Area:** Fundamentals **Strategy:** The critical phrase is *protect her 2-year-old from drowning.* Use knowledge of major health concerns for children in the toddler years to direct you to the option that provides appropriate safety information and guidance to parents. **Reference:** Kozier, B., Erb, G., Berman, A., & Snyder, S. J. (2004). *Fundamentals of nursing: Concepts, process, and practice* (7th ed.). Upper Saddle River, NJ: Pearson Education, p. 379.

6 **Answer: 2** To gain a client's trust, respect must be conveyed even if there is disagreement with the belief expressed. Introductions and further assessment are important but ineffective if respect is not conveyed. Notifying the provider does not have priority at this time.
Cognitive Level: Application **Client Need:** Psychosocial Integrity **Integrated Process:** Caring **Content Area:** Fundamentals **Strategy:** Awareness of nursing interventions to promote spiritual health will assist you in selecting the option that aids in establishing a positive relationship with the client. Recall that religion may provide a framework for a client's health beliefs.
Reference: Kozier, B., Erb, G., Berman, A., & Snyder, S. J. (2004). *Fundamentals of nursing: Concepts, process, and*

practice (7th ed.). Upper Saddle River, NJ: Pearson Education, p. 1002.

7 **Answer: 2** Culturally competent care includes providing clients with items from their culture, such as food choices. The nurse must understand the culture to provide this type of care. Unless the nurse knows the client's fluency in the English language, it would be difficult to make an appropriate choice between options 3 and 4. Thus, there is no basis for selecting them as the answer to this question. Rabbis are not the spiritual head of the Chinese religious community.
Cognitive Level: Application **Client Need:** Psychosocial Integrity **Integrated Process:** Nursing Process: Planning **Content Area:** Fundamentals **Strategy:** The critical terms in the question are *culturally competent* and *Chinese American.* Knowledge of culturally based characteristics will direct you to select actions that will be useful to clients from a specified culture. **Reference:** Kozier, B., Erb, G., Berman, A., & Snyder, S. J. (2004). *Fundamentals of nursing: Concepts, process, and practice* (7th ed.). Upper Saddle River, NJ: Pearson Education, p. 215.

8 **Answer: 1** A nursing diagnosis of spiritual distress is appropriate for this client. Therefore the most important goal is to restore his spiritual well-being. Relationships and walking are not related to this diagnosis. The rosary is a Catholic aid to prayer.
Cognitive Level: Analysis **Client Need:** Psychosocial Integrity **Integrated Process:** Nursing Process: Planning **Content Area:** Fundamentals **Strategy:** Critical phrases in this question are *punishment for past sin* and *outcome goal.* Use knowledge of nursing diagnoses related to spirituality to assist in setting appropriate goals for client outcomes. **Reference:** Kozier, B., Erb, G., Berman, A., & Snyder, S. J. (2004). *Fundamentals of nursing: Concepts, process and practice* (7th ed.). Upper Saddle River, NJ: Pearson Education, p. 1003.

9 **Answer: 3** It is important that independence be maintained in the client with a terminal illness as long as possible to convey control and dignity. Options 2 and 4 may or may not be true; there is insufficient information in the stem to determine this. Option 1 is a false statement.
Cognitive Level: Application **Client Need:** Psychosocial Integrity **Integrated Process:** Teaching/Learning **Content Area:** Fundamentals **Strategy:** Use awareness of the stages of grief to enable you to select the option that best provides guidance to family members in time of loss. **Reference:** Kozier, B., Erb, G., Berman, A., & Snyder, S. J. (2004). *Fundamentals of nursing: Concepts, process, and practice* (7th ed.). Upper Saddle River, NJ: Pearson Education, p. 1048.

10 **Answers: 1, 3, 4** Characteristics of spiritual distress include losing hope and developing feelings of despair, re-

questing spiritual assistance, and doubting or abandoning religious beliefs and practices. Options 2 and 5 do not relate to spiritual concerns.
Cognitive Level: Analysis **Client Need:** Psychosocial Integrity **Integrated Process:** Nursing Process: Analysis **Content Area:** Fundamentals **Strategy:** Critical words in the question are *spiritual distress* and *validate diagnosis.* Recall the characteristics of spiritual distress to make an accurate diagnosis. **Reference:** Kozier, B., Erb, G., Berman, A., & Snyder, S. J. (2004). *Fundamentals of nursing: Concepts, process, and practice* (7th ed.). Upper Saddle River, NJ: Pearson Education, p. 1001–1002.

Posttest

1 **Answer: 1** To assess body image, the nurse must gather the client's perception of his body. Option 3 is not related to body image. Options 2 and 4 are objective data.
Cognitive Level: Application **Client Need:** Psychosocial Integrity **Integrated Process:** Nursing Process: Assessment **Content Area:** Fundamentals **Strategy:** The critical words in the question are *subjective data* and *body image.* Remember, whenever asked for subjective data you are looking for client perceptions, opinions, or concerns. **Reference:** Kozier, B., Erb, G., Berman, A., & Snyder, S. J. (2004). *Fundamentals of nursing: Concepts, process, and practice* (7th ed.). Upper Saddle River, NJ: Pearson Education, p. 959.

2 **Answers: 1, 2, 3, 5** A cultural assessment should include information on the person's land of origin, the person's health beliefs and practices, the healthcare practitioners the person usually consults, and the person's beliefs regarding the origin of illness. The person's reason for dressing in a particular manner is not relevant to this situation and the question may be viewed as rude or intrusive.
Cognitive Level: Analysis **Client Need:** Psychosocial Integrity **Integrated Process:** Nursing Process: Assessment **Content Area:** Fundamentals **Strategy:** Awareness of cultural influences on health care beliefs and practices will enable you to assess a client's needs for culturally competent care. **Reference:** Kozier, B., Erb, G., Berman, A., & Snyder, S. J. (2004). *Fundamentals of nursing: Concepts, process, and practice* (7th ed.). Upper Saddle River, NJ: Pearson Education, p. 217.

3 **Answer: 2, 5** Antihypertensives, narcotics, diuretics, antipsychotics, antidepressants, antihistamines, and others decrease sexual desire. Propranolol is an antihypertensive while sertraline is an antidepressant. Azithromycin is an antibiotic. Ascorbic acid is a water-soluble vitamin. Warfarin is an anticoagulant.
Cognitive Level: Application **Client Need:** Physiologic Integrity: Pharmacological and Parenteral Therapies

Integrated Process: Teaching/Learning **Content Area:** Fundamentals **Strategy:** The critical phrase is *decreased sexual desire.* Recall common side effects of frequently prescribed groups of medications to assist you in eliminating the incorrect options. **Reference:** Kozier, B., Erb, G., Berman, A., & Snyder, S. J. (2004). *Fundamentals of nursing: Concepts, process, and practice* (7th ed.). Upper Saddle River, NJ: Pearson Education, p. 980.

4 **Answer: 3** Option 3 indicates that the client is not alone, which can enhance communication by affirming the client's feelings. Adolescents will feel more willing to discuss private issues if parents are not present (option 2) and if they understand that their concerns are common with other teens. Questions should be sensitively worded rather than intrusive (option 4). Written instructions should supplement teaching rather than being the primary vehicle for teaching (option 1).
Cognitive Level: Application **Client Need:** Psychosocial Integrity **Integrated Process:** Health Promotion and Maintenance **Content Area:** Fundamentals **Strategy:** The critical phrase is *facilitate communication with the adolescent.* Use knowledge of psychosocial development throughout the lifespan to choose the option that allows effective communication with adolescents. **Reference:** Kozier, B., Erb, G., Berman, A., & Snyder, S. J. (2004). *Fundamentals of nursing: Concepts, process, and practice* (7th ed.). Upper Saddle River, NJ: Pearson Education, p. 387.

5 **Answer: 1** Developmental readiness for toilet training is demonstrated by standing and walking well, dressing self, recognizing the need for elimination, and having the physical ability to delay elimination. Lack of these abilities can indicate that the toddler needs additional time before attempting toilet training.
Cognitive Level: Analysis **Client Need:** Health Promotion and Maintenance **Integrated Process:** Teaching/Learning **Content Area:** Fundamentals **Strategy:** The critical term in the question is *demonstrates readiness.* Use knowledge of the sequence of physical development in early childhood to select the option that has the greatest likelihood for success. **Reference:** Kozier, B., Erb, G., Berman, A., & Snyder, S. J. (2004). *Fundamentals of nursing: Concepts, process, and practice* (7th ed.). Upper Saddle River, NJ: Pearson Education, p. 1228.

6 **Answer: 2** The extended family is considered a source of strength, support, and emotional stability for the Mexican American family. Alternative healers and specific foods also may be important to the state of health, so these should not be banned or limited.
Cognitive Level: Application **Client Need:** Psychosocial Integrity **Integrated Process:** Caring **Content Area:** Fundamentals **Strategy:** Key words are *Mexican Ameri-*

can and *considering the client's culture.* Use knowledge of family roles within different cultures to assist you in selecting culturally competent interventions for this client. **Reference:** Kozier, B., Erb, G., Berman, A., & Snyder, S. J. (2004). *Fundamentals of nursing: Concepts, process, and practice* (7th ed.). Upper Saddle River, NJ: Pearson Education, p. 212.

7 **Answer: 1** Nonverbal behavior may have varied meaning among different cultures; therefore, the nurse must validate meaning. There is insufficient information to determine the need for a translator (option 2). Option 3 is unnecessary and option 4 is premature because the nurse has insufficient data.
Cognitive Level: Analysis **Client Need:** Psychosocial Integrity **Integrated Process:** Communication and Documentation **Content Area:** Fundamentals **Strategy:** Recall that the Italian culture may utilize nonverbal communication and behavior and therefore you need to select the option that seeks to interpret that behavior. **Reference:** Kozier, B., Erb, G., Berman, A., & Snyder, S. J. (2004). *Fundamentals of nursing: Concepts, process, and practice* (7th ed.). Upper Saddle River, NJ: Pearson Education, p. 214.

8 **Answer: 2** Assessment of religious practices that the client would find comforting should be accomplished first in order to assist the client with spiritual distress. Option 1 would be done if indicated as an answer to option 2. Option 3 may or may not be appropriate; there is insufficient data in the stem of the question to support it. Option 4 may be needed if other options are unsuccessful.
Cognitive Level: Analysis **Client Need:** Psychosocial Integrity **Integrated Process:** Communication and Documentation **Content Area:** Fundamentals **Strategy:** Recall common nursing interventions to promote spiritual health and use the process of elimination to select actions that aid in identifying and helping clients meet their spiritual needs. **Reference:** Kozier, B., Erb, G., Berman, A., & Snyder, S. J. (2004). *Fundamentals of nursing: Concepts, process, and practice* (7th ed.). Upper Saddle River, NJ: Pearson Education, p. 1002.

9 **Answer: 1** The nurse should always offer self to the client by being physically present, attentive, and listening to the client's feelings and concerns. In option 2 the nurse should always analyze the reason for sharing personal beliefs. Option 3 is not therapeutic. In times of distress clients may not be able to pray. Option 4 is not appropriate because the client is displaying depression, not anxiety.
Cognitive Level: Application **Client Need:** Psychosocial Integrity **Integrated Concept:** Communication and Documentation **Content Area:** Fundamentals **Strategy:** Recall that the

nurse should be present to the client and aid the client in achieving spiritually desired outcomes. **Reference:** Kozier, B., Erb, G., Berman, A., Snyder, S. J. (2004). *Fundamentals of nursing: concepts, process, and practice* (7th ed.). Upper Saddle River, NJ: Pearson Education, p. 1002.

10 **Answer: 3** Nurses have a moral and legal responsibility to report all suspected child abuse to the authorities. Failure to report suspected abuse can result in liability for the nurse. The mother's feelings about the child are of little relevance since she may not be the abuser. Referring the child to another center may be indicated, but only after the case has been investigated. Noting suspicions on the chart will not protect the child from harm. **Cognitive Level:** Analysis **Client Need:** Safe Effective Care Environment: Safety and Infection Control **Integrated Process:** Communication and Documentation **Content Area:** Fundamentals **Strategy:** The critical terms are *nurse suspects* and *victim of abuse.* Recall common patterns of child abuse to aid in identifying possible victims and reporting their concerns. **Reference:** Kozier, B., Erb, G., Berman, A, & Snyder, S. J. (2004). *Fundamentals of nursing: Concepts, process, and practice* (7th ed.). Upper Saddle River, NJ: Pearson Education, p. 374.

References

Ball, J. & Bindler, R. (2006). *Child health nursing: Partnering with children and families.* Upper Saddle River, NJ: Pearson Education.

Berman, A. J., Snyder, S., Kozier, B., & Erb, G. (2008). *Fundamentals of nursing: Concepts, process, and practice* (8th ed.). Upper Saddle River, NJ: Pearson Education pp. 146–209.

Bickley, L. S. (2006). *Bates' guide to physical examination and history taking* (9th ed.). Philadelphia: Lippincott Williams & Wilkins.

Harkreader, H. & Hogan, M. (2007). *Fundamentals of nursing: Caring and clinical judgment* (3rd ed.). St. Louis, MO: Elsevier Science, pp. 322–427, 1230–1270.

Lemone, P. & Burke, K. (2008). *Medical-surgical nursing: Critical thinking in client care* (4th ed.). Upper Saddle River, NJ: Pearson Education.

Davidson, M., London, M., & Ladewig, P. (2008). *Maternal-newborn nursing and women's health across the lifespan* (8th ed.). Upper Saddle River, NJ: Pearson Education.

Spector, R. (2004). *Cultural diversity in health and illness* (6th ed.). Upper Saddle River, NJ: Pearson Education.

Pender, N., Murdaugh, C., & Parsons, M. (2006). *Health promotion in nursing practice* (5th ed.). Upper Saddle River, NJ: Pearson Education, pp. 14–36, 66–94, 113–191.

U. S. Dept. of Health and Human Services. Office of Disease Prevention and Health Promotion. (2000). *Healthy people 2010.* Washington, DC: Author.

ANSWERS & RATIONALES

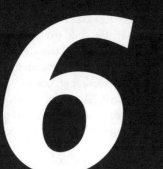

6

Overview of Skills Necessary for Safe Practice

Chapter Outline

Principles of Asepsis and Infection Control

Medical Asepsis versus Surgical Asepsis

Overview of Vital Signs

Overview of Body Mechanics

Overview of Cardiopulmonary Resuscitation

NCLEX-RN® Test Prep

Use the CD-ROM enclosed with this book to access additional practice opportunities.

Objectives

➤ Describe the infectious process, modes of transmission, risk factors, and diagnostic tests used to detect infection and inflammation.

➤ Compare and contrast medical and surgical asepsis and the principles associated with each.

➤ Explain the significance of and techniques for measuring vital signs.

➤ Identify the scientific principles and guidelines for use of proper body mechanics.

➤ Describe the procedures used to provide basic life support for both the adult and child client.

Review at a Glance

aerobic requiring oxygen to live

afebrile a condition in which the body temperature is not elevated

anaerobic an ability to live without oxygen

apnea absence of breathing

blood pressure the force of blood against an arterial wall

body mechanics efficient use of the body as a machine and as a means of locomotion

bradycardia slow heart rate, less than 60 beats per minute

bradypnea slow respiratory rate

diastolic pressure the least amount of pressure exerted on arterial walls, which occurs when the heart is at rest between ventricular contractions

dyspnea difficulty breathing

endogenous infection one in which the causative organism comes from the person's own microorganisms

eupnea normal respiration

exogenous infection an infection in which the causative organism is found outside the host

febrile a condition in which the body temperature is elevated

hypertension blood pressure elevated above the upper limit of normal

hypotension blood pressure below the lower limit of normal

iatrogenic infection an infection that occurs as a result of a treatment or diagnostic procedure

infection a disease state resulting from pathogens in or on the body

medical asepsis practice designed to reduce the number and transfer of pathogens; synonym for clean technique

orthostatic hypotension a temporary fall in blood pressure associated with assuming an upright position; synonym for postural hypotension

pathogen a disease-producing organism

pulse a wave produced in the wall of an artery with each beat of the heart

surgical asepsis a set of practices that render and keep objects and areas free from all microorganisms; synonym for sterile technique

systolic pressure highest point of pressure on arterial walls when the ventricles contract

tachycardia elevated heart rate above 100 beats per minute in an adult

tachypnea elevated respiratory rate

PRETEST

1 A client has been identified as having a very virulent bacterial infection that is spread through close physical contact. To decrease the chance of spreading this organism, the nurse would implement which infection control precautions?

1. Airborne precautions
2. Droplet precautions
3. Contact precautions
4. Protective isolation

2 A nurse needs to make rounds on four clients who are stable. Using the principle of medical sepsis, which client should be seen first?

1. A postsurgical cardiac client with hypostatic pneumonia
2. A client with a draining wound
3. A client who is severely neutropenic
4. A child with chicken pox

3 A client develops a bloodstream infection from a central venous access device that has been in place for several months. The culture reports indicate that the infection is endogenous. The nurse concludes that which of the following would be a potential source of the infectious organism?

1. Hands of a caregiver
2. Client's skin flora
3. Airborne bacteria from another client
4. Bacteria from contaminated IV fluids

4 The nurse needs to bathe a client who has an infection spread by droplets, and the client has been placed on droplet precautions. Prior to reporting to work, the nurse's hands were scratched by a pet cat. The nurse puts on which of the following pieces of protective equipment before caring for this client? Select all that apply.

1. Mask
2. Gown
3. Goggles
4. Gloves
5. Head cover (cap)

5 A nurse is preparing to take vital signs on an alert client admitted to the hospital with dehydration secondary to vomiting and diarrhea. What is the best method to assess this client's body temperature?

1. Oral
2. Axillary
3. Rectal
4. Heat-sensitive tape

6 A nursing intershift report has indicated that a client's pulse volume is described as one. After receiving the report, the initial action of the nurse should be to do which of the following?

1. Notify the health care provider.
2. Assess client right away.
3. Document that pulse volume is normal.
4. Change the client's position.

7 A client has an elevated temperature. The nurse assesses the client and finds the skin flushed and very warm. The client is oriented to person, place, and time and expresses severe fatigue. What would be the most appropriate action by the nurse at this time?

1. Place ice bags on the client's skin.
2. Remove blankets and offer fluids.
3. Increase the client's activity.
4. Decrease the client's oral fluid intake.

8 Which of the following findings would be of greatest concern to the nurse taking a client's pulse?

1. Mild tachycardia in a febrile client
2. Mild bradycardia in a young otherwise healthy male who is asleep
3. 18-month-old with a heart rate of 120 beats per minute (6pm)
4. Pulse deficit with an apical rate of 84 bpm and a peripheral pulse of 72

9 While eating in a restaurant, a nurse notices a male patron choking on food. The individual is coughing loudly, his face is red, and he is unable to answer questions. Which of the following actions should the nurse take?

1. Place arms around the choking individual's waist and exert fist pressure on the abdomen.
2. Lay the individual on the floor and straddle the individual's legs to position self for the Heimlich maneuver.
3. Stand by and further observe the individual's response.
4. Slap the choking individual firmly on the back three times before attempting chests thrusts.

10 A nurse is evaluating a nurse orientee's performance during a mock code blue. The nurse concludes that chest compressions for the adult receiving CPR are adequate when the orientee depresses the sternum to a depth of no more than _____ inches.

Answer: _____

➤ *See pages 158–159 for Answers & Rationales.*

I. PRINCIPLES OF ASEPSIS AND INFECTION CONTROL

A. Chain of infection

1. The chain of infection refers to those elements that must be present to cause an infection from a microorganism

2. Basic to the principle of infection control is to interrupt this chain so that an **infection** from a microorganism does not occur in clients

3. *Infectious agent:* a microorganism capable of causing infections are referred to as an infectious agent or a **pathogen**

   a. Examples of infectious agents or pathogens are bacteria, viruses, yeast, fungi, and protozoa

b. In order for an infectious agent to produce an infection, the following circumstances must apply:

1) The organism needs to be virulent

2) The length of exposure needs to be sufficient

3) The host must be susceptible

c. If the pathogen does not produce symptoms in the host, the infection is called asymptomatic or subclinical; an opportunistic pathogen only causes an infection in a susceptible host

d. A local infection is an infection that is limited to a certain area of the body

e. A systemic infection occurs when microorganisms spread to different parts of the body

f. Colonization refers to a microorganism in the body that becomes resident flora that grows and reproduces but does not produce disease

4. *Mode of transmission:* the microorganism must have a means of transmission to get from one location to another, called direct and indirect (see next section)

5. *Susceptible host:* describes a host (human or animal) with inadequate resistance against a particular pathogen to prevent disease or infection from occurring when exposed to the pathogen; in humans this may occur if the person's resistance is low because of poor nutrition, lack of rest, lack of exercise, or a coexisting illness that weakens the host

6. *Portal of entry:* the means of a pathogen entering a host; the means of entry can be the same as one that is the portal of exit (gastrointestinal, respiratory, genitourinary tract); may also occur through a break in skin integrity

7. *Reservoir:* the environment in which the microorganism lives to ensure survival; it can be a person, animal, arthropod, plant, soil, or a combination of these things; reservoirs that support organisms that are pathogenic to humans include inanimate objects, food and water, and other humans and animals

8. *Portal of exit:* the means by which the pathogen escapes from the reservoir and can cause disease; there is usually a common escape route for each type of microorganism; in humans, common escape routes are the gastrointestinal, respiratory, and the genitourinary tracts, and may also be the skin

Practice to Pass

Identify assessment data that indicate a client may have increased susceptibility to infections.

B. Modes of transmission

1. Direct contact: the way in which microorganisms are transferred from person to person through biting, touching, kissing, or sexual intercourse; droplet spread is also a form of direct contact but can occur only if the source and the host are within 3 feet from each other; transmission by droplet can occur when a person coughs, sneezes, spits, or talks

2. Indirect contact: can occur through fomites (inanimate objects or materials) or through vectors (animal or insect, flying or crawling); the fomites or vectors act as a vehicle for transmission; examples of fomites are handkerchiefs, toys, cooking utensils, surgical instruments or dressings, water, and food; examples of vectors are flies, mosquitoes, fleas, bats, cows, and cats

3. Airborne: involves droplets or dust; droplet nuclei can remain in the air for long periods and dust particles containing infectious agents can become airborne, infecting a susceptible host generally through the respiratory tract

C. Course of infection

1. Incubation: the time interval between initial contact with an infectious agent and the first signs or symptoms of host infection; the incubation period varies for different pathogens; microorganisms are growing and multiplying during this stage

2. Prodromal stage: the time period from the onset of nonspecific symptoms to the appearance of specific symptoms related to the causative pathogen; symptoms range from being fatigued to having a low-grade fever with malaise; during this phase it is still possible to transmit the pathogen to another host

3. Full stage: the time during which specific signs and symptoms of the infectious agent are evident; this is also referred to as the acute stage; during this stage, it may be possible to transmit the infectious agent to another, depending on the agent's virulence

4. Convalescence: the time period during which the host returns to the pre-illness state, also called the recovery period; the host defense mechanisms have responded to the infectious agent and the manifestations of the disease disappear; the host, however, is more vulnerable to other pathogens at this time; an appropriate nursing diagnostic label related to this process would be *Risk for infection*

D. Inflammation

1. Definition: the protective response of body tissues to injury or infection; the physiological reaction to injury or infection is the inflammatory response; it may be acute or chronic

2. Body's response

   a. The inflammatory response begins with vasoconstriction that is followed by a brief increase in vascular permeability; the blood vessels dilate, allowing plasma to escape into the injured tissue

   b. White blood cells (neutrophils, monocytes, and macrophages) migrate to the area of injury and attack and ingest the invaders (phagocytosis); this process is responsible for the signs of inflammation

   c. Redness occurs when blood accumulates in the dilated capillaries; warmth occurs as a result of the heat from the increased blood in the area; swelling occurs from fluid accumulation; and pain occurs from pressure or injury to the local nerves

E. Immune response

1. The immune response involves specific reactions in the body to antigens or foreign material

2. This specific response is the body's attempt to protect itself, and involves activating two types of lymphocytes, the T-lymphocytes and B-lymphocytes

3. Cell-mediated immunity: T-lymphocytes are responsible for cellular immunity

   a. When fungi, protozoa, bacteria, and some viruses activate T-lymphocytes, they enter the circulation from lymph tissue and seek out the antigen

   b. Once the antigen is found they produce proteins (lymphokines) that increase the migration of phagocytes to the area and keep them there to eradicate the antigen

   c. After the antigen is gone, the lymphokines disappear

   d. Some T-lymphocytes remain and keep a memory of the antigen and are reactivated if the antigen appears again

4. Humoral response: the ability of the body to develop a specific antibody to a specific antigen (antigen-antibody response)

    a. B-lymphocytes provide humoral immunity by producing antibodies that convey specific resistance to many bacterial and viral infections

    b. Active immunity is produced when the immune system is activated either naturally or artificially

        1) Natural immunity involves acquisition of immunity through developing the disease

        2) Active immunity can also be produced through immunizations, which introduce into the body weakened or killed antigens (artificially acquired immunity)

        3) Passive immunity does not require a host to develop antibodies, rather it is transferred to the individual; passive immunity occurs when a mother passes antibodies to a newborn or when a person is given antibodies in the form of immune globulins from an animal or person who has had the disease; this type of immunity only offers temporary protection from the antigen

F. Hospital-acquired infection

    1. Hospital-acquired infections are those that are experienced as a result of a healthcare delivery system

    2. Clients become exposed to an infectious agent while in a healthcare agency even if the infection may not be apparent at the time

    3. Iatrogenic infection: these hospital-acquired infections are directly related to the client's treatment or diagnostic procedures; an example is a bacterial infection that results from an intravenous line or *Pseudomonas aeruginosa* pneumonia as a result of respiratory suctioning

    4. Exogenous infection: these hospital-acquired infections are a result of the healthcare facility environment or personnel; an example would be an upper respiratory infection resulting from contact with a caregiver who has an upper respiratory infection

    5. Endogenous infection: can occur from clients themselves or from reactivation of a previous dormant organism such as tuberculosis; an example of endogenous infection would be a vaginal yeast infection arising in a woman receiving antibiotic therapy; the yeast organisms are always present in the vagina, but with the elimination of the normal bacterial flora, the yeast flourish

G. Factors increasing susceptibility to infection

    1. Age: young infants and older adults are at greater risk of infection because of reduced defense mechanisms

    a. Young infants have reduced defenses related to immature immune systems

    b. In older adults, physiological changes occur in the body that make them more susceptible to infectious disease; some of these changes are:

        1) Altered immune function (specifically, decreased phagocytosis by the neutrophils and by macrophages)

        2) Decreased bladder muscle tone resulting in urinary retention

        3) Diminished cough reflex, loss of elastic recoil by the lungs leading to reduced ability to evacuate normal secretions

        4) Gastrointestinal changes resulting in decreased swallowing ability and delayed gastric emptying

2. Heredity: some people have a genetic predisposition or susceptibility to some infectious diseases

3. Cultural practices: healthcare beliefs and practices, as well as nutritional and hygiene practices, can influence a person's susceptibility to infectious disease

4. Inadequate nutrition: nutritional practices that do not supply the body with the basic components necessary to synthesize proteins affect the way the body's immune system can respond to a pathogen

5. Stress: physical and emotional stressors affect the body's ability to protect against invading pathogens; stressors affect the body by elevating blood cortisone levels; if elevation of serum cortisone is prolonged, it decreases the anti-inflammatory response and depletes energy stores, thus increasing the risk of infection

6. Rest, exercise, and personal health habits: altered rest and exercise patterns decrease the body's protective mechanisms and may cause physical stress to the body, resulting in an increased risk of infection; personal health habits such as poor nutrition and unhealthy lifestyle habits increase the risk of infections over time by altering the body's response to pathogens

7. Inadequate defenses: any physiological abnormality or lifestyle habit can influence normal defense mechanisms in the body, making the client more susceptible to infection; the immune system functions throughout the body and depends on the following:

    a. Intact skin and mucous membranes

    b. Adequate blood cell production and differentiation

    c. A functional lymphatic system and spleen

    d. An ability to differentiate foreign tissue and pathogens from normal body tissue and flora; in autoimmune disease, the body has difficulty recognizing its own tissue and cells; people with autoimmune disease are at increased risk of infection because of their immune system deficiencies

8. Environmental: an environment that exposes individuals to an increased number of toxins or pathogens also increases the risk of infection; pathogens grow well in warm moist areas with oxygen (**aerobic**) or without oxygen (**anaerobic**) depending on the microorganism

9. Immunization history: inadequately immunized people have an increased risk of infection specifically for those diseases for which vaccines have been developed

10. Medications and medical therapies: examples of therapies and medications that increase risk for infection include radiation treatment, antineoplastic drugs, anti-inflammatory drugs, and surgery

H. Diagnostic tests used to screen for infection

1. Signs and symptoms of localized infection are associated with the area infected; for instance, symptoms of a local infection on the skin or mucous membranes are localized swelling, redness, pain, and warmth

2. Symptoms of systemic infection include fever, increased pulse and respirations, lethargy, anorexia, and enlarged lymph nodes

3. Certain diagnostic tests are ordered to confirm the presence of an infection (see Table 6-1)

Table 6-1	Test	Normal Values/ Conventional Units	Purpose/Indication
Diagnostic Tests Related to the Infectious Process	White blood cell count (WBC)	4,000 to 10,000/mL	A nonspecific blood test that indicates a response to either an infectious agent or to therapy; an elevation can indicate infection, tissue necrosis, stress, or neoplastic changes in bone marrow; an abnormally low count may also signal an increased risk for infection
	White blood cell count with differential	Total neutrophils: 60–70% Bands: 0–5% Lymphocytes: 20–40% Monocytes: 2–8% Eosinophils: 1–4% Basophils: 0.5–1.0%	The total WBC is differentiated according to the various leukocytes; elevation of immature neutrophils (granulocytes or bands) indicates a bacterial infection (shift to the left); eosinophil elevation indicates an allergic disorder or a parasitic infestation; lymphocytes are elevated in viral or chronic infections; monocytes are elevated in viral infections and chronic inflammatory disorders; basophils are elevated in acute or severe infection
	Erythrocyte sedimentation rate (ESR)	Male: 40–54% Female: 38–47%	ESR measures the rate at which red blood cells settle in unclotted blood; marked elevation of the ESR may occur in acute or severe bacterial infections; ESR can also provide information about the course of an infectious disease and the client's response to treatment
	Culture and sensitivity (C&S)	Dependent upon source; findings will indicate organism present as well as antibiotics to which the organism is sensitive	Cultures are obtained from body fluids (urine, blood, wound exudate, cerebrospinal fluid); tissue cells are differentiated from microorganisms; stains are added to identify the organism structure; gram stains can broadly classify the organism; this information is useful for prescribing antibiotic therapy before sensitivity results are completed

II. MEDICAL ASEPSIS VERSUS SURGICAL ASEPSIS

> **A. Medical asepsis:** a clean technique that involves healthcare practices that limit the number of pathogens present that could cause infections; application of barrier techniques to break the infectious cycle is a major nursing responsibility

> 1. Centers for Disease Control guidelines (see Box 6-1); the CDC has designated two tiers of precautions:

  a. Standard precautions are standards used for all clients regardless of medical diagnosis

  b. Transmission-based precautions are used for suspected and documented infections; isolation procedures or precautions are practices that healthcare personnel use to prevent the spread of microorganisms and are based on CDC recommendations; in some cases where the client's immune system is altered (leukopenia or low white blood cell count [WBC]), protective isolation practices are used to protect the client from microorganisms

Box 6-1	**Standard Precautions**
Summary of CDC Guidelines	➤ Perform hand hygiene between client contact and after removing gloves using non-microbial soap or hand rub for routine handwashing. Use antimicrobial soap if hands may be contaminated with body secretions or a specific infectious disease is present.

Standard Precautions

➤ Perform hand hygiene between client contact and after removing gloves using non-microbial soap or hand rub for routine handwashing. Use antimicrobial soap if hands may be contaminated with body secretions or a specific infectious disease is present.

➤ Wear clean gloves and appropriate type of personal protective equipment (such as gowns, face protection) when contact with various body secretions is expected.

➤ Change gloves between tasks on the same client.

➤ Handle used client equipment and soiled linen carefully to prevent the spread of mircoorganisms and follow procedures for cleaning equipment that is obviously contaminated with body fluids.

➤ Avoid recapping used needles. Place used needles and sharps in a puncture-resistant container.

➤ Clients who are likely to contaminate their environment should be placed in private rooms.

➤ Ensure that environmental controls such as room cleaning and disinfection procedures are followed.

Transmission-Based Precautions

➤ Are recommended in addition to Standard Precautions to prevent the spread of microorganisms based on route of transfer.

Airborne Precautions

➤ Used for clients with infections spread through the air (tuberculosis, varicella, rubeola).

➤ Provide a private room with monitored negative air pressure, 6 to 12 air changes per hour with air discharged to the outside or through a filter system, in relation to surrounding areas.

➤ Keep client in the room with door closed.

➤ Use respiratory protective equipment when entering room for clients with tuberculosis and if healthcare worker is not immune to varicella or rubeola.

➤ Transport client out of room, if required, wearing a surgical mask.

Droplet Precautions

➤ Used for clients with an infection that is spread by large-particle droplets (rubella, mumps, diphtheria, and adenovirus infection in children).

➤ Place client in a private room if possible or with other clients with same infection (cohorting).

➤ Wear respiratory protective equipment when providing care or if within 3 feet of client.

➤ Visitors should wear respiratory protective equipment if within 3 feet of client.

➤ Transport client after giving client a surgical mask to wear.

Contact Precautions

➤ Used for clients with an infection that is spread by direct or indirect contact or who are colonized with microorganisms like methcillin-resistant staphylococcus aureus (MRSA), or vancomycin-resistant enterococcus (VRE).

➤ Provide a private room or place with other clients who have the same microorganisms.

➤ Wear gloves when entering the room. Remove gloves in client's room and wash hands with an antiseptic or antimicrobial agent.

➤ Wear personal protective equipment when in contact with infected body secretions.

➤ Limit movement of the client outside the room.

2. Standard precautions: include specific behaviors and use of personal protective equipment by healthcare workers to protect themselves from acquiring pathogens from the clients in their care and to protect the clients from any pathogens the healthcare worker may have; generally no special technique is involved in the removal of equipment unless there is a reason to suspect garments or hands of the healthcare worker may become soiled; hands are always washed after removal of equipment

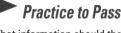

   a. Handwashing or hand hygiene: should occur before healthcare workers handle food, before and after eating, before and after each client contact, and after removing gloves; hand hygiene is considered the first line of defense against the spread of microorganisms and should be done frequently

   b. Gloves: are worn by healthcare workers to protect the hands when likely to be in contact with any body fluids/secretions (blood, urine, feces, sputum, mucous membranes, and nonintact skin); are worn by healthcare workers when any condition exists that may cause transfer of endogenous microorganisms to the client; for example, microorganisms on healthcare worker's hands may infect a client's nonintact skin; gloves also reduce the risk of the transmitting microorganisms from one client to another

   c. Gowns: clean gowns or disposable waterproof gowns are worn when there is a risk of the healthcare worker's clothing becoming soiled from the client's body secretions

   d. Masks: are worn when there is a risk of infection from the airborne route, droplet contact, or by splatters of body secretions; there are different types of masks depending on the suspected pathogen; single-use disposable masks should be discarded when becoming wet or soiled, and generally are effective during client care procedures; particulate respiratory masks are used for disease spread by airborne transmission such as tuberculosis

   e. Protective eyewear: eyeglasses, goggles, or face shields are used if there is a risk of body secretions being splattered in the face

3. Soiled equipment/supplies: each healthcare facility has policies related to the disposal and decontamination of reusable supplies and equipment; healthcare workers should follow the facility's policies and apply general principles of medical asepsis

   a. Sharps: needles, syringes, and sharps (lancets, razors, scalpels, broken glass) are placed into a puncture-resistant container; needles should never be detached from the syringe or re-capped before disposal

   b. Dishes: if the client has a condition where there is a high risk of transmission of pathogens, most agencies use disposable dishes; handling of non-disposable dishes is minimized after client's meals by using trays to transport dirty dishes from client rooms

   c. Trash: garbage and soiled disposable equipment are placed in a plastic bag that lines the waste container

      1) If articles are contaminated, they are placed in a bag that is impervious to microorganisms before removal

      2) Articles that have infective material on them such as blood, pus, body fluid, or respiratory secretions are handled according to CDC's bloodborne pathogen guidelines

▶ **Practice to Pass**

What information should the nurse provide to parents of a chronically ill child to reduce the risk of infection while promoting normal growth and development?

      3) If the facility does not have impervious bags, it is necessary to double-bag soiled equipment before removing it from the client's room

      4) Healthcare workers and clients should never retrieve articles from any waste container

   d. Thermometers: most agencies use disposable thermometers that are disposed of in the client's waste container; nondisposable thermometers are disinfected after use

   e. Linen: all soiled linen should be handled as little as possible; it should be placed in a linen bag and closed prior to removal from the client's room; laundry bags that are impervious to microorganisms are used by most agencies

4. Laboratory specimens: are placed in a leak-proof container with a secure lid; many agencies also require that they be placed in a sealed plastic bag labeled with a "biohazard" logo for transport to the laboratory

5. Transporting persons with infections: when transporting a client with an infection, the nurse must take precautions to prevent the spread of the pathogen; for instance, if the client has a respiratory infection a mask may be needed for transport; the nurse should notify the receiving department of the situation

6. Routine cleaning: all healthcare facilities have procedures for routine cleaning of clients' rooms

   a. Generally all equipment is disinfected before a new client is admitted to the room; this includes the bed, bathroom, tables, trays, telephones, call lights, remote controls, and any medical equipment kept in the room

   b. Care is taken to prevent spread of organisms from one client to another by the use of barriers

   c. For clients on isolation precautions, items used to monitor the client condition such as thermometers, stethoscopes, and blood pressure cuffs should not be removed from the room until discharge; agency policy for disinfecting these items must be followed before using them on any other client

B. Surgical asepsis

1. General principle: surgical asepsis involves those techniques that keep objects and areas free from all microorganisms, and are used for certain diagnostic procedures, and in operating rooms and labor and delivery areas (see Table 6-2); surgical aseptic (sterile) technique is indicated for procedures that require penetration of a client's skin such as with injections and IV catheter insertion

2. Sterilization, disinfection, and cleaning: these procedures interrupt the chain of infection and are used in healthcare facilities and by healthcare workers to decrease the spread of infectious organisms

   a. Sterilization: kills all microorganisms, including spores and viruses; four commonly used methods are moist heat, gas, boiling water, and radiation; the nurse should follow facility policies relating to the method of sterilization associated with different objects to be sterilized

   b. Disinfection: takes place through the use of chemicals on objects; these chemicals may be toxic to tissues and are both bactericidal and bacteriostatic; when disinfecting articles, the nurse must follow the facility policies and manufacturer's recommendations for the disinfectant used; it is important that the disinfectant come in contact with the surface of the object and be exposed for the recommended time

Table 6-2	Principles	Practices
Principles and Practices of Surgical Asepsis	All objects used in a sterile field must be sterile.	All articles are sterilized appropriately by dry or moist heat, chemicals, or radiation before use.
		Always check a package containing a sterile object for intactness, dryness, and expiration date. Sterile articles can be stored for only a prescribed time; after that, they are considered unsterile. Any package that appears already open, torn, punctured, or wet is considered unsterile.
		Storage areas should be clean, dry, off the floor, and away from sinks.
		Always check chemical indicators of sterilization before using a package. The indicator is often a tape used to fasten the package or contained inside the package. The indicator changes color during sterilization, indicating that the contents have undergone a sterilization procedure. If the color change is not evident, the package is considered unsterile. Commercially prepared sterile packages may not have indicators but are marked with the word *sterile.*
	Sterile objects become unsterile when touched by unsterile objects.	Handle sterile objects that will touch open wounds or enter body cavities only with sterile forceps or sterile gloved hands.
		Discard or resterilize objects that come into contact with unsterile objects.
		Whenever the sterility of an object is questionable, assume the article is unsterile.
	Sterile items that are out of vision or below the waist level of the nurse are considered unsterile.	Once left unattended, a sterile field is considered unsterile.
		Sterile objects are always kept in view. Nurses do not turn their backs on a sterile field.
		Only the front part of a sterile gown, from shoulder to waist (or table height, whichever is higher), and the cuff of the sleeves to 2 inches above the elbows are considered sterile.
		Always keep sterile gloved hands in sight and above waist level; touch only objects that are sterile.
		Sterile draped tables in the operating room or elsewhere are considered sterile only at surface level.
		Once a sterile field becomes unsterile, it must be set up again before proceeding.
	Sterile objects can become unsterile by prolonged exposure to airborne microorganisms.	Keep doors closed and traffic to a minimum in areas where a sterile procedure is being performed, because moving air can carry dust and microorganisms.
		Keep areas in which sterile procedures are carried out as clean as possible by frequent damp cleaning with detergent germicides to minimize contaminants in the area.
		Keep hair clean and short or enclose it in a net to prevent hair from falling on sterile objects. Microorganisms on the hair can make a sterile field unsterile.
		Wear surgical caps in operating rooms, delivery rooms, and burn units.
		Refrain from sneezing or coughing over a sterile field. This can make it unsterile because droplets containing microorganisms from the respiratory tract can travel 1 m (3 ft). Some agencies recommend that masks covering the mouth and the nose should be worn by anyone working over a sterile field or an open wound.
		Nurses with mild upper respiratory tract infections refrain from carrying out sterile procedures or wear masks.
		When working over a sterile field, keep talking to a minimum. Avert the head from the field if talking is necessary.
		To prevent microorganisms from falling over a sterile field, refrain from reaching over a sterile field unless sterile gloves are worn and refrain from moving unsterile objects over a sterile field.

Table 6-2	Principles	Practices
Principles and Practices of Surgical Asepsis (continued)	Fluids flow in the direction of gravity.	Unless gloves are worn, always hold wet forceps with the tips below the handles. When the tips are held higher than the handles, fluid can flow onto the handle and become contaminated by the hands. When the forceps are again pointed downward, the fluid flows back down and contaminates the tips. During a surgical hand wash, hold the hands higher than the elbows to prevent contaminants from the forearms from reaching the hands.
	Moisture that passes through a sterile object draws microorganisms from un-sterile surfaces above or below to the sterile surface by capillary action.	Sterile moistureproof barriers are used beneath sterile objects. Liquids (sterile saline or antiseptics) are frequently poured into containers on a sterile field. If they are spilled onto the sterile field, the barrier keeps the liquid from seeping beneath it. Keep the sterile covers on sterile equipment dry. Damp surfaces can attract microorganisms in the air. Replace sterile drapes that do not have a sterile barrier underneath when they become moist.
	The edges of a ster-ile field are con-sidered unsterile.	A 2.5 cm (1 in) margin at each edge of an opened drape is considered unsterile because the edges are in contact with unsterile surfaces. Place all sterile objects more than 2.5 cm (1 in) inside the edges of a sterile field. Any article that falls outside the edges of a sterile field is considered unsterile.
	The skin cannot be sterilized and is unsterile.	Use sterile gloves or sterile forceps to handle sterile items. Prior to a surgical aseptic procedure, wash the hands to reduce the number of microorganisms on them.
	Conscientiousness, alertness, and hon-esty are essential qualities in main-taining surgical asepsis.	When a sterile object becomes unsterile, it does not necessarily change in appearance. The person who sees a sterile object become contaminated must correct or report the situation. Do not set up a sterile field ahead of time for future use.

Source: Berman, A., Snyder, S., Kozier, B. & Erb, G., (2008). *Fundamentals of nursing: Concepts, process, and practice* (8th ed.). Upper Saddle River, NJ: Prentice Hall, p. 696.

    c. Cleaning: reduces the growth of microorganisms but does not totally remove them; rinsing the visible organic material with cold water then washing in hot soapy water and rinsing to remove the soap can clean most equipment and objects; it may be necessary to use a stiff brush to clean equipment with grooves and corners

III. OVERVIEW OF VITAL SIGNS

A. Accurate measurement of vital signs (VS) is a basic nursing skill (taking temperature, pulse, respiration, and blood pressure)

    1. VS measurement provides objective data used to assess client's health conditions and the need for intervention

    2. Accuracy is essential because subtle changes in VS measurements may indicate a change in client condition

    3. Changes in one VS measurement often cause a change in another; for instance, one degree of body temperature elevation can cause an increase of 4–6 heartbeats per minute

4. Most healthcare facilities have policies related to when vital sign measurements are taken on a client; these policies set the minimum standards of the healthcare facility

5. When and how often to measure vital signs is mainly a nursing decision

6. Vital sign measurements need to be taken on admission, before and after any invasive procedure, and when a client's condition changes

7. Nursing evaluation of vital sign measurements depends on the client's baseline data, client vital sign trends, and cause-and-effect relationship between nursing intervention and client response

B. Temperature

1. Regulation: body core temperature remains within a constant range due to the physiological balance between heat production and heat loss

   a. This process is regulated by a thermostatic arrangement in the brain's hypothalamus

   b. The body's surface temperature is the temperature of the skin and is directly related to the environment

   c. Heat production occurs through metabolism, muscle activity, thyroxine production, chemical thermogenesis (norepinephrine, epinephrine, and sympathetic stimulation), and fever

   d. Heat loss occurs through radiation, conduction, convection, and vaporization (evaporation)

2. Normal ranges: normal range for oral temperature in the adult is 36.7°C (98°F) to 37°C (98.6°F); a client with a normal temperature is said to be **afebrile**

3. Measuring: the type of measuring device and route determines the procedure to follow when taking a client's temperature; the common routes used to evaluate temperature are oral, axillary, tympanic, and rectal; internal methods to evaluate core body temperature may be used in critical care areas

   a. The client's age and condition will determine the route used; for instance, a client who has had oral surgery should not have the temperature measured using the oral method; a client with diarrhea should not have the temperature evaluated using the rectal method

   b. Current literature indicates the rectal or tympanic (external) routes and the bladder (internal) route are closest to the body's core temperature, making them the optimal routes when a client has an elevated temperature (fever) unless contraindicated

4. Alterations: body temperature can vary according to the client's age, sex, activity, time of day and emotions

   a. Newborn body temperature regulatory mechanisms are imperfect and as a result the temperature is influenced by environmental temperature

   b. Older adults have a slightly lower body temperature

   c. Women have a slightly higher temperature than men related to hormone activity

   d. Exercise and activity can increase the body temperature because of an increase in muscle activity

   e. Variations in time of day temperature are related to client activity and metabolism of food; generally speaking, the body temperature is lower when clients are sleeping

   f. Heightened emotions increase body temperature by action of the sympathetic nervous system

g. Altered body temperature may also be associated with injury to the hypothalamus (temperature regulatory centers) such as with head injury or tumors

h. Pyrexia and hyperthermia are other similar terms used to describe a fever, and this state is often referred to as being **febrile**

1) Hyperpyrexia is a body temperature above 41°C (105.8°F)

2) A deviation from normal body temperature in this range indicates a disease process is occurring that has caused an increase in heat production and a decrease in heat loss

3) Clinical signs and symptoms of elevated body temperature are associated with the body's temperature regulatory mechanisms trying to maintain balance (see Table 6-3)

4) The clinical signs of fever are associated with the hypothalamic thermostatic changes from a normal level to a higher level in response to tissue destruction, pyrogenic substances, or dehydration

5) Elevation of the body temperature is considered a normal defense mechanism in response to pathogens; it interferes with the pathogen's ability to replicate and grow

6) An elevated body temperature should be treated with antipyretic medication and other nursing interventions when the elevated temperature interferes with body system functioning (see Table 6–3 again)

Table 6-3	Period	Clinical Symptoms	Nursing Interventions (any phase)
Signs of Fever and Nursing Interventions	Onset (cold or chill phase)	Increased heart rate and respiratory rate; feeling cold with shivering; pale cold skin with "gooseflesh"; cessation of sweating	Monitor vital signs, intake and output, and skin color and temperature. Monitor white blood cell count, hematocrit, or other laboratory indicators of dehydration or infection. Remove excess blankets when client feels warm but provide warmth when chilled. Provide adequate nutrition and fluids (e.g., 2500–3000 mL daily) to meet increased metabolic demands and prevent dehydration.
	Course (plateau phase)	Increased pulse and respiratory rate; absence of chills; skin feels warm; photosensitivity; aching muscles, malaise and weakness; increased thirst; lethargic, may be disoriented; may become dehydrated	Administer antipyretic medicine as prescribed. Limit physical activity to prevent heat production. Provide tepid bath to increase heat loss by conduction. Monitor for signs of dehydration. Provide safety measures if client disoriented from fever.
	Defervescence (fever abatement/ flush phase)	Skin warm and flushed; diaphoresis; decreased shivering; possible dehydration	Provide dry bedding and clothing. Provide oral care to keep mucous membranes moist.

Adapted from Berman, A., Snyder, S., Kozier, B. & Erb, G. (2008). *Fundamentals of nursing: Concepts, process, and practice* (8th ed.). Upper Saddle River, NJ: Prentice Hall, pp. 530–531.

Practice to Pass

Identify conditions that cause heat loss in a client and nursing interventions to prevent or control this problem.

7) The four commonly occurring types of fever are constant, remittent, intermittent, and relapsing

i. Hypothermia describes a body temperature below normal; nursing measures for clients with hypothermia are associated with decreasing heat loss and promoting heat production, such as providing blankets, heat shields, and raising environmental temperature

C. Pulse

1. Basic information about the client's circulatory system can be obtained by assessing the pulse

2. The **pulse** is caused by contraction of the left ventricle of the heart moving blood into the arteries; this produces a pulse wave that can be palpated

3. In healthy people, the pulse rate is the same as the rate of ventricular contractions; in some types of heart disease, they differ

4. In a client with heart disease, it is important to measure both the apical pulse rate and the peripheral pulse rate for comparison (should be equal)

5. Pulse sites: peripheral pulse sites may be important to evaluate depending on client condition or age; the radial pulse is the most common site assessed due to accessibility (see Figure 6-1 and Table 6-4)

a. Assess the apical pulse when there is a variation from normal rate in a peripheral pulse, if the client has cardiovascular disease or is taking a cardiac glycoside or beta blocker medication, or for children under the age of 3

b. To assess the apical rate, place a clean stethoscope over the apex of the heart (left 5th intercostal space, midclavicular line, point of maximum impulse) and count the heart beats for 1 minute

Figure 6-1

Peripheral pulse sites.

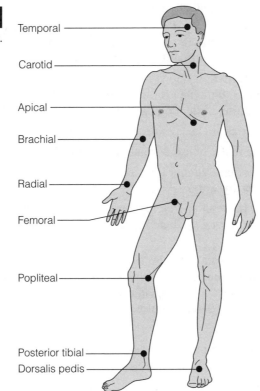

Temporal

Carotid

Apical

Brachial

Radial

Femoral

Popliteal

Posterior tibial

Dorsalis pedis

Table 6-4	Site	Location	Nursing Implications
Specific Pulse Sites and Nursing Implications	Temporal	Above and lateral to the eye over the temporal bone	Easy accessibility especially for children
	Carotid	Medial edge of the sternocleidomastoid muscle in the neck	Use when peripheral sites not palpable, such as with shock
	Apical	Fourth to fifth intercostal space; left mid-clavicular line	Auscultate apical pulse routinely for children under 3
	Brachial	Groove between biceps and triceps muscle at the antecubital fossa	Assess BP; measure during infant cardiac arrest
	Radial	Thumb side of wrist	Evaluates hand circulation
	Ulnar	Ulnar side of forearm at the wrist	Evaluates hand circulation
	Femoral	Midway between symphysis pubis and anterior superior iliac spine	Used when peripheral sites not palpable, during CPR and with shock; for infants and children; to evaluate lower limb circulation
	Popliteal	Behind the knee in the popliteal fossa	Evaluate lower leg circulation, when taking a thigh BP
	Dorsalis pedis	Top of foot; between extension tendons of great and first toe	Evaluates circulation to foot

   c. A difference between the radial pulse (peripheral) and apical pulse is referred to as a **pulse deficit;** an apical rate greater than the radial rate needs to be reported promptly, as it may indicate vascular disease or cardiac dysrhythmia

6. Rate: pulse rate can vary depending on the client's health status, age, sex, activity, medication, body build and position, stress and emotional factors, and pain

   a. A client experiencing stress or pain will have an elevated pulse whereas an athletic client's pulse may be lower; it is important to consider these factors when evaluating pulse rate, rhythm, and volume

   b. Assess rate, rhythm, and volume by compressing an artery against an underlying bone with the pads of three fingers; using too much pressure may obliterate the pulse, while too little pressure may make it difficult to feel the pulse

   c. Specific terms are used to describe variation in rate

      1) A pulse that is below normal rate (60 in adults) is referred to as **bradycardia**

      2) A pulse that is higher than normal rate (greater than 100 in adults) is called **tachycardia**

7. Rhythm: the pulse should be regular with an equal time interval between beats; a variation in rhythm is labeled as irregular and could indicate an arrhythmia or dysrhythmia

8. Pulse volume: also called pulse force, refers to the quality of the pulsation felt from the force of blood with each beat; the volume should remain constant with moderate pressure of the fingers and is obliterated with greater pressure; a scale of 0 to 3 is used to describe pulse volume

   a. 0: pulse is absent

   b. 1: pulse is difficult to feel; thready or weak

   c. 2: normal

   d. 3: bounding pulse that is difficult to obliterate

    e. Some healthcare facilities may use a different scale to measure pulse volume; be familiar with agency policy and use the scale provided by the agency

D. Respirations

1. The respiratory rate is the number of breaths per minute and includes inspiration (breathing in) and exhalation (breathing out)

2. Client factors that affect the respiratory rate include age, activity, environmental temperature and body temperature, emotions, stress, body position, medication, and disease process

3. Control of respiration occurs in several areas:
   a. Respiratory centers in the medulla oblongata
   b. The pons in the brain
   c. Chemoreceptors located centrally in the medulla and peripherally in the carotid and aortic bodies that respond to oxygen, carbon dioxide, and hydrogen ion concentrations in the arterial blood

4. Techniques for assessing the respiratory rate are measuring the rate and evaluating depth and rhythm by watching the movement of the client's chest wall and/or placing a hand on the client's chest wall
   a. Ensure that the client is relaxed and unaware of the assessment and in a position that supports maximum lung expansion, unless contraindicated by the client's condition
   b. Count the rate for 30 seconds (then multiply by 2) unless it is irregular; then it should be counted for 1 full minute
   c. Consider findings in relation to the client's normal breathing patterns, position, health problems, medications or therapies, and cardiovascular function

5. Quality: evaluate respirations for the amount of effort and sound occurring with each cycle; normally there is no sound and respirations are effortless
   a. **Dyspnea** describes difficult and labored breathing
   b. Orthopnea describes ability to breathe only when the head and chest are elevated; clients that have difficulty breathing in a prone or supine position may breathe better when sitting up
   c. Sounds are described such as stridor (harsh sound with inspiration), wheezing (high-pitched musical sound heard on expiration) and bubbling (gurgling sounds); these adventitious sounds may be present if the airway is partially obstructed on inspiration

6. Rate, depth, and pattern: normally respirations are evenly spaced at an adult rate of 12 to 20 per minute (called **eupnea**)
   a. A respiratory rate that it below normal is referred to as **bradypnea,** while a rate above normal is called **tachypnea**
   b. Depth of respiration is described as normal, deep, or shallow
   c. Terms used to describe abnormal patterns are hyperventilation (increased amount of air in the lungs characterized by prolonged deep breaths), hypoventilation (decreased in amount of air in lungs caused by shallow breathing), and Cheyne-Stokes breathing (gradual increase in depth of respirations followed by gradual decrease)
   d. Chest movements: abnormal movements include intercostal retractions, substernal retractions, and flail chest; these signs indicate a problem with air exchange due to an inflammatory response of the bronchioles (asthma), fluid consolidation in lung fields, or a chest injury

E. Blood pressure (BP)

1. Is a measure of the force of the blood as it flows through the arteries

2. Assessment of BP provides information about the circulatory system, specifically the elasticity of the arterial walls, efficiency of the heart as a pump, and volume of circulating blood (cardiac output, peripheral vascular resistance, blood volume and viscosity)

3. The movement of the blood in waves causes two pressure measurements; the **systolic pressure** (resulting from contraction of the heart's ventricles) and **diastolic pressure** (resulting from relaxation of the heart ventricles)

4. BP equipment: measures BP in millimeters of mercury (mmHg) and is recorded as a fraction, with the systolic pressure written over the diastolic pressure; equipment to measure BP may include:

   a. A sphygmomanometer with an attached BP cuff and a stethoscope; two types of sphygmomanometers are available

      1) An aneroid manometer which consists of a calibrated dial

      2) A calibrated cylinder filled with mercury (older, not often seen)

   b. An electronic sphygmomanometer is utilized without a stethoscope and does not require listening to the sounds of the client's BP

   c. A doppler ultrasound stethoscope may also be used for assessment when the sounds are difficult to hear, such as in infants and clients in shock; when a doppler stethoscope is utilized, the systolic BP is usually recorded with a large letter D (for doppler) beside the numeric value

   d. A BP cuff comes in a variety of sizes and the cuff size is determined by the size of the client; the bladder of the cuff must be the correct width and length for the client's arm (the bladder cuff encircles at least 2/3 of the upper arm); if the cuff is too wide, the resulting measurement may be low, and if it is too narrow the resulting measurement will be high

5. Measurement: adults and children

   a. The BP can be measured directly (catheter placed in artery shows waves representing arterial pressure on a monitor) or indirectly (auscultated and palpated)

   b. The auscultatory (auscultated) method is the most frequently used

      1) Apply the BP cuff to the client's left arm at heart level

      2) The right arm may be used if the left arm is contraindicated because of a surgical procedure, cast, paralysis, mastectomy, or hemodialysis graft/fistula

      3) When establishing a client's baseline, measure BP in both arms

      4) Palpate over the brachial pulse site and inflate the cuff until it is 30 mmHg above where the client's pulse disappeared

      5) Then place the stethoscope over the brachial artery and deflate the cuff 2 to 3 mmHg/second while simultaneously watching the manometer and listening to the sounds heard through the stethoscope; these sounds are called Korotkoff's sounds and consist of five phases

         a) Phase 1: the first faint tapping or thumping sound heard; the first tapping sound heard is the systolic BP

         b) Phase 2: the period during deflation when the sounds have a muffled quality

    c) Phase 3: the period when the sound becomes crisper and again assumes a thumping sound

    d) Phase 4: the time when the sound becomes muffled and has a soft blowing quality; the American Heart Association recommends this sound be recorded as the diastolic blood pressure in children; in some instances, three numbers may be recorded, phase 1, 4, and 5

    e) Phase 5: the last sound heard; this is the diastolic BP in adults

  6) If the sounds cannot be heard, palpate the BP

  7) An elevated BP is referred to as **hypertension;** a BP that is below normal is referred to as **hypotension**

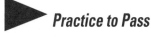

Practice to Pass

What assessment criteria will assist the nurse in determining if a newly admitted client's blood pressure is normal, although it is not consistent with established norms?

  8) **Orthostatic hypotension** refers to a significant drop in BP when the client stands from a sitting position, or sits up from a recumbent position

  9) Factors affecting BP are age, exercise, stress, race, obesity, gender, medications, diurnal variations, and disease process

  10) The average BP in a healthy adult is 120/80 mmHg; it is important when providing care for clients to consider the client's BP trends and client factors that affect BP

6. Causes for error: most errors in taking the BP are related to an improperly fitting BP cuff and improper procedure

  a. Elevating the client's arm above the heart can cause a low BP reading

  b. Deflating the cuff too slowly will cause a high diastolic reading

  c. Deflating too fast will cause a low systolic with a high diastolic reading

  d. An improperly fitting cuff can provide erroneous results as previously outlined

  e. Healthcare workers responsible for BP assessment must ensure accuracy of the results obtained; many clinical judgments are made based on BP readings

7. Interpreting abnormal findings: consider the variation in client trends, if the BP's elevated on more than two occasions, and whether there are client factors that could affect the BP

F. Special procedures/equipment

1. Cardiac monitor: provides information associated with cardiac function including rate, rhythm, and quality of heart contraction

2. Doppler: an instrument that amplifies sound and is useful when assessing pulses that are difficult to palpate or a BP that is difficult to hear; this device has an ultrasound transducer and an audio unit that transmit the sound of blood as it moves through blood vessels

3. Pulse oximeter: a noninvasive device placed on a client digit or earlobe that provides information about oxygen saturation (SaO_2) (normal = 95–100%)

4. Arterial line: provides information directly about a client's arterial BP; a catheter is inserted into an artery and the tip senses the pressure and transmits this information to a machine that displays the BP

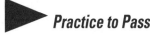

Practice to Pass

What variations in a client's pulse and respirations could be anticipated if the blood pressure was low because of bleeding?

5. Hemodynamic monitoring: is used to assess a critically ill client's cardiovascular status; it is indicated when vital sign measurements are not adequate to evaluate a client's cardiac status; information received from this monitoring includes heart rate, arterial BP, central venous pressure, pulmonary pressures, and cardiac output (CO)

IV. OVERVIEW OF BODY MECHANICS

A. Scientific principles

1. **Body mechanics** are associated with the action and function of muscles that are used to maintain the balance and posture of the body during all the activities involved in daily living

2. In nursing practice, these principles are used to protect both the nurse and client from injury to the musculoskeletal and nervous system

3. These principles involve the concepts of the center of gravity, line of gravity and the base of support

    a. The body is more stable with a greater base of support

    b. Holding an object close to the body requires less energy

    c. When a person moves, the center of gravity shifts continuously in the direction of moving body parts

    d. Facing the direction of work and using the pelvic tilt before an activity decreases the chance of injury

    e. Balance depends on the interrelationship between the center of gravity, line of gravity, and base of support; if all the body parts are balanced, less energy is used

B. Correct body alignment

1. The bones and muscles of the musculoskeletal system and central and peripheral nerves are responsible for body shape, form, and movement

2. Related concepts

    a. Correct body alignment and posture require that the weight of the body is centered and forces of gravity are balanced; when the joints and muscles are not experiencing an extreme flexion or extension, or unusual stress, alignment is achieved and structures and internal organs are supported

    b. The usual line of gravity begins at the top of the head and bisects the shoulders, trunk, and weight-bearing joints; the base of support is slightly anterior to the sacrum

    c. Maintaining proper body alignment promotes functioning of the respiratory, circulatory, renal, and gastrointestinal systems

C. Effective body movement

1. Balance and movement occur with coordinated muscle activity and neurologic integration; reticular formation integrates neural input that helps maintain the body's balance

2. Equilibrium is a function of the vestibular apparatus of the ear

3. The cerebellum coordinates motor activities of movement, the cerebral cortex begins voluntary movement, and the basal ganglia maintain posture

D. Methods to protect the back

1. Nurses need to be mindful of proper body mechanics when providing care to clients

2. Measures to prevent back injury

    a. Maintain a wide base of support when assisting clients with position changes

    b. Avoid twisting movements of the spine

    c. Adjust the height of the work area when working

    d. Bend hips and knees to alter position of the body

    e. When lifting, use the large muscle groups of the legs

    f. Hold objects close to the body when lifting

    g. Employ mechanical devices when appropriate

    h. Use smooth and coordinated motions when working

V. OVERVIEW OF CARDIOPULMONARY RESUSCITATION

A. Cardiopulmonary resuscitation (CPR) is a basic emergency procedure for life support

    1. It consists of artificial respiration and manual external cardiac massage

    2. It is used to establish circulation and ventilation to prevent irreversible brain damage resulting from anoxia

    3. Guidelines were most recently revised in 2005

B. Basic life support (BLS)

    1. BLS or CPR does not require the use of any equipment, although mechanical devices may be used

    2. It can be done with one or two people and involves three interrelated activities: opening airway, restoring breathing, and restoring circulation

    3. Most healthcare facilities require personnel to be trained in BLS

    4. The three signs of cardiac arrest are **apnea** (absence of respirations), *asystole* (absence of carotid or femoral pulse), and dilated pupils

C. One- and two-person adult CPR for healthcare providers

    1. Begin CPR after calling for help (if an automatic external defibrillator [AED] is available, obtain and use it once first if victim is unresponsives)

    2. Turn the client on his/her back and place on a board or hard surface

    3. Open the airway using the head/chin-lift maneuver or the modified jaw thrust method if flexing the client's neck is contraindicated

    4. Place an ear over the client's mouth, observing the chest for normal respirations for 3 to 5 seconds

    5. If respirations are absent or agonal, seal the mouth and nose and ventilate the client with two breaths, over 1 second each; chest should rise with each breath

    6. Assess for a carotid pulse for no more than 10 seconds while maintaining head-tilt position

    7. If the client is pulseless, begin chest compressions; with correct hand position, the sternum is depressed 1.5 to 2 inches in an adult

    8. The ratio of chest compressions to ventilations is 30:2

    9. Once an advanced airway (endotracheal tube, laryngeal mask airway [LMA], or esophageal-tracheal combitube) is in place, deliver 100 compressions per minute continuously ("push hard, push fast"), without pauses for ventilation

    10. When there are 2 or more rescuers and client has an advanced airway, switch roles every 2 minutes to prevent fatigue; switch as quickly as possible (less than 5 seconds) to minimize interruptions in chest compressions

    11. Deliver rescue breaths when a pulse is present at a rate of 10 to 12 per minute for adults (one breath every 5 or 6 seconds)

    12. Reassess pulse every 2 minutes

13. Keep to a minimum any interruptions in CPR

! 14. Performance errors/complications of CPR: complications associated with CPR include the following:

   a. Improper hand position during cardiac compressions can cause rib fracture

   b. Failure to adequately ventilate the client due to improper head position can lead to hypoxia and gastric distention

   c. Poor oxygen profusion to vital organs may result in brain and tissue damage

   d. The body attempts to maintain homeostasis by shunting circulation to vital organs, resulting in less perfusion to the periphery, which can result in distal tissue damage

! **D. Infant/child resuscitation for healthcare providers**

1. Variations in CPR are required when performing the procedure on infants (less than 1 year old) and children (age 1 year to adolescence or puberty—about 12 to 14 years)

2. With a sudden collapse of a victim (more likely caused by a cardiac arrhythmia), determine unresponsiveness, call for help, and get an AED if available; if the victim has a likely asphyxial cause of arrest (drowning), provide 5 cycles (approximately 2 minutes) of 30 compressions to 2 ventilations, before leaving to call for help

3. Take care not to overextend the infant's head when opening the airway

4. The rescuer may be required to place the mouth over the mouth and nose of an infant to establish an airtight seal

5. In infants, assess the pulse in the brachial or femoral sites because their short necks make palpation of the carotid artery difficult

6. For infants up to 1 year in age, visualize an imaginary line between the nipples and place the index finger on the sternum just below this line; place the middle and fourth finger next to the index finger locating the site for cardiac compressions; the depth of chest compressions for an infant is ⅓ to ½ its depth and compression to ventilation ratio is 15:2, with a compression rate of about 100 per minute

7. For children 1 to 8 years, hand placement on the sternum is the same as for the adult; the heel of one or two hands, depending on child size, is used to compress the sternum; the depth of chest compression is ⅓ to ½ of the chest's depth; the rate of compressions is about 100 per minute, with a compression to ventilation ratio of 30:2 (1 rescuer) or 15:2 (2 rescuers)

8. Rescue breathing for both infants and children is at a rate of 12 to 20 breaths per minute

E. Termination of basic life support

1. CPR should be maintained until there is a return of respiration and a pulse or until directed by a physician to discontinue basic life support

2. The only other acceptable reason for discontinuing CPR, once begun, is physical exhaustion of the rescuer

F. Foreign body airway obstruction

1. Airway obstruction is a medical emergency that requires immediate attention

2. Common causes

   a. A common cause of airway obstruction is the tongue falling back and blocking the airway; for this problem, the rescuer should position the unconscious, but breathing, client on either side to relieve the obstruction

b. In other cases, food or other foreign objects can be aspirated into the airway resulting in obstruction; procedures to evacuate the foreign object are based on the client's age and body size

c. Client education in the prevention of airway obstruction is an important nursing function

1) Remind adults to chew food slowly and thoroughly before attempting to swallow

2) When assisting older clients with eating, present foods with a consistency that facilitates swallowing and at an appropriate temperature

3) Instruct parents to teach their children not to run and play while eating, and not to put foreign objects in their mouths

4) Keep small objects away from children under the age of three

5) Avoid feeding peanuts, popcorn, and raisins (and other small non-dissolving or hard items) to children under the age of three

6) Cut all other food products small enough for the child to easily swallow

3. Recognition

a. When a client's airway is partially obstructed he or she may cough, have high-pitched sounds, and indicate there is trouble breathing by holding hands to the throat area

1) As long as the client is coughing strongly and vs are stable, no interventions are necessary

2) It is important not to slap the client on the back because this may move the foreign object further into the client's airway

b. If the client is producing a high-pitched inspiratory stridor, the airway is almost obstructed; in this situation, the client may only be able to produce a weak cough, as well as be unable to speak, appear cyanotic, and have irregular shallow breathing

c. If the client is not making any sound, the airway is totally obstructed and requires immediate action

4. Management for adults: performing the Heimlich maneuver should remove the foreign object

a. If the client is conscious and coughing, ask if he or she is choking; if client nods yes, ask if he or she wants help; intervene only if cough becomes silent, or respiratory difficulty is increased or is accompanied by stridor

b. Stand behind the client and wrap the arms around the client's waist; make a fist with one hand and place the thumb side of the fist against the client's abdomen above the navel and below the xiphoid process, grasp the fist with the other hand and press the fist into the abdomen while thrusting upward; repeat this sequence rapidly until the object is expelled, or the client becomes unconscious (then support client to ground, activate emergency medical system, and begin CPR)

c. When discovering unconscious client on the ground, call for help and use the tongue-jaw lift method to open the mouth and inspect for presence of a foreign object causing obstruction; perform a finger sweep only if object is visualized; perform abdominal thrust to evacuate the object; straddle the client's thighs and place the heal of one hand on the epigastric region below the xiphoid process, then place the second hand on top of the first quickly thrusting upward; repeat 6 to 10 times; if the object is not removed try to ventilate the client; if unsuccessful, repeat abdominal thrusts or try chest thrusts (see below)

         d. Clients who are obese or pregnant require chest thrusts instead of abdominal thrusts; make a fist and place the thumb side against the middle of the client's sternum and grasp the fist with the other hand to deliver a quick backward thrust

!   **5.** Management for children: for children over the age of 1, the procedure is the same as for adults only performed more gently

!   **6.** Management for infants: to dislodge a foreign object from an infant's airway; do the following:

         a. Hold the infant over the arm with the head lower than the trunk supporting the head by holding the jaw firmly in the hand, then rest the infant's body on the forearm

         b. Deliver 5 back blows with the heel of the hands between the infant's scapula

         c. If the object is not evacuated, turn the infant to a supine position and place two fingers over the sternum (position for chest compressions) and deliver 5 chest thrusts

         d. Continue to alternate between back blows and chest thrusts until the object is expelled

         e. Should the infant become unconscious from lack of oxygen, add attempts to ventilate to the sequence; do not perform blind finger sweeps

Case Study

A 35-year-old client with type 1 diabetes mellitus was admitted to the medical unit with an ulcer on the bottom of the foot that is not healing. The client injured the foot two weeks prior to admission by stepping on a stick while gardening. The client's vital signs are oral temperature 39°C (102.2°F), pulse 110, respirations 24, and blood pressure 130/90. There is a large amount of purulent drainage from the circular wound on the bottom of the right foot measuring approximately 7 cm. The affected foot is swollen, red, and warm to touch. The client states it is very painful.

1. What diagnostic tests are likely to be ordered for this client?

2. Based on the information given, describe the body's defense mechanism initiated in response to injury.

3. Identify possible nursing diagnoses that may be applicable for this client and the criteria to support the diagnoses.

4. Identify expected outcome criteria based on the nursing diagnoses identified.

5. Describe nursing interventions related to the prevention of the spread of microorganisms.

For suggested responses, see pages 336–337.

POSTTEST

1 A client had oral surgery following a motor vehicle accident, and the nurse assessing the client finds the skin flushed, warm, and diaphoretic. Which of the following would be the best method to assess the client's body temperature?

1. Oral
2. Axillary
3. Forehead temperature strip
4. Rectal

2 The nurse has taught surgical aseptic technique to the family of a surgical client in anticipation of the family changing the surgical dressings on discharge. The nurse observes a family member changing the dressing and concludes that further education is needed after observing which behavior of the family member?

1. Verbally describing to the nurse and client each phase of the dressing change process while performing it
2. Checking that sterile dressing packages are intact before opening
3. Opening gauze pads packages before putting on sterile gloves
4. Ensuring that the table that will hold the sterile field is dry

3 Which action would the nurse take to use a wide base of support when assisting a client to get up from a chair?

1. Bend at the waist and place arms under the client's arms and lift.
2. Face the client, bend knees, and place hands on client's forearms and lift.
3. Spread the feet apart before touching the client.
4. Tighten the pelvic muscles before assisting the client.

4 The nurse is changing an abdominal dressing for a client. To prevent back injury while leaning over the client, the nurse should do which of the following?

1. Narrow the base of support.
2. Raise the bed to a comfortable position.
3. Move the client to the opposite side of the bed.
4. Position self near the client's head.

5 Using the principles of standard precautions, the nurse decides to apply gloves when performing which of the following nursing interventions?

1. Providing a back massage
2. Feeding a client
3. Providing hair care
4. Providing oral hygiene

6 A nurse finds a client unresponsive in bed and is preparing to open the client's airway. Which of the following methods to open the airway would be most appropriate to use?

1. The jaw-thrust method
2. The head tilt-chin lift technique
3. The chest thrust method
4. The chin to sternum method

7 After correctly positioning a client for a urinary catheterization procedure, the nurse sets up a sterile field and places the kit supplies on the area. The nurse hears a page to respond to another client who has fallen in the hallway. Which of the following would be the most appropriate nursing action?

1. Ensure the client's safety, cover the field with a sterile towel, and respond to the other client.
2. Continue quickly with the procedure, then assist the other client, checking back with the first client as soon as possible.
3. Ensure the client's safety, discard the sterile equipment, and respond to the other client.
4. Explain the situation to the client needing catheterization, leave the sterile supplies in place, and attend to the other client.

8 The nurse is unable to palpate a client's pedal pulse in an edematous right lower extremity. Which of the following would be the best nursing action at this time?

1. Notify the physician of the inability to detect pedal pulses.
2. Check the temperature of the lower extremities.
3. Use a Doppler to check for the pedal pulse.
4. Measure the right leg circumference and compare it to the left.

9 Several clients are being admitted to the hospital unit at one time. There is only one private room available. Which client has the highest priority for being admitted to this private room?

1. A client admitted for elective surgery who requested a private room prior to admission
2. A client with a large infected abdominal wound
3. A client who has a communicable respiratory infection
4. A client under the age of 12

POSTTEST

10 A nurse is preparing a teaching plan for a family member who will be caring for a client with an abdominal incision. Which of the following concepts would have the first priority in the teaching plan?

1. Surgical asepsis
2. Demonstration in sterile gloving technique
3. Handwashing
4. Signs of healing

See pages 159–161 for Answers & Rationales.

ANSWERS & RATIONALES

Pretest

1 **Answer: 3** For infections spread by direct contact or by contact with infected items, the nursing staff would implement contact precautions. All other precautions listed are not necessary. Standard precautions, which is not listed as an option, would also be used.
Cognitive Level: Application **Client Need:** Safe, Effective Care Environment: Safety and Infection Control **Integrated Process:** Nursing Process: Implementation **Content Area:** Fundamentals **Strategy:** The critical phrase is *spread through close physical contact.* Use knowledge of Centers for Disease Control (CDC) guidelines to assist in selecting appropriate infection control measures. **Reference:** Kozier, B., Erb, G., Berman, A., & Snyder, S. J. (2004). *Fundamentals of nursing: Concepts, process, and practice* (7th ed.). Upper Saddle River, NJ: Pearson Education, p. 649.

2 **Answer: 3** Using the principle of medical asepsis, the client who should be assessed first is the client most at risk for infection. A client who is severely neutropenic has lost normal body defense mechanisms for resisting infection. The nurse should then see the post-surgical cardiac client, followed by the client with the draining wound. The client with chicken pox is seen last.
Cognitive Level: Analysis **Client Need:** Safe, Effective Care Environment: Safety and Infection Control **Integrated Process:** Nursing Process: Planning **Content Area:** Fundamentals **Strategy:** The core issue of the question is knowledge of medical asepsis. Recall that knowledge of medical asepsis is essential to safe nursing practice. **Reference:** Kozier, B., Erb, G., Berman, A., & Snyder, S. J. (2004). *Fundamentals of nursing: Concepts, process, and practice* (7th ed.). Upper Saddle River, NJ: Pearson Education, pp. 641–642.

3 **Answer: 2** An endogenous infection is one in which the source is the client. An exogenous source would be from the hospital or hospital personnel, other clients, or contaminated IV fluids.
Cognitive Level: Application **Client Need:** Safe, Effective Care Environment: Safety and Infection Control **Integrated Process:** Nursing Process: Assessment **Content Area:** Fundamentals **Strategy:** The critical word in the question is *endogenous.* Recall potential sources of infection and use the process of elimination in making a selection about this type of infection. **Reference:** Kozier, B., Erb, G., Berman, A., & Snyder, S. J. (2004). *Fundamentals of nursing: Concepts, process, and practice* (7th ed.). Upper Saddle River, NJ: Pearson Education, p. 633.

4 **Answers: 1, 2, 4** Goggles are worn only when there is danger of splashing of body fluids. Head covers are commonly used in surgery. All of the other equipment would be appropriate for the nurse in this situation to prevent the spread of the organism.
Cognitive Level: Application **Client Need:** Safe, Effective Care Environment: Safety and Infection Control **Integrated Process:** Nursing Process: Implementation **Content Area:** Fundamentals **Strategy:** The critical phrases are *infection spread by droplets* and *hands were scratched.* Use knowledge of medical asepsis and CDC precaution guidelines to select appropriate protection when caring for clients. Remember that droplet precautions recommend use of a mask when within 3 feet of a client. **Reference:** Kozier, B., Erb, G., Berman, A., & Snyder, S. J. (2004). *Fundamentals of nursing: Concepts, process, and practice* (7th ed.). Upper Saddle River, NJ: Pearson Education, p. 649.

5 **Answer: 1** The oral temperature would be the most appropriate method for this client. Although the rectal method is the most accurate way to assess a client's temperature, this client has diarrhea, and insertion of a thermometer may further stimulate the bowel. The axillary method and using heat-sensitive tape may not provide as precise a measurement as the oral route.
Cognitive Level: Application **Client Need:** Safe, Effective Care Environment: Safety and Infection Control **Integrated Process:** Nursing Process: Assessment **Content Area:** Fundamentals **Strategy:** The critical phrase is *vomiting and diarrhea.* To make a selection, recall the indications for use of the various routes and their accuracy. **Reference:** Kozier, B., Erb, G., Berman, A., & Snyder, S. J. (2004). *Fundamentals of nursing: Concepts, process, and practice* (7th ed.). Upper Saddle River, NJ: Pearson Education, p. 491.

6 Answer: 2 The nurse should recognize that a pulse volume of 1 indicates the client's pulse is difficult to feel, thready, and the client's circulatory status is altered. The first action is to check the client's condition and circulatory status. If the nurse notified the physician first, the nurse would be reporting on another nurse's assessment, which is not an appropriate nursing practice. The other options are not applicable to this situation.
Cognitive Level: Application **Client Need:** Physiological Integrity: Reduction of Risk Potential **Integrated Process:** Nursing Process: Assessment **Content Area:** Fundamentals **Strategy:** The critical phrase is *pulse volume of 1*. To choose correctly, recall that a pulse with a volume of 1 is thready, 2 is weak, 3 is normal, and 4 is bounding. **Reference:** Kozier, B., Erb, G., Berman, A., & Snyder, S. J. (2004). *Fundamentals of nursing: Concepts, process, and practice* (7th ed.). Upper Saddle River, NJ: Pearson Education, pp. 498–499.

7 Answer: 2 Removing blankets from the client will assist in heat loss through the skin. Offering fluids will prevent dehydration. Placing ice bags on the client is likely to cause shivering, which would increase heat production and reduce local circulation. Restricting fluid intake is not an appropriate nursing intervention for treating a fever.
Cognitive Level: Application **Client Need:** Physiological Integrity: Reduction of Risk Potential **Integrated Process:** Nursing Process: Implementation **Content Area:** Fundamentals **Strategy:** The core issue of the question is the most effective method of treating an elevated temperature. Use knowledge of appropriate nursing interventions for clients with alterations in body temperature to select the correct action to take with febrile clients. **Reference:** Kozier, B., Erb, G., Berman, A., & Snyder, S. J. (2004). *Fundamentals of nursing: Concepts, process, and practice* (7th ed.). Upper Saddle River, NJ: Pearson Education, p. 489.

8 Answer: 4 Options 1, 2, and 3 are expected findings and should not be considered cause for concern. A pulse deficit, with an apical rate greater than the peripheral pulse rate, may be a sign of significant vascular disease or cardiac dysfunction and should be reported immediately.
Cognitive Level: Application **Client Need:** Physiological Integrity: Reduction of Risk Potential **Integrated Process:** Nursing Process: Assessment **Content Area:** Fundamentals **Strategy:** The critical words in the question are *greatest concern*. Recall the significance of common variations in pulse rates and volumes to enable you to recognize significant changes and take appropriate action. **Reference:** Kozier, B., Erb, G., Berman, A., & Snyder, S. J.

(2004). *Fundamentals of nursing: Concepts, process, and practice* (7th ed.). Upper Saddle River, NJ: Pearson Education, p. 499.

9 Answer: 3 When the choking individual is able to cough, the nurse should do nothing to interfere with the individual's attempt to clear the obstruction. The nurse needs to intervene when air exchange is compromised.
Cognitive Level: Application **Client Need:** Physiological Integrity: Physiological Adaptation **Integrated Process:** Nursing Process: Planning **Content Area:** Fundamentals **Strategy:** The critical words are *coughing loudly*. To make a selection, recall the steps in recognition and management of foreign body airway obstruction. Remember not to interfere with the cough efforts of a client when the cough is strong. **Reference:** Kozier, B., Erb, G., Berman, A., & Snyder, S. J. (2004). *Fundamentals of nursing: Concepts, process and practice* (7th ed.). Upper Saddle River, NJ: Pearson Education, p. 685.

10 Answer: 2 The depth of chest compressions for an adult is 1.5 to 2 inches. Thus the correct answer is 2, which is the maximum depth of compressions in the adult client.
Cognitive Level: Application **Client Need:** Physiological Integrity: Physiological Adaptation **Integrated Process:** Nursing Process: Evaluation **Content Area:** Fundamentals **Strategy:** The critical words in the question are *depth* and *adult.* Use knowledge of CPR to arrive at the correct answer. **Reference:** Kozier, B., Erb, G., Berman, A., & Snyder, S. J. (2004). *Fundamentals of nursing: Concepts, process, and practice* (7th ed.). Upper Saddle River, NJ: Pearson Education, p. 1347.

Posttest

1 Answer: 4 A client who has undergone oral surgery should not have the temperature taken by the oral method. The client is exhibiting signs and symptoms of elevated body temperature, and the rectal method is the best choice. A forehead temperature strip and the axillary method does not give as precise measurements as the rectal route in a client at risk for infection or other causes of hyperthermia.
Cognitive Level: Application **Client Need:** Physiological Integrity: Basic Care and Comfort **Integrated Process:** Nursing Process: Assessment **Content Area:** Fundamentals **Strategy:** The critical words are *oral surgery* and *best method.* Recall accurate measurement of vital signs as a basic nursing skill to make a selection. **Reference:** Kozier, B., Erb, G., Berman, A., & Snyder, S. J. (2004). *Fundamentals of nursing: Concepts, process, and practice* (7th ed.). Upper Saddle River, NJ: Pearson Education, p. 491.

ANSWERS & RATIONALES

2 Answer: 1 While working over a sterile field, talking should be kept to a minimum and the head should be averted from the field if talking is necessary. The other options represent correct actions when using sterile or surgical aseptic technique.

Cognitive Level: Analysis **Client Need:** Safe, Effective Care Environment: Safety and Infection Control **Integrated Process:** Teaching/Learning **Content Area:** Fundamentals **Strategy:** The critical words are *surgical aseptic technique.* Recall the principles and practices of surgical asepsis to enable you to provide safe care and appropriate family education. **Reference:** Kozier, B., Erb, G., Berman, A., & Snyder, S. J. (2004). *Fundamentals of nursing: Concepts, process, and practice* (7th ed.). Upper Saddle River, NJ: Pearson Education, p. 656.

3 Answer: 3 A wide base of support is achieved by spreading the feet apart to lower the center of gravity. The other responses either put the nurse at risk for injury (option 1) or do not address the issue of the wide base of support (options 2 and 4).

Cognitive Level: Application **Client Need:** Safe, Effective Care Environment: Safety and Infection Control **Integrated Process:** Nursing Process: Implementation **Content Area:** Fundamentals **Strategy:** The critical term is *wide base of support.* Recall knowledge of scientific principles of body mechanics to enable you to select effective measures to protect the back and prevent injury. **Reference:** Kozier, B., Erb, G., Berman, A., & Snyder, S. J. (2004). *Fundamentals of nursing: Concepts, process, and practice* (7th ed.). Upper Saddle River, NJ: Pearson Education, pp. 1078–1079.

4 Answer: 2 To prevent back strain for the nurse, the bed should be raised to a comfortable position. A nurse should stand with a wide base of support, work as closely as possible to an object, and avoid twisting motions.

Cognitive Level: Application **Client Need:** Safe, Effective Care Environment: Safety and Infection Control **Integrated Process:** Nursing Process: Implementation **Content Area:** Fundamentals **Strategy:** The core issue of the question is how to prevent back injury while leaning over. Recall scientific principles of body mechanics to select effective measures to protect the back and prevent injury. **Reference:** Kozier, B., Erb, G., Berman, A., & Snyder, S. J. (2004). *Fundamentals of nursing: Concepts, process, and practice* (7th ed.). Upper Saddle River, NJ: Pearson Education, p. 1079.

5 Answer: 4 Providing oral hygiene is a procedure that exposes the nurse to a client's body fluids. The other responses do not require the use of gloves because contact with body fluids is not a concern.

Cognitive Level: Application **Client Need:** Safe, Effective Care Environment: Safety and Infection Control **Integrated Process:** Nursing Process: Implementation **Content Area:** Fundamentals **Strategy:** The core issue of the question is basic knowledge of standard precautions. Understanding of CDC guidelines for precautions will assist you in selecting appropriate infection control measures. **Reference:** Kozier, B., Erb, G., Berman, A., & Snyder, S. J. (2004). *Fundamentals of nursing: Concepts, process, and practice* (7th ed.). Upper Saddle River, NJ: Pearson Education, p. 642.

6 Answer: 2 The method of choice for opening the airway is the head tilt-chin lift method. The jaw thrust method should be used when neck injury is possible. Option 3 is one method for treating airway obstruction by a foreign body. Option 4 is fictitious.

Cognitive Level: Application **Client Need:** Physiological Integrity: Physiological Adaptation **Integrated Process:** Nursing Process: Implementation **Content Area:** Fundamentals **Strategy:** The critical words are *unresponsive* and *open the airway.* Recall the correct techniques for cardiopulmonary resuscitation to enable you to correctly manage common airway emergencies. **Reference:** Kozier, B., Erb, G., Berman, A., & Snyder, S. J. (2004). *Fundamentals of nursing: Concepts, process, and practice* (7th ed.). Upper Saddle River, NJ: Pearson Education, p. 1298.

7 Answer: 3 A client fall is a potential medical emergency; however, the nurse's first responsibility is ensuring the safety of the client being attended to. Sterile equipment is considered contaminated if left unattended and therefore must be thrown away (options 1 and 4). The nurse needs to prioritize care appropriately; thus the nurse needs to respond to the client who fell rather than continue with the catheterization.

Cognitive Level: Application **Client Need:** Safe, Effective Care Environment: Safety and Infection Control **Integrated Process:** Nursing Process: Implementation **Content Area:** Fundamentals **Strategy:** The critical phrase is *most appropriate action.* This tells you that there may be more than one way to proceed but that one has a better rationale than the others. Understanding rules of surgical asepsis would enable you to know that sterile supplies cannot be unattended, and critical thinking skills would direct you to correctly prioritize care for the 2 clients. **Reference:** Kozier, B., Erb, G., Berman, A., & Snyder, S. J. (2004). *Fundamentals of nursing: Concepts, process, and practice* (7th ed.). Upper Saddle River, NJ: Pearson Education, p. 655.

8 Answer: 3 To ensure that lower extremity circulation is intact, the nurse should verify the presence of the pedal pulse. Although checking the lower extremity temperature and measuring circumference will provide data on circulation, it does not ensure a pedal pulse is present. It is inappropriate to notify the physician without first gathering all appropriate data.

Cognitive Level: Application **Client Need:** Physiological Integrity: Reduction of Risk Potential **Integrated Process:** Nursing Process: Assessment **Content Area:** Fundamentals **Strategy:** The critical words are *best nursing action.* Recall that the use of a Doppler to assess peripheral pulses is an essential skill related to physical assessment. **Reference:** Kozier, B., Erb, G., Berman, A., & Snyder, S. J. (2004). *Fundamentals of nursing: Concepts, process, and practice* (7th ed.). Upper Saddle River, NJ: Pearson Education, p. 498.

9 **Answer: 3** The client with the airborne or droplet infection can spread this infection simply by breathing and requires isolation in a private room. The client with the abdominal wound (option 2) would not be as likely to spread this organism when the wound is dressed. The clients in options 1 and 4 have no medical need for a private room.

Cognitive Level: Application **Client Need:** Safe, Effective Care Environment: Safety and Infection Control

Integrated Process: Nursing Process: Implementation **Content Area:** Fundamentals **Strategy:** The critical term is *highest priority.* Recall CDC precaution guidelines to enable you to make safe room assignments. **Reference:** Kozier, B., Erb, G., Berman, A., & Snyder, S. J. (2004). *Fundamentals of nursing: Concepts, process, and practice* (7th ed.). Upper Saddle River, NJ: Pearson Education, p. 649.

10 **Answer: 3** Handwashing technique is the single most important procedure in reducing the spread of microorganisms. The other options may also be part of the teaching plan but have a lesser priority if they are used compared to basic handwashing.

Cognitive Level: Application **Client Need:** Safe, Effective Care Environment: Safety and Infection Control **Integrated Process:** Teaching/Learning **Content Area:** Fundamentals **Strategy:** The critical term is *first priority.* Recall basic principles of infection control to direct you to set handwashing as the priority for client and family education. **Reference:** Kozier, B., Erb, G., Berman, A., & Snyder, S. J. (2004). *Fundamentals of nursing: Concepts, process, and practice* (7th ed.). Upper Saddle River, NJ: Pearson Education, pp. 641–642.

References

American Heart Association (2005). 2005 American Heart Association guidelines for cardiopulmonary resuscitation and emergency, cardiovasular care. *Circulation, 112,* [Supplement I], pp. IV-12–IV-34, IV-167–IV-187.

Berman, A., Snyder, S. Kozier, B., & Erb, G. (2008). *Fundamentals of nursing: Concepts, process, and practice* (8th ed.). Upper Saddle River, NJ: Prentice Hall, pp. 526–563, 668–708, 1419–1420.

Craven, R. & Hirnle, C. (2006). *Fundamentals of nursing: Human health and function* (5th ed.). Philadelphia: Lippincott Williams & Wilkins.

Harkreader, H., & Hogan, M. (2007). *Fundamentals of nursing: Caring and clinical judgment* (3rd ed.). St. Louis, MO: Elsevier Science, pp. 113–137, 496–535, 1271–1310.

Potter, P. & Perry, A. (2005). *Fundamentals of nursing* (6th ed.). St. Louis, MO: Mosby, Inc., pp. 617–670, 772–820.

Taylor, C., Lillis C., LeMone, P. & Lynn, P. (2006). *Fundamentals of nursing: The art and science of nursing care* (6th ed.). Philadelphia: Lippincott Williams & Wilkins, pp. 521–557, 649–682, 1106–1108.

7

Meeting Basic Human Needs

Chapter Outline

Safety: Risks According to Developmental Level

Use of Restraints

Maintaining Hygiene

Meeting Oxygenation Needs

Meeting the Client's Need for Sleep

Meeting Nutritional Needs

Meeting Urinary Elimination Needs

Meeting Bowel Elimination Needs

NCLEX-RN® Test Prep

Use the CD-ROM enclosed with this book to access additional practice opportunities.

Objectives

➤ Identify principles of safety promotion based on an individual's developmental level.

➤ Describe the different types of restraints and their appropriate use.

➤ Review basic fire safety prevention measures for use in both the home and hospital setting.

➤ Discuss the importance of and methods for promoting hygiene.

➤ Identify factors that affect oxygenation, alterations in oxygenation, and nursing interventions that promote adequate air exchange.

➤ Describe sleep alterations and associated health promotion activities.

➤ Describe basic nutritional requirements, therapeutic diets, and clinical signs of altered nutrition.

➤ Specify the common problems, diagnostic tests, and health promotion activities for urinary elimination.

➤ Specify the common problems, diagnostic tests, and health promotion activities for bowel elimination.

Review at a Glance

aerobic capacity ability of the body to take in oxygen and transport it to the various organs of the body

anemia a condition in which the blood is deficient in red blood cells or oxygen

atherosclerosis buildup of fatty plaques along the walls of the arteries

cardiac output amount of blood pumped by the heart each minute (usually 4–8 liters in an adult)

catalyze accelerate a chemical reaction

cerumen wax-like substance secreted by the glands of the external ear

circadian synchronization status of being awake when physiologic and psychologic rhythms are most active and asleep when they are most inactive

clubbing a condition in which the base of the nails become swollen, the angle between the nail and the base is 180 degrees or greater, and the ends of the fingers and toes increase in size

diffusion movement of gases or other particles from an area of greater pressure or concentration to an area of lower concentration or pressure

epidermis outer epithelial layer of skin

hyperventilation increased respirations accompanied by decreased carbon dioxide levels associated with pathologies including asthma, pulmonary embolism, or edema

hypoventilation reduced rate and depth of respirations

intercostal retraction indrawing chest movement between the ribs

Kegel exercises pelvic floor muscle exercises that can reduce episodes of incontinence

Kussmaul's breathing a particular type of breathing that includes deep, pauseless respirations associated with diabetic acidosis

oxyhemoglobin compound of oxygen and hemoglobin

paronychia infection of the tissue surrounding the nail

petechiae pinpoint red areas or bleeding in the skin

polysaccharides branched chains of glucose molecules (e.g., starches)

pressure ulcer erosion of the skin occurring over a bony prominence

pruritus itching

sedentary state characterized by little physical exercise or exertion

substernal retraction indrawing chest movement beneath the sternum

PRETEST

1 Parents of a group of toddlers are participating in a safety education class to prevent accidents. Which of the following topics should the nurse include in the health teaching session?

1. Child's physical capacities and curiosity
2. Child's slow reflexes
3. Child's difficulty in reading
4. Child's social and personality development

2 A nurse on the unit observes that the night shift nurse has placed restraints on all of the following clients. In which situation(s) would the nurse conclude that the use of restraints is appropriate? Select all that apply.

1. Child who is hyperactive
2. Infant that has just had a cleft palate repair and is trying to suck his thumb
3. Developmentally disabled client who is alert but still weak
4. Client who is severely anxious about test results
5. Young client who is cognitively impaired and fell 3 times even with a bed alarm on

3 An elderly client on bed rest for a few days has been incontinent. The client now reports pruritis and excessively dry skin, particularly in the area of the lower back. To which of the following skin problems is this client most susceptible?

1. Erythema
2. Ammonia dermatitis
3. Contact dermatitis
4. Petechiae

4 A client has been instructed on the use of an incentive spirometer. The nurse evaluates that the client understood the instructions if the client performs which of the following actions?

1. Maintains a supine position while using the spirometer
2. Inhales rapidly, exhales into spirometer to reach the indicator, and waits 10 seconds before repeating the process
3. Exhales completely, places mouth around mouthpiece before inhaling slowly to reach the indicator, removes mouthpiece, holds breath, and exhales slowly
4. Purses lips tightly around mouthpiece, inhales slowly and deeply, and exhales slowly into the device until spirometer reaches indicator mark

5 A client reports to the nurse that he has had difficulty sleeping since being admitted to the hospital. Which nursing interventions would the nurse use for this client? Select all that apply.

1. Provide client with a warm beverage such as coffee or tea before bedtime.
2. Promote a bedtime routine as similar to client's home routine as possible.
3. Dim lighting in the client's room and close the door to the hallway at bedtime.
4. Change client's gown, offer a back rub, and straighten the bed linens prior to bedtime.
5. Encourage a long, brisk walk in the hallway.

6 A client is being discharged with oxygen therapy via a cannula. Which of the following instructions should the nurse give to the client and family?

1. Use battery-operated equipment instead of electrical equipment.
2. Use petroleum jelly for the nares to prevent chafing.
3. Wear cotton clothing to avoid static electricity.
4. Use baby oil to protect the facial skin.

7 A client reports inability to sleep through the night since admission 3 days ago. Which of the following factors is most likely to negatively affect the client's sleep patterns?

1. Presence of pain
2. Absence of unfamiliar stimuli
3. Ability to talk about day's events
4. Moderate fatigue

8 An elderly bedridden client reports being constipated but cannot understand why. What instruction should the nurse give to assist this client?

1. Decrease fluid intake before bedtime.
2. Encourage bland and low-residue foods.
3. Avoid beverages with caffeine.
4. Drink hot liquids and increase intake of water and fruit juices.

9 A client reports occasional urinary urgency and incontinence. The nurse has worked with the client with regard to bladder training. The nurse would evaluate that the client has achieved the expected outcome when the client is able to do which of the following?

1. Void every time there is an urge.
2. Practice deep, slow breathing until the urge to void diminishes.
3. Use adult disposable briefs continuously.
4. Use protector pads only when going out.

10 A client is on a full liquid diet following gastric surgery. The nurse evaluates the health teaching to be successful when the family brings in which of the following for the client to eat?

1. Homemade clam chowder with potatoes
2. Custard
3. Soft cake
4. Chopped vegetables

➤ *See pages 199–200 for Answers & Rationales.*

I. SAFETY: RISKS ACCORDING TO DEVELOPMENTAL LEVEL

A. Infant, toddler, and preschooler

1. Home accidents

   a. In infants, common accidents are suffocation, falls, and burns; infants are completely dependent on caregivers and are unaware of dangers in environment

   b. Among toddlers and preschoolers, common accidents include poisoning, falls, burns, playground and street-related injuries; because of their increased activity, curiosity, and immaturity, they are more susceptible to injury

2. Health education for parents is a high priority and should include several elements

   a. Knowledge of the child's developmental abilities (e.g., toddler's mobility and curiosity, preschooler's increased activity and clumsiness)

   b. Control of environment (cover electric outlets, coil electrical cords out of reach, keep cleaning supplies and medicines locked)

   c. Supervision (swimming, playgrounds)

   d. First aid measures

3. Safety education for the child should include playing in safe areas, dangers of playing with matches, avoiding strangers, and obeying traffic signals

B. School-age child

1. Transportation-related injuries: not wearing seatbelts or life-preservers; school-age children are active and may not pay attention to directions

2. Sports-related injuries: drowning, accidents while biking, skateboarding, or playing ball—usually related to intense competition and not obeying rules

C. Adolescent

1. Substance abuse: experimentation with drugs and risk-taking, often because of peer pressure

2. Volatile behavior and sometimes violence

3. Recklessness in driving, sports, and lifestyle choices such as unprotected sex, which are often influenced by the following:

   a. Feelings of immortality

   b. A distortion in adolescent egocentric thinking

   c. A notion they are invulnerable to risks that affect others

4. Safety education includes importance of seatbelts, avoiding drinking and driving, and solving problems without violence

D. Adult

1. Lifestyle habits: exposure to the sun, not wearing a seatbelt, or driving while intoxicated

2. Stress-related illnesses: inability to cope with stress can precipitate suicide, road rage, and accident proneness

3. Safety education includes health screenings, exercise, preventive care, and diet

E. Older adult

1. Accidents from falls, driving, and thermal injuries

   a. Visual difficulties, decreased hearing, slower reflexes, poor balance and coordination, impaired mobility, and changes in depth perception contribute to falls and driving accidents

          b. Neurologic disorders such as Parkinson's disease or stroke lead to difficulty with movement and weakness, predisposing the person to falls

          c. Diseases of the spinal cord interfere with the ability to feel discomfort and can lead to thermal injuries

          d. Safety education includes home safety (no throw rugs, adequate lighting, no clutter), proper temperature control on hot water heater, assessment of ability to drive, and importance of diet and exercise to maintain health and strength

    2. Change in mental status related to multiple medications

          a. Older clients taking antihypertensives or diuretics may have postural hypotension; narcotics, hypnotics, sedatives, and tranquilizers cause drowsiness and impaired awareness of the surroundings

          b. Elderly clients are more at risk for polypharmacy—mixing of multiple medications, leading of any of the following:

              1) Additive effects (similar effects used together)

              2) Potentiating effects (effects of two drugs taken together are greater than the singular effect of each drug)

              3) Paradoxical effects (effects opposite those that are expected)

          c. Safety education includes importance of using one pharmacy and telling all healthcare providers about all prescription, over-the-counter, and herbal products used

F. Risks in the healthcare agency

    1. Falls account for the majority of injuries in a hospital: clients who have disease processes that cause weakness, mobility difficulties, or who take multiple medications are more likely to experience a fall; clients in unfamiliar environments need frequent safety information

    2. Client-inherent accidents: self-inflicted cuts and injuries, setting fires, burns; these can be related to psychological dysfunction, risk-taking behaviors, cognitive deficits, and developmental disabilities; smoking in restricted places such as when oxygen is in use leads to fires

    3. Ingestion of foreign substance or poisoning: can be related to improper disposal or storage of substances or lack of precautionary measures

    4. Equipment: caused by malfunction, disrepair, misuse; accidents can result from electrical equipment not properly grounded or with frayed cords, wheelchairs or beds not properly maintained, and improper use of lifting devices; take safeguards in administering medications; follow staff protocols to prevent accidents

G. Fire safety

    1. Preventive measures for home

          a. Focus on teaching: emergency phone numbers, maintenance of smoke alarms and fire extinguishers, importance of family "fire drills;" careful disposal of burning cigarettes or use of matches; grease fire prevention

          b. If there is a fire, teach precautions such as: close windows and doors to contain fire, cover nose and mouth with damp cloth when leaving a smoke-filled area, and stay as close to the ground as possible

    2. Preventive measures for hospital or agency

          a. Be aware of safety precautions and fire prevention practices; know categories of fire and the correct type of extinguisher to use for each; participate in practice fire drills and evacuation procedures

    b. Use the acronym RACE to recall what to do in an actual fire

      1) Remove clients from danger

      2) Activate the fire alarm

      3) Contain the fire

      4) Evacuate the area (horizontal evacuation should be done if possible before vertical evacuation)

II. USE OF RESTRAINTS

A. Overall objectives

1. Reduce the risk of client injury from falls: for example, a postoperative client being transported on a stretcher or a client who is confused, agitated, and climbing out of bed might need restraints if alternatives to restraints have been exhausted

2. Prevent interruption of therapy such as traction, IV infusions, or drainage tubes; e.g., a child who pulls at sterile dressings may need to have a restraint

3. Prevent the confused or agitated client from removing therapeutic devices, e.g., a client who keeps taking off an oxygen mask or pulling out a gastric feeding tube

4. Reduce the risk of injury to others by the client; e.g., ingestion of illicit substances causes a client to become combative when hallucinating

B. Guidelines for using restraints

1. Follow regulations; use restraints as a last resort and apply only under a physician's written order; always check orders; document necessity of restraints, observations, and care given; reevaluate use according to policy

2. For all restraints, maintain a snug fit by making sure there are one to two finger-widths between client's body parts and the restraint; check adequacy of circulation and skin condition at least every hour; ensure call bell is within reach

3. Remove restraints every 2 hours to allow for exercise, toileting, and to check the condition of skin and circulation; attach restraints to the bed frame but never to a movable part of the bed; do not use restraints in place of nursing supervision; use the least restrictive restraint

4. Use caution if removing all restraints simultaneously to prevent injury to client or staff if the client is agitated

C. Types of restraints

1. Side rails: used to confine clients in bed

    a. Ensure that there is a written physician order before using in healthcare facilities

    b. Explain to the client and family the purpose of side rails; do not use them as a punishment

    c. Half or three-quarter rails may be better than full-length ones for confused or agitated clients who might be injured climbing over the rails or falling at the end of the bed; keep bed in lowest position

2. Bed restraint

    a. Requires an order

    b. Has a top and zippered sides to keep client in the bed while allowing full movement in the bed

3. Jacket: vest or chest restraint

    a. Select correct size; explain purpose to client and family; place restraint over the client's gown and follow manufacturer's recommendations

    b. Tie straps to nonmovable parts of the bed or wheelchair; do not tie vest to the head of the bed or side rails

    c. Ensure safe positioning of client for proper breathing

4. Belt or waist restraint

    a. Check that belt is in good condition; attach belt around the waist; if belt has a buckle, place it so it does not interfere with client's comfort

    b. Tie strap to nonmovable part of the bed or chair; use belts when transporting clients in stretchers or wheelchairs

5. Extremity: may be a mitt or hand, wrist, ankle, or elbow restraint; always follow manufacturer's recommendations for application

    a. Mitt: ensure client can flex fingers slightly and circulation is maintained; secure wrist ties and attach to bed frame or chair

    b. Wrist or ankle: follow recommendations and pad bony prominences when using commercial restraints

    c. Elbow: check that tongue blades in pockets are intact and ends are covered or padded; wrap restraint snugly around arm and secure properly; for small infants or children, pin restraints to shirt

D. **Alternatives to restraints**

1. Orient client and families to surroundings; explain all procedures and treatments to them

2. Encourage family and friends to stay, or utilize constant companions for clients who need supervision; familiarity with caregivers may reduce agitation

3. Assign confused or disoriented clients to rooms near the nurse's station; observe frequently and identify factors that precipitate client's confusion or agitation

4. Provide appropriate/meaningful visual and auditory stimuli; avoid overstimulating the client; offer diversionary activities such as preschool sewing cards, picture books, or ask client to fold face cloths or small towels as a simple repetitive task

5. Eliminate bothersome therapies and treatments as soon as possible, for example, catheters and drains

6. Use relaxation techniques; approach client in a calm, nonthreatening manner

7. Institute exercise and ambulation schedules as condition allows

8. Maintain toileting routines to decrease falls related to elimination needs

9. Consult with physical and occupational therapists to enhance client's ability to carry out activities of daily living (ADLs), which help increase client's sense of accomplishment

10. Evaluate all client medications to determine if each is having the desired effect; check for adverse effects such as restlessness, confusion, perceptual difficulties, and dizziness

11. Conduct ongoing assessment and evaluation of client's care and the ongoing response to care; factors such as the client's environment and presence of familiar faces may promote relaxation or precipitate agitation; try to determine causes of sundowner's syndrome (nocturnal wandering and disorientation when darkness falls, associated with dementia), such as poor eyesight, hearing, and pain

III. MAINTAINING HYGIENE

A. Functions of the skin

1. Protection: body's first line of defense is the skin because it covers the underlying tissues and acts as a barrier to microorganisms

2. Sensation: pain, temperature, and pressure are transmitted as sensations through nerve receptors

3. Temperature regulation: when body temperature drops and heat must be conserved, superficial skin blood vessels constrict; cooling of the body occurs through evaporation and when the blood vessels dilate, heat is radiated and conducted from the body

4. Excretion and secretion: sweat (composed of water, chloride, potassium, glucose, and urea) is excreted through the skin; sebum, an oily substance secreted by the skin, contains chemicals that are toxic to bacteria; the acid pH of skin secretions inhibits bacterial growth

B. Skin care

1. Developmental changes: age and ability influence one's skin care practices

   a. A newborn requires only sponge baths, not tub baths; the newborn should be dried immediately and wrapped to prevent heat loss, especially since shivering starts at a lower body temperature and there is greater body surface area for heat loss compared to adults

   b. A toddler depends on the caregiver to provide care; however, he or she may want to try doing things independently (such as brushing teeth)

   c. An older adult who is frail may be dependent but may still be able to identify skin care preferences; excessive bathing can contribute to dry skin

2. Cultural considerations

   a. Hygiene practices vary considerably among different cultures; in some cultures, daily bathing is a ritual, while in others, a weekly routine is acceptable

   b. Other examples of differences are in the use of deodorants and preference for tub bath or shower

   c. Some cultures worry about hot/cold imbalances as a cause of illness

   d. Bathing may be avoided with some body conditions; for instance, some cultures avoid bathing during menstruation and childbirth

3. Common skin problems: presence of these problems alerts the nurse to the type of skin assessment and care needed

   a. Excessive dryness: flaky and rough skin may crack; may be accompanied by **pruritus** (itching)

   b. Abrasions: **epidermis** (superficial layer of skin) is rubbed or scraped off

   c. Ammonia dermatitis (diaper rash): reddened skin that may be excoriated, caused by skin bacteria reacting to the urea in the urine

   d. Contact dermatitis: reddened skin, accompanied by pruritus that may result in infection if scratched

   e. Erythema: redness of skin associated with rashes, infections, and allergic responses

   f. **Pressure ulcer:** a skin lesion, often over bony prominences caused by decreased circulation

C. Providing specific hygiene measures

1. Partial bed bath: client may do certain portions of the bed bath as desired or as condition permits; includes only parts that may cause discomfort or odor if not washed

   a. Prepare client by explaining the procedure; provide privacy and have necessary equipment; position client for safety and easy access

   b. Wash face, rinse, and pat dry gently

   c. Assist client to immerse hands (may be one hand at a time) in wash basin to clean them; remove from basin and dry hands

   d. Wash client's chest and axilla, rinse, and pat dry; assist female clients to wash under breasts if needed; apply deodorant as desired

   e. Assist the client to turn to side or prone if able; wash, rinse, and dry the back, buttocks, and gluteal folds

   f. Assist client back to supine position; determine if client is able to do perineal care; assist as necessary; follow procedure for perineal care in a section below

   g. Assist client to put on clean gown and return client to comfortable position

   h. Document observations

2. Complete bed bath: the nurse washes the client's entire body; may use a commercial product such as bath-in-a-bag

   a. Explain procedure to the client; if desired, a family member may assist with the bath; prepare environment: close curtains and windows, elevate bed to a safe position; if appropriate, have client in a semisitting position

   b. Offer bedpan or urinal to the client

   c. Prepare equipment

   d. Place bath blanket over client and remove bed linens; remove client's gown

   e. Wash client's eyes with water only, wiping from the inner canthus to outer; use a separate corner of the washcloth for each eye; dry eyes well; wash face and use soap only as directed by client; rinse and pat gently; wash, rinse, and dry the ears and neck

   f. Place bath towel lengthwise under the arm; wash using long firm strokes starting from the wrists, rinse and dry arms, and then the axilla; repeat with the other arm

   g. Place towel on bed and put basin on top; immerse and wash client's hand in the basin; pay attention to the spaces between the fingers; dry gently

   h. Fold bath blanket down to the client's pubic area and replace it with a bath towel; wash, rinse, and dry chest and abdomen; for female clients, pay particular attention to the area under the breasts; avoid undue exposure; replace the bath blanket

   i. Fold bath blanket over one leg; place bath towel under the other leg; wash using long strokes starting from the ankle to the knee to the thigh; rinse and dry; repeat with the other leg

   j. Wash the feet by placing each foot in the basin, rinse, dry, and repeat with the other foot; clean and dry well between the toes

   k. Assist the client to a side-lying position; place a towel alongside the back and buttocks; cover the client with bath blanket; wash, rinse, and dry the back, buttocks, gluteal folds, and back of upper thighs

l. Pay particular attention to skin over bony prominences and check for beginning skin problems such as pressure ulcer or ammonia dermatitis; be aware that for older adults, a complete bath is not needed every day and could lead to dry skin

m. Change water and perform perineal care (see perineal care procedure below)

n. Assist client with other hygiene practices: use of deodorant, lotions, powder as appropriate; assist with mouth care or shaving

o. Help client put on a clean gown; remove and replace bed linens; tidy up the environment

p. Document observations such as reddened areas over bony prominences, irritation, or inflammation

3. Perineal care

   a. Explain procedure to client; ensure privacy; prepare equipment

   b. Assist client to a back-lying position with knees flexed and spread apart; drape and keep client warm

   c. Don gloves and inspect perineal area

   d. For females

      1) Using the washcloth, clean the labia majora, then spread the labia to clean the folds between the labia majora and labia minora

      2) Use separate quarters of the washcloth per stroke, wiping from the pubis down to the rectum (front to back)

      3) Rinse area well by pouring warm water over the area or use a clean washcloth; dry area gently and well

   e. For males

      1) Wash and dry the penis with firm strokes

      2) If uncircumcised, retract the foreskin or prepuce and cleanse the glans penis (tip); replace the foreskin after cleaning

      3) Wash and dry the scrotum

   f. Assist client to turn away; clean the anal area with toilet paper or disposable wipes before washing as necessary; rinse and dry; apply perineal pad or diaper as needed

   g. In some settings, a special peri-wash solution may be used to perform perineal care

   h. Document any observations such as inflammation or discharge

4. Nail and foot care

   a. Nail care: prepare equipment; do one hand at a time; soak in warm water if nails are hard; cut or file straight across to prevent ingrown nails (never cut nails of a client with diabetes); file to round the corners and push cuticles back gently; wash and dry; document observations such as **paronychia** (infection of tissue surrounding the nail) or abnormal discolorations; refer client with diabetes to a podiatrist as needed

   b. Foot care: wash each foot in the washbasin and cleanse between the toes (see total bed bath); rub callused areas with the washcloth; clean nails using a wooden stick; if agency permits, trim nails; rinse and dry gently; repeat procedure for other foot; apply lotion or powder as necessary; document observations such as breaks in the skin and pressure areas

5. Oral care

   a. For a client who can do oral care independently: prepare equipment; assist client to a Fowler's position and place towel on chest; assist as needed

   b. For a client who needs assistance

   1) Brushing teeth: place moist toothbrush bristles at a 45-degree angle against teeth; move bristles back and forth; repeat for all surfaces of the teeth; gently brush the tongue if coated; hand water cup to the client for rinsing and ask to spit into emesis basin

   2) Flossing teeth: use disposable gloves; stretch floss and move it up and down between all teeth from top of crown to gum line; have the client rinse mouth; dispose of equipment, and document any abnormalities noted such as excessive bleeding or inflammation of the gums

   3) Cleaning artificial dentures: prepare equipment and obtain a denture container and washcloth; place client in semi-Fowler's position; put on gloves; remove top dentures (move plate up and down gently to break suction then place it in container) and lower dentures (lift one side gently and then the other); clean and rinse dentures in sink carefully; dispose of equipment; document abnormalities such as irritated mucous membranes and ill-fitting dentures

   c. For a client requiring total care

   1) Assemble equipment; place client in side-lying position so fluid can easily flow out or pool in the side of the mouth for suctioning; place a towel under client's chin and a curved basin against the chin; use gloves

   2) Clean client's teeth as per procedure above; brush gently; flush client's mouth with water and let fluid drain from the mouth; ensure all fluid drains out, otherwise use gentle suction or another syringe to remove it; some agencies use mouthcare products with suction attached

   3) Inspect and clean the oral tissues; use an applicator or a tongue blade wrapped with gauze (moistened with mouthwash) to cleanse inside of cheeks, roof, and base of mouth and the tongue; rinse client's mouth

   4) Discard gloves and other equipment; reposition client and ensure comfort

   5) Lubricate client's lips with petroleum jelly

   6) Record special mouth care including any solution used; document observations such as dryness or inflammation

6. Hair and scalp care

   a. Brushing hair

   1) Use a hairbrush with soft bristles

   2) Remove tangles gently, working from ends of hair, then middle to ends, then scalp to ends

   3) Use a wide pick comb for very curly hair, such as the hair of some African Americans

   b. Shampooing hair

   1) Assist client as necessary; check whether order is necessary; if shampooing a client who is on bedrest, assemble equipment

   2) Ensure that client is warm, use a bath blanket; check the water temperature

   3) Put waterproof sheet and towel on the bed; place shampoo basin and pad where the client's neck will rest and position client's head in basin; place the receiving receptacle to collect draining water

        4) Cover client's eyes with a washcloth

        5) Shampoo hair and massage all areas of scalp working from hairline to neckline with pads of fingertips; rinse well and squeeze out as much water as possible

        6) If hair is matted or tangled with blood, consider using dry shampoo or hydrogen peroxide mixture for cleaning

        7) Rub hair thoroughly with a towel; remove shampoo basin and wrap hair with dry towel; if desired, use hairdryer and ensure client comfort

        8) In general, shampooing should be done at least once per week

  7. Care of the eyes, ears, and nose

    a. Eye care: soften dried secretions with a moistened washcloth; wipe loosened secretions from the inner to the outer canthus

    b. Ear care: wash auricles during bed bath; if **cerumen** visible, loosen it by retracting the auricles downward then remove with a damp washcloth

        1) Unconscious client: if corneal reflex impaired, apply moist compresses over the eye every 2 to 4 hours; clean each eye with a moistened washcloth; instill ordered ophthalmic ointment or artificial tears

        2) Removable prosthetic (artificial) eye: use gloves; exert slight pressure below the eyelid to overcome suction and remove the artificial eye; clean the socket and the tissues around the eye with moistened washcloth; clean the artificial eye with warm normal saline and rinse; to reinsert the prosthetic eye, retract eyelids and exert pressure on the supraorbital and infraorbital bones; hold prosthetic eye with index finger and thumb of the other hand and slip it gently into the socket

    c. Nasal care: ask if the client wishes to blow the nose using tissue; the nares or nostrils can be cleaned with damp washcloth

D. Care of the client's room environment

  1. Making the occupied bed

    a. Explain procedure and enlist the client's cooperation; gather clean linen; have a linen hamper in the room; draw curtains and place bed at a comfortable working height

    b. Remove call bell or other devices attached to the bed linens; lower rail on nearest side of bed after determining that opposite side rail is up and locked

    c. Loosen all top linen at the foot of the bed; replace top sheet with bath blanket; fold spread or blanket and place on chair

    d. Put head of bed as flat as client can tolerate; move the mattress up on the bed; ask the client to turn to distant side and adjust pillow under head; loosen old linen and fold draw sheet and bottom sheet towards the center of bed

    e. Place new bottom sheet and draw sheet on the bed and fan-fold the half to be used for the other side of the bed; tuck sheets and miter the corners if using flat sheet

    f. Raise near side rail; assist client to roll over fan-folded sheets toward nurse; move pillow towards the clean side; move to the other side and lower side rail; remove used linens and place in linen hamper

    g. Unfold fan-folded clean linen; pull sheets to prevent wrinkles and tuck under mattress or make mitered corners

    h. Reposition client at the center of the bed; remove and replace pillowcase, then reposition for client's comfort

    i. Replace bath blanket with top sheet; place blanket and then bedspread on top; tuck in sheet, blanket and spread at the foot of the bed, making room for movement of client's feet, and miter the corners

    j. Fan-fold top covers to the upper chest or waistline of the client as desired

    k. Place bed in lowest position; restore side rails to original position; replace call bell within client's reach; and put client items within safe reaching distance

2. Making the unoccupied bed

    a. Gather equipment; assist the client out of bed as necessary; assess the client and ensure safety and comfort

    b. Remove call bell or drainage equipment attached to bed linens

    c. Loosen bed linens systematically starting from the top of the bed on one side and finishing at the head of the bed on the other side; remove pillowcases, place in linen hamper and place pillows on bedside chair

    d. Fold reusable linens on the bed into fourths; roll all soiled linen and dispose directly into linen hamper

    e. Move mattress up in the bed if needed

    f. Place folded bottom sheet on top of the bed with hem side down; unfold and tuck fitted or contoured sheet on one side

    g. If needed, place a plastic or waterproof pad on top of the bed extending from approximately the client's middle back to mid-thigh; cover with a cloth draw sheet and tuck one side

    h. Place top sheet hem-side up on top of the bed, then blanket or bedspread, unfold and tuck them in at the foot of the bed and miter corner on this side

    i. Move to the other side of the bed; pull the bottom sheet, tuck the fitted bottom sheet and foot of the bed at the top and bottom of the mattress

    j. Spread remainder of the linens; make a fold in the top sheets perpendicular to the foot of the bed before tucking sheets; miter the bottom corner

    k. Fold top of the top sheet over the blanket and bedspread providing a cuff; if client is getting back to bed, fan-fold the top linens to the center; place the bed in a low position

    l. Replace pillowcases; attach call bell; place bedside table and overhead table where client can reach them; tidy the room

3. Keep area clutter-free

    a. Arrange furniture to avoid accidents, for example, no furniture in the middle of the room

    b. Remove unnecessary objects; keep obstacles out of the way

4. Keep objects needed by the client nearby; put necessary objects for daily hygiene and activities of daily living within reach, e.g., client's eyeglasses, cane, fluids, and call bell

5. Control odors

    a. Provide good ventilation

    b. Remove and dispose of offensive waste products appropriately

    c. Use room deodorizers as necessary

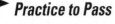

Practice to Pass

The nurse is admitting a young child with burns to the unit. What safety precautions should the nurse implement?

IV. MEETING OXYGENATION NEEDS

A. Overview of anatomy and physiology of cardiovascular and respiratory systems

1. Cardiovascular

   a. Structure

   1) Heart

   a) A hollow, cone-shaped organ within the mediastinum, bordered laterally by the lungs, posteriorly by the spine, and anteriorly by the sternum; it is covered by pericardium and has three layers: epicardium, myocardium, and endocardium

   b) Four chambers: the upper chambers (atria) and lower chambers (ventricles) are separated by the tricuspid (right) and bicuspid/mitral (left) valves; the interventricular septum separates the two sides; semilunar valves separate ventricles from the great vessels—pulmonic (right) and aortic (left) valves

   2) Blood vessels

   a) Arteries: elastic vessels that carry blood away from the heart

   b) Veins: carry blood back to the heart

   c) Capillaries: smallest vessels, form connection between **arterioles** (tiny vessels taking blood from the arteries to the capillaries) and **venules** (tiny vessels returning blood from the capillaries to the veins)

   b. Function: the heart serves as a system pump, moving oxygenated blood and nutrients through the arteries to the tissues, and deoxygenated blood and wastes from the tissues through the veins

2. Conduction system: controls electrical activity and contraction of heart

   a. Sinoatrial (SA) node: primary pacemaker located where superior vena cava enters right atrium; initiates impulses conducted throughout the heart resulting in ventricular contraction

   b. Atrioventricular (AV) node: specialized muscle tissue located in the floor of the right atrium near interatrial septum

   c. AV bundle or bundle of His and Purkinje fibers: ventricular conduction fibers

3. Respiratory system

   a. Structure

   1) Upper respiratory tract: mouth, nose, pharynx, larynx

   2) Lower respiratory tract: trachea, lungs (bronchi, bronchioles, and alveoli), pulmonary capillary network, and pleura (visceral and parietal)

   b. Function

   1) Pulmonary ventilation or breathing: inspiration (inhalation)—air flows into lungs and expiration (exhalation)—air moves out of lungs

   2) Alveolar gas exchange: after alveoli are ventilated, **diffusion** (movement) of oxygen occurs from alveoli into pulmonary blood vessels

   3) Transport of oxygen (O_2) and carbon dioxide (CO_2): O_2 is transported from lungs to tissues and CO_2 is transported from tissues back to lungs; O_2 combines with hemoglobin in red blood cells and is then carried to tissues as **oxyhemoglobin** (a compound of O_2 and hemoglobin)

*B. **Factors affecting oxygenation**

1. Environment

a. Altitude: higher altitude increases respiratory and cardiac rate and respiratory depth

b. Heat: causes peripheral vessel dilation, increased blood flow to skin and decreased resistance to blood flow; this increases cardiac output to raise blood pressure; rate and depth of breathing also increase

c. Cold: vasoconstriction occurs and blood pressure elevates; this decreases cardiac action because of reduced need for O_2

d. Air pollution: leads to symptoms such as coughing, choking, and difficulty breathing

*2. Developmental factors affecting oxygenation

a. Premature infants: inadequate respiratory function is caused by immature lungs; stimulation of respiratory center of the brain is immature; gag and cough reflexes are weak

b. Infants and toddlers: have smaller airway passages, which contributes to obstruction by foreign objects such as peanuts, coins, and small toys; diseases such as cystic fibrosis and asthma lead to difficulty breathing and affect oxygenation

c. School-age children: because of exposure to infectious agents at school and play, there is a tendency to develop upper respiratory problems

d. Adolescents: at puberty, the heart and lungs increase considerably in size and the heart rate drops

e. Young and middle-aged adults: **aerobic capacity** (ability of the individual to provide O_2 to the body's organs) and **cardiac output** (CO) (amount of blood pumped by the heart each minute [4–8L]) show age-related changes during work or exercise starting at age 35 to 40; loss of blood vessel elasticity may contribute to hypertension, which affects oxygenation; **atherosclerosis** (plaque build-up in the walls of the arteries) is a factor that decreases blood flow, particularly to the heart muscle

*f. Older adults: chest wall becomes more rigid and lungs are less elastic, so more air is retained in the lungs at expiration; cough effectiveness decreases; protective cilia become less effective so may be more prone to upper respiratory infections; decreased respiratory reserve increases risk for exercise intolerance; blood flow may be impaired because of hypertension, atherosclerosis and obstructive lung disease

3. Lifestyle factors affecting oxygenation

*a. Nutrition: high fat and salt intake may increase risk for heart disease and inadequate diet can lead to **anemia** (insufficient red blood cells)

b. Physical exercise: increases rate and depth of respirations and cardiac rate, thus increasing the supply of O_2 in the body

c. Smoking: nicotine increases heart rate, BP, and peripheral resistance; vasoconstriction occurs and decreases oxygenation to tissues

*d. Substance abuse: alcohol is a respiratory depressant and slows respirations; long-term use increases BP and tendency for malnutrition and anemia; narcotics (opioids) such as morphine decrease respiratory rate and depth

e. Anxiety: in moderate and severe anxiety, hyperventilation occurs, the arterial pressure of O_2 rises and pressure of CO_2 falls; the individual often experiences light-headedness, numbness of fingers and toes; epinephrine and norepineph-rine released under stress increase BP and heart rate

    f. Overall health status: cardiovascular disease causes compromise in O_2 transport; respiratory disease affects oxygenation of blood

C. Alterations in respiratory functioning

  1. Hyperventilation: increased movement of air into and out of the lungs

    a. Causes: stress, metabolic acidosis may cause **Kussmaul's breathing,** a type of hyperventilation

    b. Signs and symptoms: increased rate and depth of respiration, more CO_2 is eliminated than normal

  2. Hypoventilation: inadequate alveolar ventilation

    a. Causes: alveolar collapse, airway obstruction, or side effect of some drugs

    b. Signs and symptoms: inadequate alveolar ventilation; CO_2 retained in bloodstream; can lead to hypoxia

  3. Hypoxia: inadequate amount of O_2 transported to the tissues

    a. Causes: diseases such as anemia, pulmonary edema, heart failure; drugs such as anesthetics

    b. Signs and symptoms: rapid pulse; rapid shallow respirations, dyspnea; flaring of the nostrils, restlessness; **substernal** or **intercostal retractions** (retractions under and between ribs occurring with respirations), and cyanosis; in chronic hypoxia, client may experience fatigue, lethargy, and have **clubbing** (changes in the appearance of the ends of the fingers and toes with angle of nailbed to digit 180 degrees or greater; associated with hypoxia)

  4. Cyanosis

    a. Causes: severe anemia, respiratory tract obstruction, heart disease, cold environment; a very late indicator of hypoxia

    b. Signs and symptoms: bluish discoloration of skin, nail beds, and mucous membranes

  5. Pain: chest pain can impair breathing patterns and respiratory functioning

    a. Causes: respiratory diseases such as pneumonia, pulmonary embolism, advanced bronchogenic carcinoma, and heart conditions, such as coronary artery disease, and angina

    b. Signs and symptoms: complaints of pain that may be dull, aching, persistent or localized/radiating; discomfort accompanied by pallor, rapid or slowed breathing; anxiety; rapid heart rate

  6. Orthopnea: (positional breathing discomfort associated with lying down)

    a. Causes: respiratory and cardiac diseases, airway obstruction

    b. Signs and symptoms: inability to breathe except when in a sitting or upright position; **dyspnea** (air hunger) when in a reclining position

  7. Wheezing

    a. Causes: severely narrowed bronchus

    b. Signs and symptoms: high-pitched, continuous musical, rasping, or whistling sounds heard during inspiration or expiration; does not clear with coughing

  8. Cough: natural lung clearance mechanism to remove secretions

    a. Causes: excessive sputum production; allergies; pulmonary diseases

    b. Signs and symptoms: forced exhalation and clearing of the airway passages

9. Hemoptysis

   a. Causes: pulmonary infection, carcinoma (cancer) of the lungs, abnormalities of the heart or blood vessels

    b. Signs and symptoms: bright red frothy blood from the lungs mixed with sputum; initial symptoms include tickling in the throat, salty taste, a burning or bubbling sensation in the chest

D. **Nursing interventions to promote oxygenation**

   1. Positioning: Fowler's position (elevated head of bed) allows maximum chest expansion that eases respirations in clients with dyspnea; turn clients from side to side every 1 to 2 hours to allow alternate sides of chest to expand

   2. Decrease anxiety: promote relaxation techniques, alleviate pain by using distraction or guided imagery as adjuncts to analgesics

   3. Deep-breathing and coughing: teach clients breathing techniques to assist in clearing fluid from the lungs and to promote oxygenation

      a. Assume a comfortable position: sitting or supine position with knees flexed

      b. Place one hand on abdomen just below the ribs

      c. With mouth closed, breathe in deeply through the nose to a count of three; concentrate on feeling the abdomen rise

      d. Purse lips and breathe out slowly and gently; concentrate on feeling the abdomen fall and tightening the abdominal muscles; count to seven during exhalation

      e. Repeat several times (about 10 times initially) and gradually increase to 5 to 10 minutes four times a day

      f. For coughing: inhale deeply and hold breath for a few seconds, lean forward and cough rapidly, using abdominal, thigh and buttock muscles (coughing is contraindicated in postoperative eye, ear, neck, or brain surgery or in other clients who have risk of increased intracranial pressure)

   4. Suctioning: oro/nasopharyngeal, tracheal

      a. See Box 7-1 for procedure

      b. Limit suctioning to 10 seconds (some texts say 15) because no O_2 exchange occurs during this portion of the procedure; allow rest periods between suctioning to allow the client to inhale O_2

      c. Assess for dysrhythmias or cyanosis as grave indicators of inadequate oxygenation; hyperoxygenate before suctioning, between attempts, and when suctioning is complete

   5. Chest physiotherapy: percussion, vibration, postural drainage (often done by respiratory therapist unless nurse is authorized and competent to perform)

      a. Percussion or clapping: explain the procedure and encourage the client to breathe slowly and deeply; place the client in a comfortable sitting or side-lying position; cover area with a gown or towel; cup hands, alternately flex and extend wrists rapidly to percuss the affected lung segments for 1 to 2 minutes

      b. Vibration: vigorous or high-frequency quivering on the chest wall, used alternately with or after percussion; explain procedure to client and position according to lung segment to be treated; encourage client to breathe slowly and deeply; place hands one on top of the other with palms down; during exhalation, tense hand and arm and using mostly the heel of the hand, vibrate or shake hands against the client's chest; stop vibrating when the client inhales;

Box 7-1

Suctioning Technique

- Prepare equipment: portable or wall suction with tubing and collection container; sterile normal saline or water; sterile gloves; water soluble lubricant; Y-connector; sterile gauzes; disposal bag.

- Select appropriate sterile suction catheters usually #12 to #18 for adults; #8 to #10 for children; and #5 to #8 for infants.

  - Set pressure on the suction gauge.

  - For wall unit: adults: 100–120 mmHg; children: 95–110 mmHg; infants: 50 to 95 mmHg.

  - For portable unit: adults: 10 to 15 mmHg; children: 5 to 10 mmHg; infants: 2 to 5 mmHg.

- Explain procedure to the client. Position a conscious client in a semi-Fowler's or an unconscious client in a lateral position with head turned towards nurse.

- Put on sterile gloves, maintain sterility of the dominant hand and connect sterile catheter to the suction.

- Measure distance between the client's nose and earlobe (approximately 13 cm or 5 in. in adults) and mark position with the fingers of sterile gloved hand. Test pressure and patency by placing nondominant thumb or finger on port or open branch of the Y-connector.

- Hyperoxygenate the client with deep breaths or bag-valve-mask device (Ambu bag).

- Lubricate catheter tip with sterile water or saline (or for nasopharyngeal suctioning may use the lubricant).

- Insert the catheter:

  - For oropharyngeal suctioning: pull tongue forward with gauze; introduce and advance catheter along one side of mouth into oropharynx.

  - For nasopharyngeal suctioning: introduce catheter through the nostril or naris and advance to the recommended distance.

  - For tracheal suctioning, insert during inhalation because epiglottis is open; continue to advance catheter to approximately 20 cm or until resistance is met; pull back slightly (expect client to cough during insertion).

- Do not apply suction while inserting the catheter.

- Apply nondominant gloved thumb or finger to the port to start suction and gently rotate catheter between thumb and forefinger. Apply suction intermittently and release during withdrawing movement of catheter; allow 20- to 30-second intervals between each suction and limit each suctioning to 10 seconds maximum (some sources say 15).

- Hyperoxygenate the client between suction attempts and at the completion of the procedure.

- For oropharyngeal suctioning, it may be necessary to suction secretions that collect in the buccal cavity.

- Clean catheter by wiping off secretions with sterile gauze; flush catheter with sterile water; relubricate and repeat suctioning until air passage is clear. Alternate nares for repeat suctioning. Encourage client to breathe deeply and cough between suctions.

- Provide nasal or oral hygiene. Dispose of equipment.

- Assess effectiveness of suctioning: observe respiratory rate, skin color, dyspnea, and level of anxiety. Document relevant information.

after each vibration, encourage the client to cough and expectorate; vibrate five times over each lung segment

c. Postural drainage: use of gravity to drain secretions from the respiratory tract; explain procedure and position the client so the head is lower than the chest; place sputum container and wipes within client's reach; do percussion and vibration for 5 minutes and allow 5 minutes for drainage; encourage client to cough and expectorate; instruct client to turn to the other side then to the supine position, and repeat procedure; assist client to a sitting position and offer mouth care; document observations

6. Care of the client with chest tubes

a. Maintain the water seal and patency of the drainage system: tape connector sites; provide a straight line of tubing from bed to the collection system, no kinks in tubing; do not use pins or restrain tubing

b. Assess client's vital signs, respiratory and cardiovascular status regularly

c. Maintain integrity of the drainage system: disposable system or suction bottles below level of bed; maintain suction control to create gentle bubbling

d. Do not strip chest tubes unless there is a physician's order and if agency policy permits (most do not) because excessive negative pressure can damage lung tissue; if ordered, stripping is done by pinching the tube close to client's chest with one hand, lubricating thumb and forefinger to compress and sliding down toward the receptacle

e. Keep sterile water, rubber-tipped clamps (if agency policy allows) and sterile dressing materials (dry gauze, petrolatum gauze, and tape) near the client; if disconnection occurs, reattach after wiping ends quickly with alcohol or place chest tube distal end in sterile water to restore underwater seal; clamp the chest tube only if agency policy dictates (could cause tension pneumothorax); if the chest tube is pulled out inadvertently, apply a sterile occlusive dressing to the wound immediately

f. Mark drainage on the receptacle every shift and read at eye level; report if drainage exceeds 100 mL/hr

g. Document amount and color of drainage on intake and output record and progress notes, respectively

7. Oxygen therapy: when O_2 therapy is used, follow certain safety precautions (see Box 7-2)

a. Check physician's orders and assess client's respiratory and cardiovascular status

b. Explain procedure to the client and place client in a semisitting position

c. Set up O_2 equipment: attach flow meter to wall outlet or portable O_2 cylinder; fill humidifier with water and attach to base of flow meter; attach the delivery system (cannula or face mask) and tubing to the flow meter; turn on O_2 at the prescribed rate

d. Cannula: put cannula over client's face with outlet prongs fitting the nares and elastic band around the head; pad the bands over the ears and under the cheekbones as necessary

e. Face mask: guide mask toward the client's face and apply it from the nose downward; mold the mask to the face; secure elastic band around client's head and pad the band over the ears as needed

f. Assess the client's respiratory and cardiovascular status regularly; check client's nares for irritation if cannula is used, facial skin if with a face mask; document observations

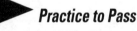

Practice to Pass

A client with chest tubes is admitted to the nursing unit. How would the nurse care for this client?

Box 7-2	➤ No smoking is allowed at any time when oxygen is in use.

Safety Precautions during Oxygen Therapy

➤ No smoking is allowed at any time when oxygen is in use.

➤ Instruct the client and visitors not to smoke and discuss possible consequences of smoking when oxygen is in use. If necessary, remove matches, lighters, and ash-trays.

➤ If O_2 therapy is used at home, instruct family members or caregivers to smoke only outside.

➤ Avoid materials that generate static electricity such as woolen blankets and synthetic fabrics; instead use cotton fabrics.

➤ Avoid use of volatile, flammable substances such as acetone in nail polish re-movers, alcohol, ether, and oils near clients using O_2.

➤ Remove any friction type or battery operated gadgets, devices, or toys.

➤ Make sure electric devices such as radios, razors, and televisions are in good work-ing order to prevent short-circuit sparks.

➤ Ensure that electric monitoring equipment and suction machines are properly grounded. Disconnect any ungrounded equipment.

➤ Personnel need to be aware of the location of fire extinguishers and be able to use them properly.

➤ Know location of O_2 meter turn-off valve on nursing unit.

    g. Check flow of O_2 and level of water in humidifier regularly

    h. Document O_2 saturation level obtained by pulse oximetry every 8 hours; also document amount of O_2 on flowsheet and client response to O_2 therapy in progress notes

  8. Incentive spirometer (IS)

    a. Check physician's orders; assist client to a sitting or Fowler's position and ex-plain procedure

    b. Assemble equipment; set marker at the recommended volume goal

    c. Instruct client to place mouth tightly around the mouthpiece

    d. Instruct client to inhale slowly and maintain a steady flow as if pulling through a straw; encourage client to raise and maintain flow rate indicator

    e. Instruct client to remove mouthpiece but hold breath for 2 to 3 seconds and then exhale slowly through pursed lips

    f. Have client repeat the procedure a few times and then cough; encourage to use 5 to 10 times hourly; keep the IS within reach of client; document IS use in client record

  9. Frequent reassessment: monitor respiratory rate, O_2 saturation, lung sounds, and other respiratory data at least once per 8 hours and more frequently as needed to detect subtle changes; monitor trends and report accordingly

V. MEETING THE CLIENT'S NEED FOR SLEEP

A. Physiology of sleep

  1. Circadian rhythm: rhythmic repetition of patterns each 24 hours; sleep is a complex biologic rhythm; if a person's biologic clock coincides with the sleep-wake patterns, the person is in **circadian synchronization**

  2. Sleep regulation: the centers in the lower portion of the brain actively inhibit wakefulness causing sleep

3. Stages of sleep: two types of sleep are NREM (non–rapid eye movement) and REM (rapid eye movement)

    a. NREM: deep and restful sleep characterized by decrease in physiologic functions: BP and pulse decreases, skeletal muscles relax, basal metabolic rate decreases, brain waves become slower; there are 4 stages of NREM

        1) Stage I: very light sleep, relaxed and drowsy, floating sensation, eyes roll from side to side, lasts only a few minutes

        2) Stage II: light sleep, easily roused, slight decrease of pulse and respirations, lasts 10 to 15 minutes

        3) Stage III: medium-depth sleep, less easily aroused, pulse and respirations and other physiologic functions such as BP and temperature continue to fall; skeletal muscles are relaxed, reflexes diminished, and snoring may occur

        4) Stage IV: called the delta sleep; deepest sleep stage, difficult to arouse, rarely moves and muscles completely relaxed; dreaming may occur; may last about 30 minutes

    b. REM sleep: usually occurs every 90 minutes and lasts 5 to 30 minutes; active dreaming occurs and dreams are remembered; the brain is highly active and the person is difficult to arouse or may wake up spontaneously; rapid eye movements and irregular muscle movements take place; muscle tone is depressed and heart and respiratory rates are irregular

B. Normal sleep requirements and patterns

1. Neonates: newborns sleep an average of 16 to 18 hours per day, divided into about 7 sleep periods; most sleep is spent in Stages III and IV of the NREM and nearly 50% is in the REM sleep

2. Infants: range of sleep is from 12 to 22 hours; periods of wakefulness increase with age; by 4 months, infants sleep through the night and nap during the day; at the end of the first year, sleep about 14 of every 24 hours; half of the time, infants have light sleep, and 20 to 30% is REM sleep

3. Toddlers: normal sleep wake cycle established by 2 to 3 years; generally sleep for 10 to 12 hours, still require a mid-afternoon nap, but morning nap needs decrease; still 20 to 30% is REM sleep

4. Preschoolers: need 11 to 12 hours sleep but may fluctuate because of activity and growth spurts; older preschoolers do not need a nap; continue to have 20 to 30% of REM sleep

5. School-age: most school-age children sleep 8 to 12 hours without daytime naps; REM sleep decreases to about 20%

6. Adolescents: amount of time for sleeping declines but adolescents still need 8 to 10 hours sleep; changes in pattern occur as some adolescents have a need for daytime napping

7. Young adults: generally, young adults require 7 to 8 hours but because of life style changes they may have erratic sleep patterns

8. Middle-age adults: sleep pattern established earlier is maintained, and the middle aged adult sleeps 6 to 8 hours/night and about 20% is REM sleep; the amount of Stage IV NREM sleep decreases

9. Older adults: sleep about 6 hours a night with about 20 to 25% REM sleep and a marked decrease in Stage IV NREM sleep; they awaken more frequently and have difficulty returning back to sleep, hence having less restorative sleep

C. Factors affecting sleep

1. Illness: increases the requirement for sleep; however, the illness may cause pain, difficulty breathing, or discomfort with movement that interferes with sleep; elevated body temperature can cause a reduction in the Stages III and IV NREM and REM sleep

2. Drugs and substances: excessive alcohol disrupts REM sleep, although it may accelerate onset of sleep; alcohol-tolerant individuals may have difficulty with sleep and when drug effects wear off, there may be nightmares; caffeine-containing beverages and amphetamines act as stimulants and interfere with sleep; nicotine has a stimulating effect and smokers have more difficulty falling asleep

3. Lifestyle: shift work may interfere with the person's ability to adjust sleeping patterns; inactivity or boredom may contribute to sleep problems

4. Usual sleep patterns and excessive daytime sleepiness: individuals commonly refer to themselves as morning or night people; these are their sleep patterns; excessive daytime sleepiness may be caused by night-time sleep deprivation

5. Emotional stress: anxiety makes it difficult for the person to fall asleep; depression may result in difficulty falling asleep or premature awakening

6. Environment: any change in noise level may inhibit sleep—people are habituated to a certain noise; ventilation and environmental temperature can affect sleep

7. Various prescribed drugs: decongestants, narcotics, sedatives, beta-blockers, and antidepressants may cause drowsiness and may disrupt REM sleep

8. Exercise and fatigue: moderate exercise is conducive to sleep but if excessive, may delay sleep; moderate fatigue may lead to a restful sleep

9. Food/calorie intake: weight loss is associated with reduced quantity of sleep, broken sleep, and earlier awakening, while weight gain is associated with increased total sleep time, less broken sleep, and later waking; eating a heavy meal just prior to bedtime could interfere with sleep

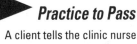

Practice to Pass

A client tells the clinic nurse that she is having difficulty falling asleep at night. What common factors that interfere with sleep should the nurse assess for?

D. Overview of sleep disorders

1. Insomnia: inability to obtain an adequate amount or quality of sleep; can be initial (difficulty falling asleep), middle or intermittent (difficulty maintaining sleep because of frequent or prolonged waking), or terminal (early or premature awakening), which may be associated with depression or medications, such as HIV drugs; treatment is usually directed at developing new sleep-inducing/maintaining behaviors such as modifying the environment or relaxation techniques

2. Sleep apnea: periodic cessation of breathing during sleep; the episode lasts from 10 seconds to 2 minutes and the incidence may range from 50 to 600 episodes per night

   a. It is suspected when the person snores loudly, has frequent nocturnal awakening, excessive daytime sleepiness, fatigue, irritability, and personality changes

   b. Incidence of sleep apnea is high in elderly men

   c. Is also more common among obese clients

   d. Complications of prolonged sleep apnea may be increased blood pressure, cardiac arrhythmias, and left-sided heart failure

   e. Treatment is directed at the cause: if obstructive, enlarged tonsils or adenoids may be removed

    f. The use of a nasal continuous positive airway pressure (CPAP) device may be effective, because it keeps alveoli and small airways open, permitting better gas exchange because alveoli cannot collapse

3. Narcolepsy: sudden wave of overwhelming sleepiness during the day, where the person may nod off in the middle of the day while involved in activities; treatment is with the use of stimulants, such as amphetamines

4. Parasomnias: abnormal behavioral or physiologic events associated with the stages of sleep and interfere with sleep; treatment consists of relaxation techniques and sleep hygiene practices

    a. Somnambulism: sleepwalking that occurs in the Stage III and IV NREM sleep; it is episodic and occurs 1 to 2 hours after falling asleep; the sleep-walker does not notice dangers such as stairs

    b. Sleeptalking: talking occurs during NREM sleep before REM sleep

    c. Nocturnal enuresis: bedwetting, more common in male children over 3 years old; often occurs 1 to 2 hours after falling asleep, when rousing from Stage III to IV of the NREM sleep

    d. Nocturnal erections: both erections and emissions start around adolescence and occur during REM sleep

    e. Bruxism: clenching and grinding teeth that occur during Stage II of the NREM sleep

5. Sleep deprivation: syndrome where the individual's prolonged disturbance results in a decrease in the amount, quality, and consistency of sleep

    a. REM sleep deprivation can be caused by use of alcohol, shift work, jet lag, or extended ICU hospitalization and can result in excitability, confusion, and emotional lability; delay procedures or medications when possible to avoid waking a client during REM sleep

    b. NREM sleep deprivation can be caused by the same factors as REM deprivation as well as hypothyroidism, depression, sleep apnea, and age (common in the elderly) and can result in withdrawal, excessive sleepiness, and hyporesponsiveness

    c. An individual who has both REM and NREM sleep deprivation may have difficulty with concentration, judgment, and attention, marked fatigue, and perceptual distortions

E. Health promotion to improve sleep

1. Environmental controls: ensure appropriate lighting, ventilation, and temperature; keep noise level to a minimum

2. Promote bedtime routines: respect client's customary rituals or routines in order to promote relaxation and encourage sleep; provide hygienic routines such as washing face, brushing teeth, and voiding; listening to music or praying; children's bedtime stories; adult's conversations with their caregivers or family members if possible

3. Promote comfort: backrubs, change of linen/clothing, positioning for comfort, as well as administering medications for pain can promote and help maintain sleep; listening to the client's concerns can alleviate emotional stress and promote relaxation; avoid heavy meal 3 hours before bedtime, decrease fluid intake 2 hours before sleep, and avoid alcohol, caffeine, or heavily spiced foods

4. Promote activity: get adequate exercise during the day to reduce stress; engage in a nonstrenuous activity prior to sleep

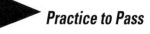

Practice to Pass

The nurse is providing health teaching to a group of clients about promoting sleep. What specific instructions would be appropriate for the nurse to provide?

5. Pharmacological sleep aids: may be prescribed for short-term treatment of insomnia; however, they generally should be used as a last resort and be taken on PRN (as necessary) basis; clients need to be aware of the actions, desired and adverse effects of sleep aids; sedatives and hypnotics have different onset and duration of their actions; regular use may lead to tolerance of the drug and may lead to rebound insomnia

VI. MEETING NUTRITIONAL NEEDS

A. Principles of nutrition

1. Digestion: process by which food substances are changed into forms that can be absorbed through cell membranes
2. Absorption: the taking in of substances from GI tract into bloodstream
3. Metabolism: sum of all physical and chemical processes by which a living organism is formed and maintained and by which energy is made available
4. Storage: some nutrients are stored when not used to provide energy; e.g., carbohydrates are stored either as glycogen or as fat
5. Elimination: process of discarding unnecessary substances through evaporation, excretion

B. Nutrients

1. Carbohydrates: the primary sources of carbohydrates are plant foods
   a. Types of carbohydrates
      1) Simple (sugars) such as glucose, galactose, and fructose—all water soluble
      2) Complex ones, which are insoluble; starches (which are **polysaccharides**) and fibers (supplies bulk or roughage to the diet) are complex carbohydrates
   b. Digested carbohydrates are absorbed in the small intestines; insulin (a hormone secreted by the pancreas) augments glucose transport through the cell membrane
   c. Some glucose continues to circulate in the bloodstream for energy, and the remainder gets converted to fat or stored as glycogen in the liver and skeletal muscles
2. Proteins: organic substances made up of amino acids; complete proteins are found in animal products such as eggs, milk, and meat; incomplete ones are found in legumes, nuts, grains, cereals, and vegetables
   a. Most protein is digested in the small intestine where enzymes break it down into smaller molecules and finally into amino acids, where they are actively transported into the portal blood circulation
   b. The liver uses amino acids to synthesizes specific proteins
   c. Other amino acids are transported to cells and tissues to make proteins for cell structure
3. Lipids: organic substances that are insoluble in water but soluble in alcohol and ether
   a. Fatty acids are the basic structural units of all lipids and are either saturated (all the carbon atoms are filled with hydrogen) or unsaturated (could accommodate more hydrogen than it presently contains)
   b. Lipids are primarily digested in the small intestine by bile, pancreatic lipase, and enteric lipase (enzymes) with end products of glycerol, fatty acids, and

cholesterol; these products are reassembled in the small intestines and then broken down into soluble compounds called lipoproteins

    c. Food sources for lipids are animal products (milk, egg yolks, and meats) and plants and plant products (seeds, nuts, oils)

4. Vitamins: organic compounds not manufactured in the body and needed in small quantities to **catalyze** metabolic processes

    a. Water-soluble vitamins include C and the B-complex vitamins: B_1 (thiamine), B_2 (riboflavin), B_3 (niacin or nicotinic acid), B_6 (pyridoxine), B_9 (folic acid), B_{12} (cobalamin), pantothenic acid, and biotin; the body cannot store water-soluble vitamins, so a daily supply through the diet is needed

    b. Fat-soluble vitamins include A, D, E, and K, and these can be stored in limited amounts in the body

5. Minerals: compounds that work with other nutrients in maintaining structure and function of the body

    a. An adequate supply of calcium, phosphorus, sodium, potassium, chloride, magnesium, and sulfur (known as macrominerals), and trace elements such as iron, iodine, copper, zinc, manganese, and fluoride (known as microminerals) are necessary for health

    b. The best sources are vegetables, legumes, milk, and some meats

6. Water: the body's most basic nutrient need; it serves as a medium for metabolic reactions within cells and transports nutrients, waste products, and other substances

C. MyPyramid: a graphic guide in making daily food choices; it suggests that people eat a variety of foods to obtain the necessary nutrients and is individualized to individual client needs (see Figure 7-1)

D. Anthropometry: non-invasive measurements that measure changes in body composition; such changes reflect chronic rather than acute changes in nutritional status

1. Skinfold measurement: uses special calipers to measure the thickness of the fold in the triceps (TSF—triceps skin fold) at the back of the upper arm

2. Mid-arm circumference (MAC): a measure of fat, muscle, and skeleton

3. Mid-arm muscle circumference (MAMC): estimate of lean body mass or skeletal muscle reserves; the formula is:

[MAMC [cm] = MAC[cm] minus (3.14 multiplied by the TSF[mm] divided by 10)]

4. Body mass index: correlates weight with height using a nomogram or chart; normal range is considered to be 18.5 to 24.9; smaller number corresponds with underweight status while a larger number indicates overweight or obese status

E. Laboratory values associated with nutrition (see Table 7-1)

F. Components of a diet history

1. Usual eating patterns and habits: Does the client eat regularly, have snacks, and eat alone? Has the client been on any diets?

2. Frequency, types, amounts, or quantities of foods consumed: How much food and what types of food has the client consumed in the last 24 hours? In the last 7 days?

3. Food preferences, allergies, and intolerances: Does the client have strong preferences for specific food groups? Are the allergies and intolerances affecting the amount of intake?

Figure 7-1

MyPyramid.

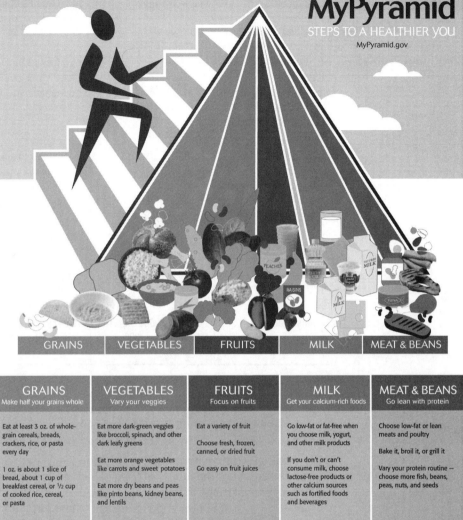

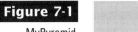

MyPyramid
STEPS TO A HEALTHIER YOU
MyPyramid.gov

GRAINS	VEGETABLES	FRUITS	MILK	MEAT & BEANS

GRAINS Make half your grains whole	**VEGETABLES** Vary your veggies	**FRUITS** Focus on fruits	**MILK** Get your calcium-rich foods	**MEAT & BEANS** Go lean with protein
Eat at least 3 oz. of whole-grain cereals, breads, crackers, rice, or pasta every day 1 oz. is about 1 slice of bread, about 1 cup of breakfast cereal, or ½ cup of cooked rice, cereal, or pasta	Eat more dark-green veggies like broccoli, spinach, and other dark leafy greens Eat more orange vegetables like carrots and sweet potatoes Eat more dry beans and peas like pinto beans, kidney beans, and lentils	Eat a variety of fruit Choose fresh, frozen, canned, or dried fruit Go easy on fruit juices	Go low-fat or fat-free when you choose milk, yogurt, and other milk products If you don't or can't consume milk, choose lactose-free products or other calcium sources such as fortified foods and beverages	Choose low-fat or lean meats and poultry Bake it, broil it, or grill it Vary your protein routine -- choose more fish, beans, peas, nuts, and seeds

For a 2,000-calorie diet, you need the amounts below from each food group. To find the amounts that are right for you, go to MyPyramid.gov.

Eat 6 oz. every day	Eat 2½ cups every day	Eat 2 cups every day	Get 3 cups every day; for kids aged 2 to 8, it's 2	Eat 5½ oz. every day

Find your balance between food and physical activity
- Be sure to stay within your daily calorie needs.
- Be physically active for at least 30 minutes most days of the week.
- About 60 minutes a day of physical activity may be needed to prevent weight gain.
- For sustaining weight loss, at least 60 to 90 minutes a day of physical activity may be required.
- Children and teenagers should be physically active for 60 minutes every day, or most days.

Know the limits on fats, sugars, and salt (sodium)
- Make most of your fat sources from fish, nuts, and vegetable oils.
- Limit solid fats like butter, stick margarine, shortening, and lard, as well as foods that contain these.
- Check the Nutrition Facts label to keep saturated fats, *trans* fats, and sodium low.
- Choose food and beverages low in added sugars. Added sugars contribute calories with few, if any, nutrients.

MyPyramid.gov
STEPS TO A HEALTHIER YOU

U.S. Department of Agriculture
Center for Nutrition Policy and Promotion
April 2005
CNPP-15

USDA is an equal opportunity provider and employer.

Table 7-1	Laboratory Test	Normal Values	Abnormal Findings
Lab Values Associated with Nutritional Problems	Hematocrit: A comparison of the volume of RBCs to plasma in the blood	Men: 40–50% Women: 37–47%	Decreased in iron deficiencies and undernutrition
	Hemoglobin: Measurement of the iron-containing pigment in RBCs	12–16.5 grams/dL	Iron-deficiency anemia
	Serum potassium	3.5–5.0 mEq/L	Depletion seen in severe malnutrition
	Albumin	3.5–5 grams/dL	A low serum albumin level is a useful indicator of prolonged protein depletion; altered liver function and poor hydration may lower albumin levels
	Transferrin	230–400 mg/dL	Reduced numbers indicates protein deficiency, hepatitis, liver dysfunction
	Total lymphocyte count	1500–4000/mm^3	Reduced numbers may indicate malnutrition
	Blood urea nitrogen (BUN)	5 to 20 mg/dL	Elevated levels may be associated with increased protein catabolism caused by destruction or with dehydration
	Urinary creatinine	Men: 800–2000 mg/24 hr Women: 600–1800 mg/24 hr	When skeletal muscles atrophy because of malnutrition, creatinine excretion decreases

4. Social, economic, ethnic, or religious factors that influence nutrition: Is the client suffering from economic hardship? Is there an adequate facility for food preparation? Is there an adequate food storage facility?

5. Health factors that may affect nutrition: Does the client have a disease that interferes with the intake of food? Does the client have problems complying with special diets? Has the client recently gained or lost weight? Can the client see, taste, or smell the food? Does the client have any physical disability that may affect nutrition?

G. Clinical signs of poor/altered nutrition

1. General appearance: appears tired and fatigued; listless

2. Weight: overweight or underweight

3. Posture: stooped or rigid

4. Behavior/motor/perceptual function: slowing of reflexes; motor restlessness; confusion, disorientation

5. Gastrointestinal (GI) function: lack of appetite (anorexia), nausea, vomiting, overeating, indigestion, constipation

6. Hair: dry, dull, sparse, loss of color, brittle

7. Skin: dry, flaky, or scaly; pale or pigmented; presence of **petechiae** (pinpoint red areas) or bruising; lack of subcutaneous fat; poor skin turgor

8. Face/neck: facial edema; any swelling in the neck (enlarged lymph nodes)

9. Lips: swollen, red cracks at side of mouth (angular stomatitis), vertical fissures (cheilosis)

10. Mouth/oral membranes: dry buccal cavity

11. Tongue: swollen, beefy-red or magenta-colored; coated; smooth appearance; increase or decrease in size

12. Teeth: dental caries; gums inflamed (gingivitis), spongy, bleed easily

13. Eyes: pale or red conjunctiva; dryness (xerophthalmia); soft cornea (keratomalacia); dull cornea

14. Nails: brittle; pale; ridged; spoon-shaped

15. Legs/feet: numbness, tingling, edema

16. Musculoskeletal: underdeveloped flaccid, soft, wasting muscles

H. **Therapeutic diets:** special diets prescribed for different reasons: for example, to treat a disease process or modified in texture, consistency, nutrients, or kilocalories (see Table 7-2); the regular diet is a balanced diet that supplies the metabolic requirements of a person who is sedentary (low activity); light diets have foods that are plainly cooked

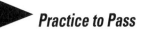

Practice to Pass

The nurse is evaluating a client for nutritional deficiencies. What are the signs of altered nutrition?

VII. MEETING URINARY ELIMINATION NEEDS

A. **Normal urinary function**

1. The normal output of urine is 60 mL/hr or 1500 mL/day; should remain $\geq$ 30 mL/hr to ensure continued normal kidney function

2. Urine normally consists of 96% water

3. Solutes found in urine include:

   a. Organic solutes, including urea, ammonia, uric acid, and creatinine

   b. Inorganic solutes, including sodium, chloride, potassium, sulfate, magnesium, and phosphorus

4. Table 7-3 describes the characteristics of normal urine as well as possible abnormal findings

B. **Common assessment findings**

1. Urgency: strong desire to void may be caused by inflammations or infections in the bladder or urethra

2. Dysuria: painful or difficult voiding

3. Frequency: voiding that occurs more than usual when compared with the person's regular pattern or the generally accepted norm of voiding once every 3 to 6 hours

4. Hesitancy: undue delay and difficulty in initiating voiding

5. Polyuria: a large volume of urine voided at any given time

6. Nocturia: excessive urination at night interrupting sleep

7. Hematuria: red blood cells in the urine

8. Oliguria: reduced urine output between 100 and 500 mL/24 hr

9. Anuria: urine output less than 100 mL in 24 hr

C. **Common urinary elimination problems**

1. Urinary retention: occurs when bladder emptying is impaired, urine accumulates, and bladder becomes overdistended; causes include prostatic hyperplasia, surgery, and medications such as anticholinergics, antidepressants, antipsychotics, antiparkinsonian agents, and antihypertensives

Table 7-2 Therapeutic Diets		
Type of Diet	**Purpose of Diet**	**Examples of Foods Allowed in the Diet/ Other Recommendations**
Clear liquid	Used after certain surgeries or in acute stages of GI tract infection (to minimize stimulation and prevent dehydration)	Coffee, tea, carbonated beverages, bouillon, clear fruit juices (apple, cranberry, grape), other juices (strained), popsicles, gelatin, hard candy, sugar, honey
Full liquid	Used for clients unable to tolerate solid or semisolid foods or who have GI disturbances	All foods allowed in the clear liquid diet plus milk and milk drinks, custards, ice cream, sherbet, yogurt, vegetable juices, strained cereals (e.g., Cream of Wheat), butter
Soft	Used for clients who have difficulty chewing or swallowing	All foods in clear and full liquid plus: all lean meats chopped or shredded; scrambled or poached eggs; mashed potatoes and cooked chopped vegetables and fruits (low in fiber, without membranes or peels); rice, pasta, soft breads, cooked cereals
Pureed	See soft diet	All foods in soft diet: fluid is added to the food and blended to a semisolid consistency
Mechanical/ dental	Used when clients are edentulous, have poorly fitted dentures, or have difficulty chewing	Any food that can be broken down easily
High-fiber (high residue)	Used to treat constipation and diverticulosis	Cereals and grains such as wheat or oat bran, cooked cereals, dry cereals such as cornflakes, shredded wheat; whole grain breads; fruits such as unpeeled raw apples, peaches, or pears; oranges and berries; vegetables such as broccoli, carrots, peas, corn, beans, celery, and tomatoes
Sodium-restricted	Used to manage hypertension, hepatitis, congestive heart failure, renal insufficiency or failure, cirrhosis of the liver	Allow most fresh fruits and vegetables (except beets, celery and frozen or canned vegetables with added salt); and most meats (except processed ones such as bacon, sausage, luncheon meats, cold cuts or smoked fish); restrict salt in cooking or at the table; avoid foods naturally high in sodium: brains, kidney, clams, crab, lobster, oysters, shrimp, dried fruit, spinach, carrots, cheese, buttermilk, most dry cereals
Healthy heart	Used to help control cholesterol levels and promote weight reduction; calories may be reduced	Wide variety of foods allowed; low-fat or nonfat dairy products such as yogurt, skim milk; fish, poultry; monounsaturated fats found in canola, olive, and peanut oils; all fresh fruits and vegetables; whole grain cereals, rice, and pasta
Diabetic exchange	Structured diet to prevent hyperglycemia; exchange list diet based on person's ideal weight, activity level, age, and occupation	Distribution of foods based on exchange lists with three groups of foods; carbohydrates, meat and meat substitutes; and fats; one food portion of the list can exchanged or substituted for another with little difference in calories or amount of carbohydrates, proteins, or fats; examples of carbohydrate exchanges: ½ cup of cereal, ½ cup of pasta, ½ slice bagel, ½ hamburger bun, 1 medium pancake; examples of protein exchanges: 1 oz lean poultry no skin, 1 oz fish, ¼ cup nonfat cottage cheese, 1 egg, 1 oz cheese; examples of fat exchanges: 1 tsp margarine, 6 cashews, 2 tsp mayonnaise substitute, 1 tbsp cream cheese

Table 7-3	Characteristics of Normal and Abnormal Urine		
Characteristic	**Normal**	**Abnormal**	**Nursing Considerations**
Amount in 24 hours (adult)	1200–1500 mL	Under 1200 mL A large amount over intake	Urinary output normally is approximately equal to fluid intake. Output of less than 30 mL/hr may indicate decreased blood flow to the kidneys and should be immediately reported.
Color, clarity	Straw, amber Transparent	Dark amber Cloudy Dark orange Red or dark brown Mucous plugs, viscid, thick	Concentrated urine is darker in color. Dilute urine may appear almost clear, or very pale yellow. Some foods and drugs may color urine. Red blood cells in the urine (hematuria) may be evident as pink, bright red, or rusty brown urine. Menstrual bleeding can also color urine but should not be confused with hematuria. White blood cells, bacteria, pus, or contaminants such as prostatic fluid, sperm, or vaginal drainage may cause cloudy urine.
Odor	Faint aromatic	Offensive	Some foods (e.g., asparagus) cause a musty odor; infected urine can have a fetid odor; urine high in glucose has a sweet odor.
Sterility	No microorganisms present	Microorganisms present	Urine in the bladder is sterile. Urine specimens may become contaminated by bacteria from the perineum during collection.
pH	4.5–8	Under 4.5 Over 8	Freshly voided urine is normally somewhat acidic. Alkaline urine may indicate a state of alkalosis, urinary tract infection, or a diet high in fruits and vegetables. More acidic urine (low pH) is found in starvation, with diarrhea, or with a diet high in protein foods or cranberries.
Specific gravity	1.010–1.025	Under 1.010 Over 1.025	Concentrated urine has a higher specific gravity; diluted urine has a lower specific gravity.
Glucose	Not present	Present	Glucose in the urine indicates high blood glucose levels (> 180 mg/dL), and may be indicative of undiagnosed or uncontrolled diabetes mellitus.
Ketone bodies	Not present	Present	Ketones, the end product of fatty acid breakdown, are not normally present in the urine. They may be present in the urine of clients who have uncontrolled diabetes mellitus, who are in a state of starvation, or who have ingested excessive amounts of aspirin.
Blood	Not present	Occult (microscopic) Bright red	Blood may be present in the urine of clients who have urinary tract infection, kidney disease, or bleeding from the urinary tract.
Protein	Not present	Present	Protein may spill into urine when there is damage to glomerular membrane of kidney, such as with glomerulonephritis.

Source: Berman, A., Snyder, S., Kozier, B., & Erb, G. (2008). *Fundamentals of nursing: Concepts, process, and practice* (8th ed.). Upper Saddle River, NJ: Prentice Hall, p. 1293.

2. Urinary tract infections (UTI): infectious process leads to inflammation in any portion of the urinary tract

   a. Lower UTI: includes urethritis (inflammation of the urethra), cystitis (inflammation of the urinary bladder, most common), and prostatitis (inflammation of the prostate gland)

   b. Upper UTI: pyelonephritis (inflammation of the renal pelvis and parenchyma, the functional portion of the kidney tissue)

3. Incontinence: involuntary urination

   a. Stress incontinence: involuntary loss of urine of less than 50 mL occurring with increased abdominal pressure through coughing, laughing, or lifting

   b. Reflex incontinence: involuntary loss of urine at predictable intervals when bladder reaches a specific volume

   c. Urge incontinence: involuntary loss of urine soon after a strong urge to void

    d. Functional incontinence: involuntary unpredictable passage of urine because of inability to get to toilet as a result of physical or cognitive impairment

    e. Total incontinence: continuous and unpredictable involuntary loss of urine

D. Urinary diversion devices: ureterostomy—a surgical rerouting of urine from the kidneys to a site other than the bladder, usually when the bladder is removed or diseased

    1. Cutaneous ureterostomy: ureters brought directly to the skin surface to form small stomas; disadvantages include that stomas provide direct access for microorganisms from skin to kidneys; pouches may be difficult to fit to small stomas; stenosis of stomas may occur as a complication

    2. Ileal conduit: a segment of the ileum is separated from the small intestine and formed into a pouch with the open end brought out through the abdominal wall to form a stoma; the ureters are implanted into the ileal pouch (see Figure 7-2)

E. Common urinary tests

    1. Urinalysis: macroscopic and microscopic analysis of urine to determine physical and chemical characteristics; refer back to Table 7–3

    2. Urine culture/sensitivity: identifies an infecting organism and the most effective antibiotic; a clean-catch specimen or catheterized specimen is needed; culture requires 24 to 72 hours for organism growth and identification

    3. Intravenous pyelogram (IVP) or intravenous urogram (IVU): intravenous injection of a radiopaque contrast media that concentrates in the urine and facilitates visualization of the kidneys, ureters, and bladder

    4. Renal scan: radiotraces or isotopes injected intravenously to evaluate renal size, shape, position, and function or the blood flow to the kidneys; pictures are taken by a scintillation camera

    5. Ultrasound: high-frequency sound waves are used to create ultrasonic images of the urinary system

    6. Cystoscopy: direct visualization of the urethra and bladder with a cystoscope that is a self contained optical lens system and provides a magnified illuminated view of the bladder

    7. Bladder scan at bedside: detects amount of urine in bladder to help determine need for voiding or straight catheterization; may be done by nurses or other personnel trained to use portable device

Figure 7-2

An ileal conduit.

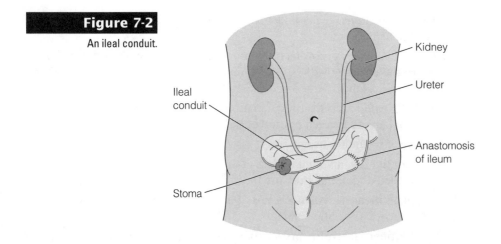

F. Teaching/health promotion for urinary elimination

1. Adequate hydration: normal daily intake of 1500 mL of measurable fluids recommended; if prone to development of stones or infections, increase fluid intake to 2000 to 3000 mL per 24 hours; if experiencing abnormal fluid losses, additional fluid intake is necessary

2. Personal hygiene: teach client to maintain cleanliness by washing perineal area with soap and water daily, and wiping after defecation; instruct female clients to wipe from front to back (urinary meatus toward the anus) after voiding and discard after each wipe; if recurrent infections are occuring, avoid tub baths

3. Emptying bladder completely: regular exercise increases muscle tone that helps maintain the ability to contract the detrusor muscle of the bladder for complete emptying; abdominal muscle contraction assists in bladder emptying; teach **Kegel exercises**—contract perineal muscles and hold for a count of 3 to 5 seconds and relax; do ten contractions five times daily

4. Infection prevention measures

   a. Drink eight 8-ounce glasses of water daily

   b. Empty bladder at least every 2 to 4 hours while awake, avoiding voluntary retention; if client is incontinent, instruct to void according to a timetable rather than the urge to void (bladder training); void at regular intervals (habit training); or supplement habit training by encouraging and reminding client to void (prompted voiding); instruct client to practice deep, slow breathing until urge to void diminishes

   c. For women: wear cotton briefs; cleanse perineal area from front to back after voiding and defecating; void before and after sexual intercourse; avoid bubble baths, feminine hygiene sprays and douches

   d. Unless contraindicated: teach client to maintain acidity in urine by drinking at least two glasses of cranberry juice per day or taking vitamin C, and avoiding excess milk products and sodium bicarbonate

   e. The client should be able to identify symptoms of urinary tract infection and preventive measures, as well as reporting symptoms promptly

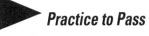

Practice to Pass

A client has a urinary tract infection. What instructions are appropriate for the nurse to give the client?

VIII. MEETING BOWEL ELIMINATION NEEDS

A. Factors that influence bowel elimination

1. Age

   a. Infants and toddlers: have immature control of bowel elimination; daytime control is achieved by age 2½ with toilet training

   b. School-age and adolescents: have similar bowel habits as adults; however, school-age children involved in play may delay elimination

   c. Older adults: are prone to constipation because of slowing down of GI motility and decreased food intake and activity

2. Diet

   a. Sufficient bulk is needed to provide fecal volume

   b. If a client is on low-residue or -fiber diet, there may be insufficient volume to stimulate reflex for defecation

   c. Irregular eating can interfere with regular elimination

   d. Certain foods can affect elimination
   1) Spicy or overly sweet foods may cause diarrhea
   2) Cabbage, onions, apples, and bananas are gas-producing
   3) Bran, prunes, figs, and alcohol have laxative effect
   4) Cheese, eggs, pasta, and lean meat have constipating effect

   3. Position: normal bowel elimination is facilitated by thigh flexion (increases intrabdominal pressure) and a sitting position, which increases the downward pressure on the rectum; using a bedpan while in a supine position is not comfortable and does not facilitate defecation, so client needs to be placed in a semisitting position

   4. Pregnancy: there is decreased intestinal secretion; colon is displaced upward, laterally, and posteriorly; peristaltic activity is decreased, causing constipation; later in pregnancy, venous pressure increases, causing hemorrhoids

   5. Fluid intake: healthy elimination requires an intake of 2000 to 3000 mL/day; inadequate fluid intake or excessive fluid output may lead to hard feces

   6. Activity: peristalsis is stimulated by adequate activity; immobility, weak muscles from lack of exercise, or impaired neurologic functioning can lead to constipation

   7. Psychological: anxiety or anger can increase peristalsis and lead to subsequent diarrhea, while depression slows intestinal activity resulting in constipation

   8. Personal habits: if an individual continually ignores the urge to defecate, water continues to be reabsorbed and feces harden; the reflexes tend to be progressively weakened and may be lost

   9. Pain: when pain or discomfort occurs upon defecation, clients may suppress the urge to defecate to avoid pain, thereby eventually leading to constipation

   10. Medications: antidepressants, antipsychotic and antiparkinsonian agents, morphine and codeine (or other opioids) may cause constipation

   11. Surgery/anesthesia: general anesthetics may slow intestinal movement, resulting in constipation; surgery in the abdominal area that involves handling of the intestines may cause cessation of intestinal movement (paralytic ileus) that lasts for 24 to 48 hours

B. Characteristics of normal stool
   1. Color: varies from light to dark brown; affected by foods and medications
   2. Odor: aromatic, affected by ingested food and person's bacterial flora
   3. Consistency: formed, soft, semi-solid, moist
   4. Frequency: varies with diet; once a day is a common pattern
   5. Amount: varies with diet (about 100 to 400 grams/day)
   6. Constituents: small amounts of undigested roughage, sloughed dead bacteria and epithelial cells, fat, protein, dried constituents of digestive juices (bile pigments), inorganic matter (calcium, phosphates)

C. Common bowel elimination problems
   1. Constipation: abnormal infrequency of defecation and abnormal hardening of stools
   2. Impaction: accumulated mass of dry feces that cannot be expelled
   3. Diarrhea: increased frequency of bowel movements (more than 3 times a day) as well as liquid consistency and increased amount; accompanied by urgency, discomfort, and possibly incontinence

4. Incontinence: involuntary elimination of feces

5. Flatulence: expulsion of gas from the rectum

6. Hemorrhoids: dilated portions of veins in the anal canal causing itching and pain and bright red bleeding upon defecation

D. Diagnostic tests

1. Abdominal film: x-ray of the abdomen taken with the client in flat and upright positions

2. Upper GI/barium swallow: fluoroscopic x-ray examination of the esophagus, stomach, and small intestines after client ingests barium sulfate

3. Barium enema: fluoroscopy x-ray examination visualizing the entire large intestine after client is given an enema of barium; outlines structural changes such as polyps and diverticulitis

4. Endoscopy: use of a flexible tube (fiberoptic endoscope) to visualize the GI tract; images produced are transmitted to a video screen

5. Upper endoscopy: a fiberoptic endoscope connected to a telescopic eyepiece can be inserted through the mouth; example is EGD—esophagogastroduodenoscopy

6. Lower endoscopy: a fiberoptic endoscope connected to a telescopic eyepiece is inserted through the rectum; example is proctosigmoidoscopy

E. Health promotion for elimination problems

1. Constipation: increase fluid intake; instruct to drink fruit juices (especially prune juice) and warm liquids; encourage to eat foods high in roughage or fiber such as raw fruits and vegetables, bran products, whole grain cereals and bread

2. Diarrhea: encourage oral intake of fluids and bland foods; avoid spicy and fatty foods, alcohol, beverages with caffeine, and high-fiber foods

3. Flatulence: limit chewing gum, carbonated drinks, drinking straws, and gas-producing foods such as cabbage, cauliflower, beans, and onions

F. Bowel diversion ostomies: an ostomy is a surgical opening in the abdominal wall for the elimination of feces or urine; bowel diversion ostomies are classified according to status (temporary or permanent), anatomic location, and the construction of the stoma

1. Permanence: colostomies can be temporary (for traumatic injuries or inflammatory conditions) or permanent (birth defect or disease such as cancer)

2. Anatomic location (see Figure 7-3): identifies the site from which the ostomy empties

   a. Ileostomy: distal end of the small intestine (ileus)

   b. Cecostomy: first part of the ascending colon (cecum)

   c. Ascending colostomy: ascending colon

   d. Transverse colostomy: transverse colon

   e. Descending colostomy: descending colon

   f. Sigmoidostomy: sigmoid colon

3. Construction of the stoma

   a. Single: one end of the bowel as the opening

   b. Loop: a loop of bowel brought out into the abdominal wall supported by a glass rod or a plastic bridge; has two openings, the proximal or active, and the distal or inactive; usually performed as an emergency procedure and situated often in the right transverse colon

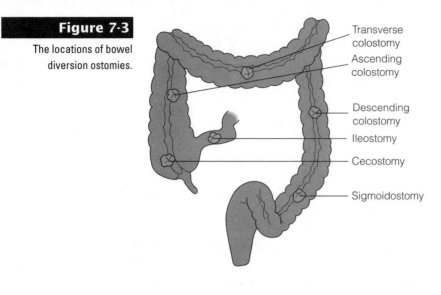

Figure 7-3

The locations of bowel diversion ostomies.

Transverse colostomy

Ascending colostomy

Descending colostomy

Ileostomy

Cecostomy

Sigmoidostomy

    c. Divided: two separated stomas; opening from the digestive end is the colostomy and the distal end is the mucus fistula (bowel continues to secrete mucus)

    d. Double-barreled: proximal and distal loops are sutured together and both ends are brought out into the abdominal wall

4. Health promotion for clients with ostomies

    a. For a client with a colostomy, dietary teaching needs to include information about:

        1) Foods that cause stool odor (asparagus, beans, eggs, fish, onions, garlic)

        2) Foods that increase gas (cabbage, onions, apples, bananas)

        3) Foods that thicken stool (applesauce, bananas, rice, tapioca, cheese, yogurt)

        4) Foods that loosen stool (chocolate, dried beans, fried foods, highly spiced foods, leafy green vegetables, raw fruits and vegetables)

    b. For a client with ileostomy, teaching to relieve food blockage should include the following:

        1) Drink warm fluids or grape juice if not vomiting

        2) Take a warm shower

        3) Assume a knee-chest position

        4) Massage peristomal area

        5) Remove pouch if stoma is swollen and apply one with a larger opening

        6) Eat a low-residue diet initially; avoid foods that cause blockage such as popcorn, nuts, cucumbers, celery, fresh tomatoes, figs, blackberries, and caraway seeds

        7) Limit high-fiber foods and chew them well if eaten

        8) Know signs of blockage: abdominal cramping, swelling of the stoma, and absence of ileostomy output for 4 to 6 hours

5. Stoma management

    a. Stoma appearance: should be bright pink or red in color, moist and raised above abdominal skin surface, and surrounded by intact skin; abnormalities include being sunken (below level of abdominal skin), abnormal in color

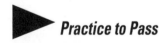

Practice to Pass

The nurse is taking care of a client with a colostomy. What health teaching is appropriate for this client?

(dusky, pale, cyanotic, or black—report immediately), stenosed (opening is narrowed), or herniated (stoma protrudes excessively above skin level)

b. Keep peristomal skin clean and dry

c. Cut stoma appliance so that opening in the skin barrier/wafer is no more than ⅛ to ¼ inch larger than the stoma itself

d. Use a one-piece or two-piece system according to client need

e. Empty pouch when it is ⅓ to ½ full to prevent weight of pouch from separating the stoma wafer from the skin

f. Pouches vary in the frequency with which they are changed; some are changed weekly (maximum length of time) and others are changed more frequently; in clients with peristomal skin that is reddened, denuded, or ulcerated, the pouch should be changed every 24 to 48 hours for skin assessment and ongoing skin care

g. Assess the client's adjustment to having an ostomy (disturbed body image), and provide referrals to certified wound and ostomy nurse as needed

Case Study

A 72-year-old female is being admitted for evaluation after a fall at home. Although x-rays revealed no fractures, the client is complaining of severe pain in the lower back, inability to sleep at night because of the pain, difficulty breathing, and lack of appetite. You are the admitting nurse in the unit.

1. What assessments does the nurse need to make about the client's ability to meet basic needs?

2. How would the nurse ensure the safety of the client?

3. What interventions will be appropriate to promote client's sleep?

4. How would the nurse assist the client have adequate air exchange?

5. What instructions will the nurse give to promote healthy urinary elimination?

For suggested responses, see pages 337.

POSTTEST

① The family member of an elderly client objects that restraints are being used to prevent the client from wandering to other clients' rooms, especially in the evening. In order to avoid the use of restraints the nurse should consider:

1. Providing visual and auditory stimuli.
2. Using antianxiety medications as prescribed.
3. Assigning client to a room near the nurse's station.
4. Locking the other clients' rooms.

② A client is hospitalized for the first time. Which of the following actions would the nurse take to ensure the safety of the client?

1. Keep unnecessary furniture out of the way.
2. Keep lights on all the time.
3. Keep side rails up at all times.
4. Keep all equipment out of view.

③ A client who is unconscious needs frequent mouth care. While performing mouth care, the nurse takes care to place the client in which of the following positions?

1. Fowler's
2. Side-lying
3. Supine
4. Trendelenburg

4 The nurse is providing health teaching to the client about lifestyle factors that affect oxygenation. The most accurate explanation the nurse should include is that:

1. Epinephrine and norepinephrine released under stress decrease blood pressure and cardiac rate.
2. Long-term use of alcohol stabilizes blood pressure and cardiac functioning.
3. Nicotine increases heart rate, blood pressure, and peripheral resistance and produces vasoconstriction, which decreases oxygenation to tissues.
4. Physical exercise decreases the depth of respirations and cardiac rate and eventually lowers the need for oxygen by the tissues.

5 A nurse is performing oropharyngeal suctioning on an unconscious client. The nurse should perform which of the following actions? Select all that apply.

1. Insert the catheter approximately 20 cm while applying suction.
2. Allow 20 to 30 second intervals between each suction attempt, and limit suctioning to a total of 15 minutes.
3. Gently rotate the catheter while applying suction.
4. Apply suction for 5 seconds while inserting the catheter and continue for another 5 seconds before withdrawing.
5. Provide oxygen to the client prior to suctioning.

6 A client with chest tubes is admitted to the nursing unit. The nurse should place the highest priority during admission on which of the following?

1. Monitoring client's vital signs, respiratory, and cardiovascular status regularly
2. Explaining the importance of deep breathing and coughing regularly
3. Reporting if drainage exceeds 100 mL/hour
4. Placing rubber-tipped clamps, sterile water, and sterile occlusive dressing materials at the bedside

7 While doing a physical assessment on a client, the nurse suspects that the client has poor nutritional status. The nurse concludes that this concern is validated when the nurse observes which of the following?

1. Delayed wound healing
2. Firm, smooth pink nails
3. Moist buccal cavity mucous membranes
4. Erect posture

8 The nurse evaluates the results of laboratory tests completed on a client. The nurse concludes that the client may have an abnormality related to nutritional status based on which of the following values?

1. Blood urea nitrogen (BUN) 15 mg/dL
2. Urinary creatinine 800 mg/24 hr. in an adult female
3. Albumin 5 grams/dL
4. Serum potassium 2.4 mEq/L

9 The nurse has taught a client measures to avoid complications associated with urinary elimination. Which of the following indicates to the nurse that the expected outcome is achieved? The client:

1. Identifies symptoms of and measures to prevent urinary tract infection.
2. Is able to perform perineal care by self.
3. Maintains proper disposal of urinary output.
4. Takes regular tub baths and appropriate personal hygiene measures.

10 A client with a colostomy asks the nurse about types of foods that may loosen stool and cause leakage into the pouch. In order to avoid leakage, the nurse should instruct the client to consume:

1. Asparagus, beans, eggs, fish, onions.
2. Applesauce, bananas, rice, tapioca, yogurt.
3. Fried foods, highly spiced foods, raw fruits and vegetables.
4. Carbonated drinks, fruit juices, greasy and pureed foods.

➤ *See pages 200–202 for Answers & Rationales.*

ANSWERS & RATIONALES

Pretest

1 Answer: 1 A toddler is mobile and naturally curious and experiments with things in the environment; therefore, the parents need to know that supervision will be necessary. Toddlers' reflexes are not necessarily slow, and reading is not a concern. Social and personality development is a good topic for health teaching but is not the main concern in regard to safety.
Cognitive Level: Application **Client Need:** Safe, Effective Care Environment: Safety and Infection Control **Integrated Process:** Teaching/Learning **Content Area:** Fundamentals **Strategy:** The critical words are *parents of toddlers* and *safety education.* Recall safety risks according to developmental level to permit you to select the option that provides key information to parents.
Reference: Kozier, B., Erb, G., Berman, A. & Snyder, S. J. (2004). *Fundamentals of nursing: Concepts, process, and practice* (7th ed.). Upper Saddle River, NJ: Pearson Education, p. 379.

2 Answers: 2, 5 One of the purposes of restraints should be to prevent interruption of therapy such as sutures or sterile dressings. The least restrictive restraint should be used even when it is indicated. Restraints should not be used for the convenience of the staff (option 1), nor should they be used just because a client is weak or developmentally disabled (option 3). The client in option 4 has no need for restraints.
Cognitive Level: Application **Client Need:** Safe, Effective Care Environment: Safety and Infection Control **Integrated Process:** Nursing Process: Assessment **Content Area:** Fundamentals **Strategy:** The critical term is *appropriate use of restraints.* Recall the overall objectives for restraint use to assist you in making correct decisions about the use of restraints. **Reference:** Kozier, B., Erb, G., Berman, A., & Snyder, S. J. (2004). *Fundamentals of nursing: Concepts, process, and practice* (7th ed.). Upper Saddle River, NJ: Pearson Education, p. 687.

3 Answer: 2 Because the client has been incontinent, the possibility of skin bacteria reacting with the urea in the urine can lead to ammonia dermatitis. Erythema (option 1) is reddening of the skin; contact dermatitis (option 3) is a possibility if a client is allergic to soaps or other substances; and petechiae (option 4) are tiny pinpoints of bleeding in the skin.
Cognitive Level: Application **Client Need:** Physiological Integrity: Basic Care and Comfort **Integrated Process:**

Nursing Process: Assessment **Content Area:** Fundamentals **Strategy:** The critical words are *incontinence, pruritis,* and *lower back.* Recognize signs and symptoms of common skin problems and their underlying causes to assist you in selecting appropriate treatment and prevention measures. **Reference:** Kozier, B., Erb, G., Berman, A., & Snyder, S. J. (2004). *Fundamentals of nursing: Concepts, process, and practice* (7th ed.). Upper Saddle River, NJ: Pearson Education, p. 858.

4 Answer: 3 The proper sequence for using a spirometer is to exhale completely, place the mouthpiece, inhale; remove the mouthpiece, hold breath, and exhale. A Fowler's or sitting position best allows full chest expansion. Slower breaths are better and deeper than fast ones. Client should remove the mouthpiece, exhale through pursed lips, and not exhale into the spirometer.
Cognitive Level: Application **Client Need:** Physiological Integrity: Basic Care and Comfort **Integrated Process:** Nursing Process: Evaluation **Content Area:** Fundamentals **Strategy:** The critical terms are *incentive spirometer* and *client understood instructions.* Recall the correct use of the incentive spirometer to answer the question and remember its benefit to the client using it. **Reference:** Kozier, B., Erb, G., Berman, A., & Snyder, S. J. (2004). *Fundamentals of nursing: Concepts, process, and practice* (7th ed.). Upper Saddle River, NJ: Pearson Education, p. 1304.

5 Answers: 2, 3, 4 Basic measures to promote sleep in hospitalized clients include maintaining their bedtime routine, decreasing light and noise levels, and promoting relaxation and general comfort. Alcohol and caffeine (option 1) as well as unusual exertion (option 5) should be avoided by clients who are trying to develop a state of relaxation to enable sleep.
Cognitive Level: Application **Client Need:** Physiological Integrity: Basic Care and Comfort **Integrated Process:** Nursing Process: Implementation **Content Area:** Fundamentals **Strategy:** The critical term is *difficulty sleeping.* Recall basic nursing care measures that promote rest and sleep to assist you in providing effective care to the client. **Reference:** Kozier, B., Erb, G., Berman, A., & Snyder, S. J. (2004). *Fundamentals of nursing: Concepts, process, and practice* (7th ed.). Upper Saddle River, NJ: Pearson Education, pp. 1127–1128.

6 Answer: 3 Electrical equipment in good condition (with no frayed wires) is acceptable for use in the vicinity of oxygen. Petroleum products and most oils have the po-

tential for being flammable when used on the body, and this is a contraindication for their use. Cotton clothing limits static.
Cognitive Level: Application **Client Need:** Safe, Effective Care Environment: Safety and Infection Control **Integrated Process:** Teaching/Learning **Content Area:** Fundamentals **Strategy:** The critical phrase is *oxygen therapy via a cannula.* Recall safety precautions needed during oxygen therapy that will help to promote client safety and improve outcomes. **Reference:** Kozier, B., Erb, G., Berman, A., & Snyder, S. J. (2004). *Fundamentals of nursing: Concepts, process, and practice* (7th ed.). Upper Saddle River, NJ: Pearson Education, pp. 1311–1312.

7 **Answer: 1** Pain can often interfere with sleep. Options 2, 3, and 4 do not negatively affect or interfere with sleep. Absence of unfamiliar stimuli (option 2) can assist with sleep; dealing with stress by talking about the day's events (option 3) promotes relaxation and eventually sleep; moderate fatigue (option 4) may lead to a restful sleep.
Cognitive Level: Application **Client Need:** Physiological Integrity: Basic Care and Comfort **Integrated Process:** Nursing Process: Assessment **Content Area:** Fundamentals **Strategy:** The critical phrase is *negatively affects sleep patterns.* Recall common factors that disrupt sleep to assist you in identifying causes of this disturbance. **Reference:** Kozier, B., Erb, G., Berman, A., & Snyder, S. J. (2004). *Fundamentals of nursing: Concepts, process, and practice* (7th ed.). Upper Saddle River, NJ: Pearson Education, p. 1117.

8 **Answer: 4** Because of limited mobility, the client is already at risk for constipation. To promote bowel function, instruct clients to drink plenty of liquids, including fruit juices such as apple and prune. In addition, foods that are high in fiber and roughage should be encouraged to avoid constipation secondary to immobility.
Cognitive Level: Application **Client Need:** Physiological Integrity: Basic Care and Comfort **Integrated Process:** Teaching/Learning **Content Area:** Fundamentals **Strategy:** The critical phrases are *bedridden client* and *constipation.* Use nursing knowledge of the common complications of immobility to allow you to select the teaching points to treat and further prevent this complication of immobility. **Reference:** Kozier, B., Erb, G., Berman, A., & Snyder, S. J. (2004). *Fundamentals of nursing: Concepts, process, and practice* (7th ed.). Upper Saddle River, NJ: Pearson Education, p. 1229.

9 **Answer: 2** When a premature urge to void occurs, focused breathing exercises may assist the client to overcome the sense of urgency. The intervals between voiding should eventually lengthen, rather than voiding every hour or more often when an urge is felt. Protector pads should be worn continuously for leakage. Adult disposable briefs are used only as a last resort.
Cognitive Level: Application **Client Need:** Physiological Integrity: Basic Care and Comfort **Integrated Process:** Teaching/Learning **Content Area:** Fundamentals **Strategy:** The critical terms are *bladder training* and *expected outcomes.* Recall essential techniques of bladder training to assist you in providing appropriate client information. **Reference:** Kozier, B., Erb, G., Berman, A., & Snyder, S. J. (2004). *Fundamentals of nursing: Concepts, process, and practice* (7th ed.). Upper Saddle River, NJ: Pearson Education, p. 1267.

10 **Answer: 2** A full liquid diet allows such items as puddings, creamed soups, sherbet, strained cereals, and all items that are liquid at room temperature. Options 1, 3, and 4 would not be appropriate.
Cognitive Level: Application **Client Need:** Physiological Integrity: Basic Care and Comfort **Integrated Process:** Teaching/Learning **Content Area:** Fundamentals **Strategy:** The critical words in the question are *successful* and *full liquid diet.* Recall information about the components of therapeutic diets to assist you in providing the client and family with appropriate guidance. **Reference:** Kozier, B., Erb, G., Berman, A., & Snyder, S. J. (2004). *Fundamentals of nursing: Concepts, process, and practice* (7th ed.). Upper Saddle River, NJ: Pearson Education, p. 1201.

Posttest

1 **Answer: 3** The client needs to be supervised and monitored and placed in a room that is more accessible. Assessment is needed to determine causes of wandering. Stimulation is not necessary for a client who is a wanderer. Antianxiety medications may cause more agitation, and locking other clients' rooms will not prevent the client from wandering.
Cognitive Level: Application **Client Need:** Safe, Effective Care Environment: Safety and Infection Control **Integrated Process:** Nursing Process: Planning **Content Area:** Fundamentals **Strategy:** Recall that alternatives to restraints include: reducing noise, alarm systems, activities, family involvement, and adequate lighting. **Reference:** Taylor, C., Lillis, C., & LeMone, P. (2005). *Fundamentals of nursing: The art and science of nursing care* (5th ed.). Philadelphia, PA: Lippincott Williams & Wilkins, p. 632.

2 **Answer: 1** The environment has to be clutter-free; therefore, unnecessary pieces of equipment or furniture have to be out of the way. Lights on and side rails up are not mandatory at all times. It is unnecessary to keep equipment out of view.

Cognitive Level: Application **Client Need:** Safe Effective Care Environment: Safety and Infection Control **Integrated Process:** Nursing Process: Planning **Content Area:** Fundamentals **Strategy:** Remember that the elderly are at great risk for falls. Recall common methods of falls prevention and use the process of elimination to make a selection. **Reference:** LeMone, P., & Burke, K. (2004). *Medical-surgical nursing: Critical thinking in client care* (3rd ed.). Upper Saddle River, NJ: Pearson Education, p. 24.

3 **Answer: 2** In the side-lying position, fluid is more likely to flow readily out of the mouth or pool in the side of the mouth where it can easily be suctioned. Fowler's position and Trendelenburg position are not appropriate since the unconscious client does not have control of the airway in those positions. The supine position is unsafe as the client may aspirate the fluids.
Cognitive Level: Application **Client Need:** Physiological Integrity: Basic Care and Comfort **Integrated Process:** Nursing Process: Implementation **Content Area:** Fundamentals **Strategy:** Recall that an unconscious client always requires airway maintenance. Next, remember that side lying prevents aspiration as well as preventing the tongue from occluding the airway. **Reference:** Taylor, C., Lillis, C., & LeMone, P. (2005). *Fundamentals of nursing: The art and science of nursing care* (5th ed.). Philadelphia, PA: Lippincott Williams & Wilkins, p. 1027.

4 **Answer: 3** Stress and long-term alcohol use increase the blood pressure. Physical exercise increases respirations and cardiac rate, increasing the supply of oxygen to the body. Nicotine increases blood pressure and vasoconstriction, which prevents oxygen from reaching the different parts of the body.
Cognitive Level: Analysis **Client Need:** Health Promotion and Maintenance **Integrated Process:** Teaching/Learning **Content Area:** Fundamentals **Strategy:** Recall general nursing knowledge related to lifestyle and its effects on the respiratory system and use the process of elimination to choose the option that could be a risk factor for the client. **Reference:** Taylor, C., Lillis, C., & LeMone, P. (2005). *Fundamentals of nursing: The art and science of nursing care* (5th ed.). Philadelphia, PA: Lippincott Williams & Wilkins, p. 1384.

5 **Answer: 3, 5** Gentle rotation ensures that all surfaces are reached and prevents trauma to any one area caused by prolonged suctioning. In oropharyngeal suctioning, the catheter should be advanced to 10 to 15 cm; 20 cm is the distance for tracheal suctioning (option 1). Fifteen minutes of suctioning (option 2) and applying suction while inserting the catheter (options 1 and 4) can cause

trauma to the mucous membranes. Oxygenating the client adds to the comfort and safety of the client.
Cognitive Level: Application **Client Need:** Physiological Integrity: Basic Care and Comfort **Integrated Process:** Nursing Process: Implementation **Content Area:** Fundamentals **Strategy:** Recall essentials of the suctioning procedure. Remember that airway maintenance of an unconscious client is essential. **Reference:** Taylor, C., Lillis, C., & LeMone, P. (2005). *Fundamentals of nursing: The art and science of nursing care* (5th ed.). Philadelphia, PA: Lippincott Williams & Wilkins, pp. 1408–1409.

6 **Answer: 4** Although all of the actions are appropriate, the highest priority on admission is to anticipate any emergency that may occur if problems with the chest tubes occur, such as disconnection or accidental removal.
Cognitive Level: Analysis **Client Need:** Physiological Integrity: Physiological Adaptation **Integrated Process:** Nursing Process: Implementation **Content Area:** Fundamentals **Strategy:** Recall that chest tubes remove air and/or fluid from the pleural space and that if dislodged they could pose a threat to the client's respiratory status. Use this knowledge to select the option that prepares for a possible emergency with the chest tube. **Reference:** LeMone, P. & Burke, K. (2004). *Medical-surgical nursing: Critical thinking in client care* (3rd ed.). Upper Saddle River, NJ: Pearson Education, p. 1148.

7 **Answer: 1** Delayed wound healing may be a sign of inadequate nutritional status. Protein is needed to heal wounds. All of the other options are signs of adequate nutritional status.
Cognitive Level: Analysis **Client Need:** Physiological Integrity: Basic Care and Comfort **Integrated Process:** Nursing Process: Assessment **Content Area:** Fundamentals **Strategy:** Recall that inadequate nutrition is manifested by muscle weakness, weight loss, decreased cognition, poor wound healing, and increased risk of infection. **Reference:** Kozier, B., Erb, G., Berman, A., & Snyder, S. J. (2004). *Fundamentals of nursing; concepts, process, and practice* (7th ed.). Upper Saddle River, NJ: Pearson Education, p. 1190.

8 **Answer: 4** Options 1, 2, and 3 are all normal levels, while option 4 is indicative of potassium depletion that occurs in severe cases of malnutrition.
Cognitive Level: Analysis **Client Need:** Physiological Integrity: Reduction of Risk Potential **Integrated Process:** Nursing Process: Evaluation **Content Area:** Fundamentals **Strategy:** Use knowledge of normal laboratory test results to make a selection. Recall that laboratory studies can predict nutritional potential or actual nutritional deficits, but it is important not to draw a conclusion based on a single laboratory value. **Reference:** Kozier, B.,

Erb, G., Berman, A., & Snyder, S. J. (2004). *Fundamentals of nursing; concepts, process, and practice* (7th ed.). Upper Saddle River, NJ: Pearson Education, p. 1198.

 Answer: 1 Symptoms and ways of preventing an infection are crucial for a client to understand. Performance of perineal care independently and disposal of urinary output are not appropriate outcomes. Tub baths are to be avoided, especially in females, as they may increase the possibility of developing lower tract infections. **Cognitive Level:** Application **Client Need:** Physiological Integrity: Physiological Adaptation **Integrated Process:** Teaching/Learning **Content Area:** Fundamentals **Strategy:** Evaluation involves assessing the attainment of goals. Teaching must always be evaluated. Recall that infections may be prevented by increasing consumption of cranberry juice, voiding frequently, and cleansing from front to back. **Reference:** Kozier, B., Erb, G., Berman, A., & Snyder, S. J. (2004). *Fundamentals of nursing; concepts, process, and practice* (7th ed.). Upper Saddle River, NJ: Pearson Education, p. 1260.

Answer: 2 The foods that thicken stools are in option 2. The foods in option 1 increase stool odor; foods in options 3 and 4 loosen stools. **Cognitive Level:** Application **Client Need:** Physiological Integrity: Basic Care and Comfort **Integrated Process:** Teaching/Learning **Content Area:** Fundamentals **Strategy:** To answer this question correctly, it is necessary to learn which foods loosen the stool and which foods thicken it. Memorize common foods and use the process of elimination to answer the question. **Reference:** Kozier, B., Erb, G., Berman, A., & Snyder, S. J. (2004). *Fundamentals of nursing; concepts, process, and practice* (7th ed.). Upper Saddle River, NJ: Pearson Education, p. 1237.

References

Berman, A. J., Snyder, S., Kozier, B., & Erb, G. (2008). *Fundamentals of nursing: Concepts, process, and practice* (8th ed.). Upper Saddle River, NJ: Pearson Education, pp. 710–730, 1231–1355.

Harkreader, H. & Hogan, M. (2007). *Fundamentals of nursing: Caring and clinical judgment* (3rd ed.). St. Louis, MO: Elsevier Science, pp. 536–611, 717–783, 891–942, 975–999.

LeMone, P. & Burke, K. M. (2008). *Medical-surgical nursing: Critical thinking in client care* (4th ed.). Upper Saddle River, NJ: Pearson Education.

Nettina, S. (Ed.) (2005). *The Lippincott manual of nursing practice* (8th ed.). Philadelphia: Lippincott, Williams, & Wilkins, pp. 39–101.

Potter, P. & Perry, A. (2005). *Fundamentals of nursing* (6th ed.). St. Louis, MO: Mosby, Inc., pp. 959–1133, 1322–1419.

Smeltzer, S. C. & Bare, B. G. (2006). *Textbook of medical surgical nursing* (11th ed.). Philadelphia: Lippincott Williams & Wilkins.

Smith, S. F., Duell, D. J., & Martin, B. C. (2004). *Clinical nursing skills: Basic to advanced skills* (6th ed.). Upper Saddle River, NJ: Pearson Education.

ANSWERS & RATIONALES

Meeting the Needs of the Client with Pain

8

Chapter Outline

Introduction

Neurophysiologic Mechanisms of Pain

Theories of Pain

Types of Pain

Barriers to Pain Relief

Pain Assessment

Pharmacological Therapies for Pain Control

Nonpharmacological Techniques for Promoting Comfort

Common Nursing Diagnoses for the Client with Pain

Objectives

➤ Define the concept of pain.

➤ Explain various theories of pain.

➤ Identify barriers to adequate pain relief.

➤ List components of a thorough pain assessment.

➤ Compare pharmacological and nonpharmacological therapies for managing pain and discomfort.

➤ Identify common nursing diagnoses associated with pain.

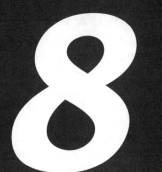

NCLEX-RN® Test Prep

Use the CD-ROM enclosed with this book to access additional practice opportunities.

Review at a Glance

addiction compulsive use of a substance despite negative consequences, such as health threats or legal problems

agonist a substance that when combined with the receptor produces the drug effect or desired effect

antagonist a substance that blocks or reverses the effects of the agonist (e.g., morphine) by occupying the receptor site without producing the drug effect

bradykinin amino acid that appears to be most potent pain-producing chemical

breakthrough pain additional pain that is of rapid onset and greater intensity than the baseline pain

ceiling doses increases beyond a certain drug dose that no longer produce relief

drug tolerance process by which the body requires a progressively larger amount of a drug to achieve the same results

endorphins naturally occurring peptides present in neurons of the brain, spinal cord, and gastrointestinal tract that bind with opiate receptors on neurons to inhibit pain impulse transmission

equianalgesia equivalent analgesia

nociceptor nerve receptors for pain

non-nociceptor nerve fibers that do not usually transmit pain

opioid morphine-like compound that produces systemic effects, including pain relief and sedation

pain tolerance amount of pain or discomfort that a person is able or willing to endure; varies from person to person

patient-controlled analgesia (PCA) self-administration of intravenous analgesics by a client instructed about the procedure

physical drug dependence biologic need for a substance; if the substance is not supplied, physiological withdrawal symptoms occur

prostaglandins chemical substances that increase the sensitivity of pain receptors by enhancing the pain-provoking effect of bradykinin

referred pain pain that is perceived in an area distant from the site of stimuli

PRETEST

1 A 30-year-old client arrives at the clinic for a diagnostic work-up related to chronic right hip pain. The nurse teaching the client about chronic pain would include which of the following items?

1. It is an unusual occurrence for younger adults.
2. It lasts longer than 12 months in duration.
3. It can be difficult to treat effectively.
4. It is often associated with nerve damage.

2 Which technique is the most effective method for the nurse to use to validate an alert client's level of pain?

1. Ask client to use a pain scale.
2. Note physiologic responses to pain.
3. Determine degree of anxiety associated with pain.
4. Observe and document client's facial expressions.

3 Which statement made by the nurse best explains to a client experiencing pain why an opioid analgesic and nonsteroidal anti-inflammatory drug (NSAID) are given together for pain relief?

1. "The NSAID will decrease the likelihood of respiratory depression caused by the opioid."
2. "The NSAID targets muscle pain while the opioid relieves central nervous system irritation."
3. "Giving the medications together reduces the need for additional pain medication during the nighttime hours."
4. "Giving the medications together will provide better relief of pain while decreasing the amount of opioid medication required."

4 A client with chronic back pain is using transcutaneous electrical nerve stimulation (TENS). Which of the following best describes the rationale for using this device that the nurse could simplify and use for client teaching? The TENS unit:

1. Works by stimulating non-nociceptors.
2. Provides an electrical current that alters cell function.
3. Primarily serves the purpose of distraction of pain perception.
4. Will decrease the amount of tissue damage associated with pain.

5 A client is placed on a patient-controlled analgesia (PCA) pump with an opioid medication following total hip replacement surgery. After the client has administered a bolus of the prescribed medication, the nurse should do which of the following as highest priority?

1. Allow client to rest uninterrupted for several hours.
2. Assess the client's level of sedation.
3. Record amount of medication the client received.
4. Monitor the client for respiratory arrest.

6 A client has had chest surgery and is using patient-controlled analgesia (PCA) with morphine to manage the pain. The nurse determines that it is most important to intervene if observing which of the following signs?

1. Respiratory rate 24 breaths per minute
2. Respiratory rate 8 breaths per minute
3. Sleeping but arousable
4. Comfortable when reading a book but uncomfortable when ambulating to rest room

7 An adult client is receiving medication through an epidural catheter for pain resulting from metastatic cancer. To provide safe care to this client, the nurse performs which of the following as an essential nursing action related to the epidural catheter?

1. Assist client to change position every 2 hours.
2. Aspirate catheter prior to administration of medication.
3. Establish baseline pulse oximetry reading.
4. Inspect catheter insertion site every hour.

8 A client has approached the nurse at a pain management clinic and relates an interest in trying biofeedback for pain relief. Which statement indicates to the nurse that the client understands this treatment?

1. "I have spent a lot of money on medication and look forward to a treatment that will not cost me anything."
2. "I am so tired of focusing on my pain. This treatment will allow me to concentrate on something else."
3. "I enjoy being around other people and feel certain a support group will be beneficial to my pain relief."
4. "I want to try to control how blood flows to different parts of my body in order to make some progress."

9 A male client has undergone bowel resection surgery and is given an oral analgesic for reported incisional pain; he reports that the analgesic has provided an acceptable degree of relief. The client's wife states, "I had a similar procedure a few years ago. I believe he needs a stronger medicine this soon after surgery." The nurse's best reply to this concern is which statement?

1. "He has intravenous medication ordered, too. I'll use that next time."
2. "The oral route is the preferred way for giving medications."
3. "A stronger analgesic may delay the return of his bowel functioning."
4. "I believe you are concerned for him, but it is your husband's perception of pain that I need to assess."

10 An elderly female client is admitted to the Emergency Department (ED) after falling on ice and sustaining a fractured hip. The client's daughter pulls the nurse aside and states, "Watch my mother carefully—she has an unbelievable tolerance for pain." Based on this information being accurate, the nurse will anticipate which client need? Select all that apply.

1. The client will be able to endure a great deal of pain.
2. The client will experience discomfort with the slightest movement.
3. The client will probably not experience significant pain.
4. The client will ask for pain medication more often than prescribed.
5. The client will not ask for pain medication and may need to be assessed more frequently for comfort.

➤ *See pages 228–229 for Answers & Rationales.*

I. INTRODUCTION

A. Definitions of pain

1. "Pain is an unpleasant sensory and emotional experience associated with actual or potential tissue damage, or described in terms of such damage" (International Association for the Study of Pain [IASP], 1979); this definition clarifies the multiple dimensions of pain; pain is more than a change in the nervous system; it also reflects the client's past pain experiences and the meaning of the pain

2. "Pain is whatever the person says it is, experienced whenever they say they are experiencing it" (McCaffery & Pasero, 1999); this definition describes the subjectivity of pain; nurses cannot know when another is experiencing pain unless it is communicated; self-report is the only valid measure of pain

B. Joint Commission for Accreditation of Healthcare Organizations (JCAHO) Standards

1. Clients have the right to pain assessment

a. The facility must provide pain assessment tools

b. If a facility cannot treat a client for pain, such as providing a PCA pump, the client must be referred to a facility that can

2. Clients must be treated for pain and involved in their own pain management

3. Discharge planning and teaching must include pain management strategies

C. At the end of life, many clients cannot communicate pain because of delirium, dementia, aphasia, motor weakness, language barriers, and other factors; if the client has any potential physical reason for discomfort, the nurse should consider the individual to have pain until proven otherwise

II. NEUROPHYSIOLOGIC MECHANISMS OF PAIN

A. Stimuli

1. The type of nerve receptor responsible for pain sensation is called a **nociceptor;** these receptors are located at the ends of small afferent neurons and are woven throughout all body tissues except the brain; they are especially numerous in the skin and muscle; a **non-nociceptor** is a nerve fiber that does not usually transmit pain

2. Pain occurs when nociceptors are stimulated by a variety of factors (see Table 8-1)

3. The intensity and duration of stimuli determine the sensation; long-lasting, intense stimulation results in greater pain than brief, mild stimulation

4. Nociceptors are stimulated either by direct damage to the cell or local release of biochemicals secondary to cell injury

Table 8-1	Causative Factor	Example
Examples of Painful Stimuli	Microorganisms (e.g., virus, bacteria)	Pneumonia
	Inflammation	Arthritis
	Impaired blood flow	Angina
	Invasive tumor	Adenocarcinoma
	Radiation	Treatment for cancer
	Heat	Sunburn
	Electricity	Electrical burn
	Obstruction	Gallstone
	Spasm	Muscle cramp
	Compression	Carpal tunnel syndrome
	Decreased movement	Skeletal traction
	Stretching/straining	Sprained ligament
	Fractures	Any bone
	Swelling	Cellulitis
	Chemicals	Skin rash

5. Biochemical sources
   a. **Bradykinin:** an amino acid, appears to be the most potent pain-producing chemical
   b. **Prostaglandins:** chemical substances that increase the sensitivity of pain receptors by enhancing the pain-provoking effect of bradykinin
   c. Histamine
   d. Hydrogen ions
   e. Potassium ions

B. **Pain pathway (see Figure 8-1)**
1. Pain is perceived by the nociceptors in the periphery of the body (e.g., skin); transmitted though small afferent A-delta and C nerve fibers to the spinal cord
   a. A-delta fibers are myelinated and transmit impulses rapidly producing sharp, acute pain sensations
   b. C fibers are not myelinated and transmit pain more slowly; impulses are generated from deeper structures such as muscle and viscera, producing more aching, chronic pain sensations
2. Secondary neurons transmit the impulses from the afferent neurons through the dorsal horn of the spinal cord; a synapse in the substantia gelatinosa occurs; impulses cross over to anterior and lateral spinothalamic tracts
3. Impulses ascend the anterior and lateral spinothalamic tracts and pass through the medulla and midbrain to the thalamus
4. Pain impulses are perceived, interpreted, and a response is generated in the thalamus and cerebral cortex

Figure 8-1

A. Cutaneous nociceptors generate pain impulses that pass via A-delta and C fibers to spinal cord's dorsal horn. B. Secondary neurons in dorsal horn pass impulses across spinal cord to anterior spinothalamic tract. C. Slow pain impulses ascend to the thalamus, while fast pain impulses ascend to the cerebral cortex. The reticular formation in the brainstem integrates the emotional, cognitive, and autonomic responses to pain.

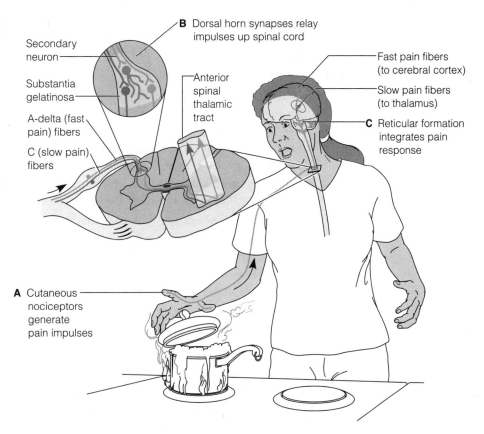

C. Inhibitory mechanisms

1. Efferent fibers run from the reticular formation and mid-brain to the substantia gelatinosa in the dorsal horns of the spinal column; along these fibers, pain transmittal may be inhibited, although the exact process of the mechanism is not understood

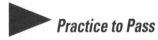
Practice to Pass

What are five distinct sources of pain stimuli?

2. **Endorphins** (endogenous morphines) are natural occurring peptides present in neurons of the brain, spinal cord, and gastrointestinal (GI) tract; they work by binding with opiate receptors on the neurons to inhibit pain impulse transmission

   a. They are released in the brain in response to afferent noxious stimuli

   b. They are released in the spinal cord in response to efferent impulses

III. THEORIES OF PAIN

A. Specificity theory

1. Proposes that body's neurons and pathways for pain transmission are specific, similar to other senses like taste

2. Free nerve endings in the skin act as pain receptors, accept input, and transmit impulses along highly specific nerve fibers

3. Does not account for differences in pain perception or psychologic variables among individuals

B. Pattern theory

1. Identifies two major types of pain fibers; rapidly and slowly conducting

2. Stimulation of these fibers forms a pattern; impulses ascend to the brain to be interpreted as painful

3. Does not account for differences in pain perception or psychologic variables among individuals

C. Gate control theory

1. Pain impulses can be modulated by a transmission blocking action within the central nervous system

2. Large-diameter cutaneous pain fibers can be stimulated (e.g., rubbing or scratching an area) and may inhibit smaller diameter fibers to prevent transmission of the impulse ("close the gate")

D. Current developments in pain theory indicate that pain mechanisms and responses are far more complex than believed to be in the past

1. Pain may be modulated at different points in the nervous system

   a. First-order neurons at the tissue level

   b. Second-order neurons in the spinal cord that process nociceptive information

   c. Third-order tracts and pathways in the spinal cord and brain that relay/process this information

2. The role of the pain experience in the development of new nociceptors and/or reducing the threshold of current nociceptors is also being investigated

IV. TYPES OF PAIN

A. Acute pain

1. Usually temporary, sudden in onset, localized, lasts for less than 6 months; results from tissue injury associated with trauma, surgery, or inflammation

2. Types of acute pain

   a. *Somatic:* arises from nerve receptors in the skin or close to body's surface; may be sharp and well-localized or dull and diffuse; often accompanied by nausea and vomiting

   b. *Visceral:* arises from body's organs; dull and poorly localized because of minimal nociceptors; accompanied by nausea and vomiting, hypotension, and restlessness

   c. **Referred pain:** pain that is perceived in an area distant from the site of stimuli (e.g., pain in a shoulder following abdominal laparoscopic procedure)

3. Acute pain initiates the "fight-or-flight" response of the autonomic nervous system and is characterized by the following symptoms:

   a. Tachycardia

   b. Rapid, shallow respirations

   c. Increased blood pressure

   d. Sweating

   e. Pallor

   f. Dilated pupils

   g. Fear and anxiety

B. Chronic pain

1. Prolonged, lasting longer than 6 months, often not attributed to a definite cause, often unresponsive to medical treatment

2. Types of chronic pain

   a. Neuropathic: painful condition that results from damage to peripheral nerves caused by infection or disease; postherpetic neuralgia (shingles) is an example

   b. Phantom: pain syndrome that occurs following surgical or traumatic amputation of a limb

      1) The client is aware that the body part is missing

      2) Pain may be result of stimulation of severed nerves at the site of amputation

      3) Sensation may be experienced as an itching, tingling, pressure, or as stabbing or burning in nature

      4) It can be triggered by stressors (fatigue, illness, emotions, weather)

      5) This experience is limited for most clients because the brain adapts to the amputated limb; however, some clients experience abnormal sensation or pain over longer periods

      6) This type of pain requires treatment just as any other type of pain does

   c. Psychogenic: pain that is experienced in the absence of a diagnosed physiologic cause or event; the client's emotional needs may prompt pain sensation

3. Depression is a common associated symptom for the client experiencing chronic pain; feelings of despair and hopelessness along with fatigue are expected findings

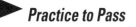

Practice to Pass

What are the psychologic symptoms generally associated with acute and chronic pain?

V. BARRIERS TO PAIN RELIEF

A. Importance of discussing barriers

1. Identify where obstacles exist; these barriers are prevalent throughout health care; nurses can work to overcome the barriers through education, quality

improvement efforts, and involvement in professional groups that advocate for those in pain

2. Recognize when and what client teaching is required; clients suffer from many of the same myths and attitudes that plague healthcare professionals; nurses empower clients through education

B. Specific barriers

1. Barriers related to healthcare professionals

   a. Inadequate or inaccurate information about pain management

   b. Inadequate or suboptimal pain assessment techniques

   c. Concern about overuse of controlled substances and subsequent client addiction

   d. Concern about excessive adverse effects

   e. Concern about clients developing tolerance to analgesics

2. Barriers related to the healthcare system

   a. Low priority given to pain treatment in relation to other client needs

   b. Inadequate reimbursement for other or costly pain management therapies

   c. Restrictive regulation of controlled substances

   d. Less than optimal availability or access to treatment; opioids may be unavailable in inner-city pharmacies as well as rural areas; nurses should work to ensure that necessary medications are available for clients, regardless of the environment

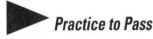

Practice to Pass

What are common barriers that prevent nurses from providing adequate pain relief measures to clients experiencing pain?

3. Barriers related to clients

   a. Reluctance to report pain or to take pain medications

   b. Fear that pain indicates the disease process is progressing

   c. Concern about being thought about as a "complainer"

   d. Reluctance to take pain medications for a variety of reasons

   e. Concern about adverse drug effects

   f. Concern about developing tolerance or addiction to pain medications

   g. Cost is a significant barrier to good analgesia; many pharmaceutical companies have programs that provide medications at reduced or no cost to clients with financial need

4. Client education

   a. Nurses can reassure clients that pain control is every client's right, health professionals rely on the client to report pain, and that good pain management will improve quality of life

   b. Proactive education of clients and family/support persons is necessary, including information about addiction, drug tolerance, and physiological dependence

   c. Clients may use such terms as "hooked" when referring to **addiction** (the compulsive use of a substance despite negative consequences, such as health threats or legal problems)

   d. Clients may express anxiety about becoming "immune" to a medication when discussing **drug tolerance** (the process by which the body requires a progressively greater amount of a drug to achieve the same results)

   e. Clients may worry about developing a **physical drug dependence** (a biologic need for a substance; if the substance is not supplied, physiological withdrawal symptoms occur)

   f. Give clients/caregivers permission to discuss concerns and fears

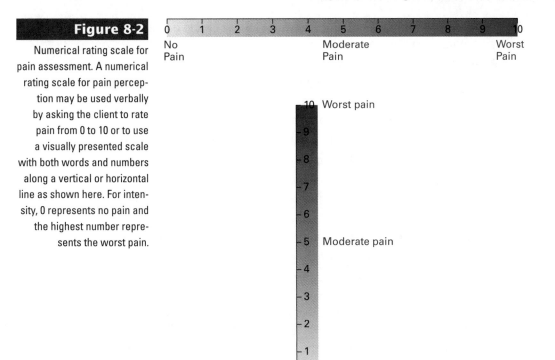

Figure 8-2

Numerical rating scale for pain assessment. A numerical rating scale for pain perception may be used verbally by asking the client to rate pain from 0 to 10 or to use a visually presented scale with both words and numbers along a vertical or horizontal line as shown here. For intensity, 0 represents no pain and the highest number represents the worst pain.

VI. PAIN ASSESSMENT

A. Tools/instruments used

1. Various pain assessment tools are available to use, which provide the client and nurse with an easy method to quantify pain (see Figure 8-2 for samples of visual analog scales)

2. A verbal report using an intensity scale is a fast, easy, and reliable method allowing the client to state pain intensity and, in turn, promotes consistent communication among the nurse, client, and other healthcare professionals about the client's pain status; the two most common scales used are "0 to 5" or "0 to 10," with 0 specifying no pain and the highest number specifying the worst pain

3. A visual analog scale is a horizontal pain-intensity scale with word modifiers at both ends of the scale, such as "no pain" at one end and "worst pain" at the other; clients are asked to point or mark along the line to convey the degree of pain being experienced

4. A graphic rating scale is similar to the visual analog scale but adds a numerical scale with the word modifiers; usually the numbers "0 to 10" are added to the scale

5. FACES pain scale: children, clients who do not speak English, and clients with communication impairments may have difficulty using a numerical pain intensity scale; the FACES pain scale may be used for these clients and for children as young as 3 years old; this scale provides facial expressions (happy face reflects no pain, crying face represents worst pain)

6. Physiologic indicators of pain may be the only means a nurse can use to assess pain in a noncommunicating client; facial and vocal expressions may be the initial manifestations of pain; expressions may include rapid eye blinking, biting

of the lip, moaning, crying, screaming, either closed or clenched eyes, or stiff unmoving body position

B. ABCDE method of pain assessment

1. This acronym was developed for cancer pain; however, it is very appropriate for clients with any type of pain, regardless of the underlying disease

2. A = Ask about pain regularly; assess pain systematically

3. B = Believe the client and family about the reports of pain and what relieves it

4. C = Choose pain control options appropriate for the client, family, and setting

5. D = Deliver interventions in a timely, logical, and coordinated fashion

6. E = Empower clients and families; enable them to control their course to the greatest extent possible

C. PQRST assessment for pain perception

1. This method is especially helpful when approaching a new pain problem

2. P = What *precipitated* the pain? Has anything *palliated* the pain? What is the *pattern* of the pain?

3. Q = What are the *quality* and *quantity* of the pain? Is it sharp, stabbing, aching, burning, stinging, deep, crushing, viselike, or gnawing?

4. R = What is the *region* of the pain? Does the pain *radiate* to other areas of the body?

5. S = What is the *severity* (or intensity) of the pain?

6. T = What is the *timing* of the pain? When does it begin, how long does it last, and how is it related to other events in the client's life?

D. Pain history

1. Involve the family/caregiver when obtaining a pain history, keeping in mind the client's self-report is the most valid measure of pain

   a. **Pain tolerance** (the ability or willingness to endure pain) varies from person to person

   b. Discrepancies may occur between the client's report and those of the other family members; explore these differences (e.g., the client may be stoic and may underreport the pain or the family member may be very distressed about the loved one's illness and overestimate the client's pain in response to personal suffering)

2. People are often unable to use the word "pain"

   a. This may be because of stoicism, concern about appearing whining or a complainer, belief that admitting to the pain makes it real (implying that the underlying disease is real and possibly advancing), cultural biases, or other causes

   b. "Discomfort" is the most frequently used alternative

   c. Other terms may include *hurt* or *ache;* some terms suggest emotion, such as *distressing* or *horrible;* explore the meaning of pain for each client and family

3. Location

   a. Many clients have multiple pain sites

   b. When clients report "pain all over," this generally refers to total pain or existential distress (unless there is an underlying physiologic reason for pain all over the body, such as myalgias); assess the client's emotional state for depression, fear, anxiety, or hopelessness

4. Intensity

    a. It is important to quantify pain using a standard pain intensity scale

    b. When clients cannot conceptualize pain using a number, simple word categories can be useful (e.g., no pain, mild, moderate, severe)

5. Quality

    a. Nociceptive pains are usually related to damage to bones, soft tissues, or internal organs; nociceptive pain includes somatic and visceral pains

        1) Somatic pain is aching, throbbing pain; arthritis is an example of somatic pain

        2) Visceral pain is squeezing, cramping pain such as the pain associated with ulcerative colitis

    b. Neuropathic pain is generally caused by damage to the nervous system; clients describe the pain as burning, tingling, electrical, or shooting; examples include diabetic neuropathy or postherpetic neuropathy (shingles)

6. Pattern

    a. Pain may be always present for a client; this is often termed baseline pain

    b. Additional pain may occur intermittently that is of rapid onset and greater intensity than the baseline pain, known as **breakthrough pain**

    c. People at end-of-life often have both types of pain

    d. Aggravating/alleviating factors: those factors that make the pain better or worse; these assessments can provide information about the etiology of the pain as well as potential treatments; for example, if massage makes the pain better, it probably has a musculoskeletal origin, rather than neuropathic

    e. Medication history: it is imperative to understand which drugs the client has already tried, whether they were effective, and what adverse effects resulted; question clients regarding what has been prescribed and what is actually being used for pain control (and the reasons for any disparity); also ask clients about use of over-the-counter drugs, recreational drugs, and herbal products

    f. Meaning of the pain: the meaning of the client's pain can profoundly affect pain perception; many see pain as punishment for something done (or left undone) earlier in life

    g. Cultural beliefs regarding the meaning of pain should be examined

    h. Client's expectations for pain relief

E. Physical examination

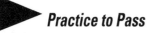

1. Observe for nonverbal cues that might suggest pain, including withdrawal, fatigue, grimaces, moans, irritability, particularly in the client unable to verbalize pain

2. Examine sites of pain for trauma, skin breakdown, changes in bony structures, etc.

3. Palpate the areas for tenderness

4. Auscultate for abnormal breath sounds that could signal pneumonia (e.g., crackles, rhonchi, decreased breath sounds) or abnormal bowel sounds that could signal bowel obstruction (e.g., hyperactive bowel sounds) or other syndromes

5. Percuss the area for fluid accumulation or gas (especially for abdominal pain to rule out obstruction, ascites, etc.)

6. Conduct a neurological examination to evaluate sensory and/or motor loss, as well as changes in reflexes

Practice to Pass

What elements should the nurse include when taking a pain history from a client who presents with end-stage cancer?

7. The information derived from the physical examination contributes to the information obtained during the history to determine the underlying cause of pain; this can lead to potential treatment decisions (e.g., laxatives/softeners if the client is constipated, antibiotics if there is an underlying infection, or radiotherapy for bone metastasis)

F. Reassessment

1. It is critical to reassess pain regularly, with any changes in pain, or with changes in the analgesic regimen; the regularity of pain assessment depends on the degree to which the client's condition or pain state is changing; more rapidly progressive disease demands more frequent assessment

2. Pain relief should be assessed using the same rating scale (such as 0 to 10) that was used to determine the intensity of pain prior to nursing intervention; using the same scale provides more objective data about the degree of relief the client obtained

3. Pain relief can be also assessed using a 0 to 100% scale, with 0 meaning no relief and 100% meaning complete relief; when clients are unable to use this scale, options include "no relief," "a little relief," "moderate relief," or "complete/total relief"

4. When attempting to determine the success of a new analgesic the client may be asked, "After taking that pill (or liquid, shot, etc.), how much pain relief did it provide?"; if the client is able to articulate the amount of relief, then ask, "How long did you get relief?" as this provides evidence regarding the duration of effect

5. Pain must be made visible (such as labeling it the fifth vital sign); adding pain intensity scores to the same part of the chart where temperature, pulse, and other vital signs are recorded has been shown to enhance pain relief efforts and effectiveness

6. A useful strategy for reassessment is asking clients/caregivers to keep a daily pain diary; nurses can teach the client or family members to record daily pain responses (e.g., intensity scores, pain relief, times and doses of breakthrough pain medications given, additional comments about activities or other factors) to determine patterns of pain

G. Clients at risk for poor pain assessment and treatment

1. Children: may be too young to verbally express pain; healthcare workers may fear overmedicating them

2. Elderly: may have decreased perception of sensory stimuli and a higher pain threshold; chronic disease processes (e.g., diabetes or peripheral vascular disease) may interfere with normal nerve impulse transmission; may believe pain is a normal part of growing older and as a result, attempt to ignore or self-medicate

3. Cognitively impaired/unconscious clients

4. Non-English-speaking clients

5. Persons of different cultures from healthcare professionals

6. Persons with a history of substance use: complaints of pain in persons with a current or past history of substance use may be disregarded or discounted as attempts to obtain additional medication

H. Communicating assessment findings

1. Clear objective communication (both verbally and in writing) of the pain assessment findings will ultimately improve pain management

!

> ## ▶ Practice to Pass
>
> A client reports pain to the right lower quadrant of the abdomen described as "aching and throbbing" and rates it numerically as an 8 on a scale of 1 to 10. What type of pain is the client experiencing?

2. It is important to describe the intensity of pain, the functional limitations that result from the pain (e.g., the client cannot tolerate radiation therapy treatments), and the response from the current analgesic regimen (e.g., 50% relief, no adverse effects); this gives other healthcare professionals essential data when modifying the treatment plan; it also allows the nurse to serve as a client advocate

VII. PHARMACOLOGICAL THERAPIES FOR PAIN CONTROL

A. Nonopioids

1. Acetaminophen (Tylenol)

   a. Has analgesic and antipyretic properties

   b. Adverse effects: can cause liver dysfunction in routine doses higher than 4,000 mg/day in clients with normal liver function and in doses of 6,000 mg/day acutely; acetaminophen is present in many analgesic products

2. Nonsteroidal anti-inflammatory drugs (NSAIDs) have anti-inflammatory, analgesic, and antipyretic effects

   a. Examples: salicylate (aspirin), ibuprofen (Motrin), naproxen (Naprosyn); these block cyclooxygenase-1 (COX-1)

   b. Mechanism of action: inhibit prostaglandins by blocking cyclooxygenase; prostaglandins are rich in the periosteum of the bone and in the uterus, as well as other locations; thus, NSAIDs are useful in relieving bone pain and dysmenorrhea; they are also useful in many other pain syndromes

   c. A cyclooxygenase-2 (COX-2) inhibitor is celecoxib (Celebrex), which selectively blocks the COX-2 enzymatic pathway; there appears to be less risk of GI bleeding, renal dysfunction, and generalized bleeding with the continuous or prolonged use of the COX-2 NSAID

   d. Unlike the opioids, the NSAIDs have a ceiling effect; increasing the dose beyond a certain point will not increase analgesia and will only increase the risk of adverse effects

   e. Adverse effects

      1) COX-1 NSAIDs produce significant gastric toxicity through local effects and systemic effects; locally, they migrate through the gastric mucus and into epithelial cells that line the stomach; once in these cells, they convert to their ionized form, causing hydrogen ions to be trapped within the cells

      2) The systemic effects of COX-1 NSAIDs are accomplished largely by inhibiting prostaglandin synthesis, which results in decreased epithelial mucus to coat the stomach, decreased mucosal blood flow, and decreased epithelial proliferation; the reduction in mucus exposes the gastroduodenal mucosal lining to injury by substances within the gut (such as acid, pepsin, and bile salts)

      3) As a result of these local and systemic factors, GI bleeding is common in COX-1 NSAIDs especially in the elderly, in persons at risk for ulceration, and when used in combination with other drugs such as corticosteroids

      4) Platelet aggregation is inhibited by NSAIDs, thus bleeding is a potential risk; this effect is reversible by stopping the NSAID; however, aspirin produces an irreversible effect on platelets so should be discontinued at least 7 days prior to an invasive procedure

5) Renal dysfunction can occur because of NSAIDs, especially when clients are dehydrated; this effect is caused by the inhibition of renal vasoactive prostaglandin, altering the blood flow within the arterioles of the kidneys; urine output diminishes; this effect is reversible by stopping the NSAID

6) The COX-2 NSAID (celecoxib) may cause indigestion, diarrhea, and stomach pain, and could lead to ulcers and GI bleeding

7) In April 2005, the FDA required that all NSAIDs include in their safety information that they potentially increase the risk of heart attack, stroke, and stomach problems

B. Opioids and adjuvant medications

1. Opioids are morphine-like compounds that produce systemic effects including pain relief and sedation

2. They can be categorized as **agonist** (a substance that, when combined with the opioid receptor [mu, kappa, or sigma], produces the drug effect or desired effect) or as a partial agonist (agonist-antagonist), which exerts effects on some types of receptors but displaces opioids from other types of receptors

3. Use of drugs in this latter category (which are more likely to be used to treat chronic pain or in previous opioid abusers) is associated with less risk of dependency

4. Selected examples of opioids

a. Codeine (generic); morphine (MS Contin, Oramorph, Kadian, Roxanol)

b. Hydrocodone (Vicodin/Lortab)

c. Hydromorphone (Dilaudid)

d. Fentanyl (Duragesic)

e. Methadone (Dolophine)

f. Oxycodone (OxyContin, Roxicodone, Roxifast)

g. Meperidine (Demerol)

5. Mechanism of action: opioids block the release of neurotransmitters involved in the processing of pain

6. Adverse effects

a. Allergic reactions to opioids are extremely rare; clients may state there is an allergy, especially if nausea and vomiting occur when given a particular opioid; this is an opportunity to educate clients regarding allergic responses versus adverse effects; the only absolute contraindication to the use of an opioid is a history of a hypersensitivity reaction (e.g., wheezing, edema)

b. Respiratory depression is greatly feared, yet rare; it is almost always preceded by sedation, thus, in most cases, the healthcare professional has adequate warning

c. If the client has true opioid-induced respiratory depression, it can be reversed parenterally using naloxone (Narcan) or nalfemene (Revex); these are classified as opioid **antagonists** (substances that block or reverse the effects of the agonist [e.g., morphine] by occupying the receptor site without producing the drug effect); naltrexone (ReVia) is a different antagonist that is used orally as adjunct treatment for detoxifying opioid-dependent clients

   d. Constipation is a significant effect of opioid therapy, often leading to discontinuation or reduction in opioid dose if not well-managed

      1) Opioids produce many effects that lead to constipation, such as reduced peristalsis and increased resorption of water from fecal contents that results in slow-moving, dry fecal material

      2) Constipation can lead to hemorrhoids or anal fissures that are painful and potential sites for infection

      3) Increased fluids, addition of fiber to the diet, activity or exercise, and use of a laxative/stool softener combination help counteract these effects

   e. Urinary retention is more common in opioid-naive clients and is most common with spinal delivery of medications (e.g., epidural or intrathecal); tolerance to this effect usually occurs within a few days; in the meantime the client may need an indwelling urinary cather or intermittent bladder catheterization every 6 to 8 hours PRN

   f. Nausea and vomiting can occur; treatment includes antiemetics or changing to a different opioid; this side effect may diminish on its own after some days of opioid therapy

   g. Pruritis occurs more commonly with spinal delivery of opioids; antihistamines may help, but sedation may occur with use of these drugs; cool packs or lotions as well as diversional activities may help; tolerance to this effect will also develop over time

   h. Addiction is a primary, chronic, neurobiological disease with genetic, psychosocial, and environmental factors influencing its development and manifestations; it is characterized by behaviors that include one or more of the following: impaired control over drug use, compulsive use, continued use despite harm, and craving

   i. Mixed agonist-antagonists: selected examples of medications in this class include butorphanol (Stadol), nalbuphine (Nubain), and pentazocine (Talwin)

      1) Adverse effects: the mixed agonist-antagonists are not recommended in the treatment of chronic pain; **ceiling doses** (when increases beyond a certain dose no longer produce increased relief) create a high rate of psychotomimetic effects (e.g., hallucinations and disorientation), and can produce the abstinence or withdrawal syndrome if clients are also taking pure agonist opioids

      2) Withdrawal symptoms from opioids include agitation, abdominal cramping, diarrhea, runny nose, tearing, yawning, and "goose bumps"; withdrawal from meperidine can also lead to seizures

   j. Adjuvant analgesics

      1) Tricyclic antidepressants as analgesics: the mechanism of analgesic effect appears to be related to inhibition of norepinephrine and serotonin; these agents are useful when treating neuropathic pain states; amitriptyline (Elavil) and nortriptyline (Pamelor) produce more sedation and other adverse effects than desipramine (Norpramin, Pertofrane), therefore, the first two should be given at bedtime and the latter given in the morning

      2) Antiepileptics as analgesics: older antiepileptics, such as carbamazepine (Tegretol) block sodium channels, which prevents the conduction of pain through sensory neurons; as a result, these compounds are believed to be useful in the treatment of neuropathic pain, especially pain described as "shooting"

3) Local anesthetics: work in a similar manner to the older antiepileptics by inhibiting the movement of sodium ions across the membrane of the sensory nerve to prevent the transmission of pain along the neuron

   a) Useful in relieving neuropathic pain, local anesthetics can be given intravenously (e.g., lidocaine)

   b) Epidural or intrathecal: bupivacaine (Marcaine)

   c) Topical where the skin is intact (Emla cream and Lidoderm)

4) Corticosteroids: inhibit prostaglandin synthesis and reduce edema surrounding many types of tissues; are useful in treating neuropathic pain, bone pain, and visceral pain; dexamethasone (Decadron) produces the least amount of mineralocorticoid effect and is often preferred for use in end-of-life care

5) Baclofen (Lioresal): a skeletal muscle relaxant useful in the relief of spasm-associated pain; doses are titrated gradually based upon client response and adverse effects; weakness and confusion occur with higher doses

6) Capsaicin (Zostrix): derived from chili peppers and believed to relieve pain by releasing, then depleting, supplies of substance P, a protein released from the nerve endings of pain neurons that is involved in pain transmission; when capsaicin is first administered, it causes pain (caused by the substance P release), and then it may relieve pain (caused by substance P depletion)

   a) Capsaicin has been shown to be useful in treating peripheral pain syndromes; examples include pain associated with postmastectomy syndrome, shingles, and postsurgical neuropathic pain in cancer; a sensation of burning is a common reason for discontinuing therapy

   b) Clients and caregivers should wash hands immediately after application of this topical medication to prevent burning on the hands or inadvertently rubbing the eyes and creating severe ocular pain

k. Routes of administration

1) Oral: tablets and liquid

   a) Immediate-release tablets/capsules

   b) Long-acting (sustained-release) tablets (e.g., MS Contin or OxyContin), capsules; "sprinkles" (currently only available in morphine preparation as Kadian); long-acting tablets allow longer periods of time between dosing (e.g., 8, 12, or 24 hours); also allow clients to obtain more consistent relief, which also provides uninterrupted sleep

   c) Sprinkles provide long-acting relief for clients who cannot swallow a tablet but can swallow small amounts of applesauce mixed with the drug

   d) There is a misconception that intravenous (IV), intramuscular (IM), or subcutaneous (SubQ) delivery is stronger than oral administration; oral delivery can provide equivalent analgesia (known as **equianalgesia**), but because of first-pass metabolism, the dose must be increased when compared to IM, IV, or SubQ routes; thus, 10 mg of morphine given IV, IM, or SubQ is approximately equal to 30 mg of oral morphine

   e) Enteral feeding tubes can be used to administer oral medications when clients can no longer swallow; however, the size of the tube should be considered, especially when placing long-acting morphine "sprinkles," to avoid tube obstruction

2) Mucosal

   a) Oral transmucosal fentanyl citrate (OTFC or Actiq) is composed of fentanyl placed on an applicator for clients to rub against the oral mucosa to provide rapid absorption of the drug; therapeutic plasma levels of the drug are achieved within 5 to 15 minutes of application

   b) Two examples of the appropriate use of OTFC might be for the relief of breakthrough pain that is of rapid onset (i.e., when traditional breakthrough medications would lead to a delay in relief) or prior to a brief, but painful, dressing change

3) Rectal (also stomal/vaginal)

   a) Thrombocytopenia or painful anorectal lesions preclude the use of these routes; additionally, delivering medications via these routes can be difficult for family members, especially when the client is obtunded or unable to assist

   b) Long-acting opioid tablets have been placed rectally when clients are no longer able to swallow

   c) Because the vagina has no sphincter, a tampon covered with a condom or an inflated urinary catheter balloon may be used to prevent early discharge of the drug

4) Transdermal

   a) Currently, the only formulation for transdermal delivery is fentanyl; the patch is placed every 72 hours over nonhairy, nonedematous skin with good capillary blood flow (often over the torso, shoulders, or upper arms)

   b) There is a delay in peak onset of approximately 17 hours after applying the first patch

   c) The effects of cachexia and fever are believed to accelerate drug distribution; although the precise mechanisms are unknown, altered fat stores and increased capillary flow may lead to these changes

5) Parenteral

   a) Intravenous (IV): useful when clients cannot swallow or when absorption through the gastrointestinal tract is altered

   b) Subcutaneous (SubQ): boluses have a slower onset and lower peak effect when compared with IV boluses; SubQ infusions may be run at up to 5 to 10 mL/hr, although 1 to 3 mL is ideal

   c) Intramuscular (IM): not recommended because of wide variability in absorption, potential delays in vascular uptake of the drug, and pain with administration

6) Nasal: currently, the only nasal preparation available is the mixed agonist-antagonist butorphanol (Stadol); this is not recommended for chronic pain management

7) Spinal

   a) Epidural or intrathecal routes allow delivery of drugs, (most often used is Duramorph, a preservative-free morphine derivative) into epidural space via a catheter inserted by an anesthesiologist

   b) Benefits: produces effective analgesia without sensory, motor or sympathetic changes

   c) Disadvantages: epidural catheter's proximity to spinal nerves and canal, along with potential for catheter migration, make correct injection technique and close assessment imperative

d) Side effects include: generalized pruritis, nausea, urinary retention, respiratory depression, and hypotension

e) Strict asepsis is necessary when injecting the epidural catheter; initially aspirated gently; if blood or greater than 1 mL of clear fluid is aspirated, withhold injection and notify MD

f) Opioid-related side effects are reversed with naloxone hydrochloride (Narcan) or nalfemene (Revex)

8) Patient-controlled analgesia (PCA): self-administration of IV analgesics by a client who has been instructed about the procedure

a) A portable PCA pump-type device delivers a preset dosage of opioid IV; an adjustable lockout interval controls the frequency of dose administration, preventing another one from being administered prematurely; a sample order might read: "Morphine 1 mg with a lock-out time of 6 minutes"

b) The client pushes a button to activate the device, and the client should control administration of the analgesic, not the family, nursing staff, or any other well-intentioned individual

c) Monitor the client's sedation level, pain rating, and vital signs while using PCA; the pump records the settings and amount of medication delivered, as well as number of demands (for example, client may push button 10 times in a 1-minute period when in severe pain, however, will receive bolus only every 6 minutes using above order)

d) Allows for less sedation during waking hours with smaller, frequent doses compared to oral/IM doses given every 3 to 4 hours

e) Provide instruction about use of PCA preoperatively whenever possible; some clients fear being overdosed by the machine and require reassurance; it is always important to reinforce postoperatively any instructions given before surgery for PCA to have greatest effect

C. Principles regarding the use of analgesics

1. The World Health Organization (WHO) three-step analgesic ladder is a guide to selecting the initial analgesic choice and dosing; continued reassessment is needed to modify the treatment plan based on the client's response

a. When clients present with mild pain (approximately 1 to 3 on the 0 to 10 scale) a nonopioid is prescribed, with an adjuvant drug if the client has neuropathic pain

b. If the pain is moderate (4 to 6), the prescriber should add an opioid in low doses; the nonopioids and adjuvants may also be continued

c. If the pain is severe (7 to 10), the prescriber should add higher dose(s) of the opioid; the nonopioids and adjuvants may be continued; if the client presents with severe pain, the prescriber should not start at the bottom rung; but should begin at the appropriate level for that client's pain

d. One limitation of the ladder is the belief that weak opioids (e.g., codeine) must be used in step 2; actually smaller doses of strong opioids, such as morphine, are just as effective and preclude later switching between drugs

2. Prevent and treat adverse effects

a. Anticipate, prevent, and treat predictable adverse effects

b. Almost all clients prescribed an opioid will also require a laxative/stool softener combination; exceptions include clients with HIV-associated diarrhea, clients with pancreatic insufficiency associated with pancreatic cancers, and other clients with preexisting diarrhea

3. Properly use long-acting and breakthrough medications

    a. Begin with immediate-release formulations available to the client as needed to relieve pain; once the client has achieved pain relief for 24 to 48 hours, calculate the 24-hour dose of opioid and convert to long acting formulation; for example, the client that has been taking 60 mg of liquid morphine in a 24-hour period may be converted to:

        1) MS Contin 30 mg po q 12 hours

        2) Kadian 60 mg po daily

        3) OxyContin 20 to 30 mg po q 12 hours

        4) Duragesic patch 25 mcg every 72 hours

    b. Sustained-release formulations and around-the-clock dosing should be used for continuous pain syndromes

    c. Immediate-release formulations should be made available for breakthrough pain; the dose of immediate-release drug is usually 10 to 20% of the total 24-hour dose of the routine opioid; therefore, if the 24-hour dose of MS Contin is 200 mg, the breakthrough dose should be 20 to 40 mg; start with the lower dose and titrate as needed; the immediate-release drug can be repeated as often as every hour, since the peak effect of oral opioids is one hour

    d. If the client is receiving a continuous infusion of an opioid (either IV or subQ), breakthrough doses are calculated as 50 to 100% of the hourly rate; therefore, if the client has a rate of 2 mg/hr of morphine, the breakthrough dose should begin at 1 mg IV bolus with appropriate titration; the peak effect of an IV bolus dose of most opioids is 15 minutes; thus, if the client is still in pain after that time, the bolus should be repeated

    e. Breakthrough pain can be incident-related (e.g., movement-induced), idiopathic (etiology unknown), or because of end-of-dose failure (increased pain prior to the next scheduled dose)

    f. Titrate analgesics based upon client goals, requirements for supplemental analgesics, pain intensity, severity of undesirable or adverse drug effects, measures of functionality, sleep, emotional state, and client/caregiver reports of the impact of pain on quality of life

4. Converting properly from one route or drug to another involves the use of an equianalgesic chart (see Table 8-2 for example)

> **Practice to Pass**
>
> In addition to opioids, what other drug classifications can be used for pain management?

VIII. NONPHARMACOLOGICAL TECHNIQUES FOR PROMOTING COMFORT

A. Cutaneous stimulation

    1. Touch: place hands on client's body or 1 inch above to realign energy; is thought to initiate gate closure to pain as well as communicate caring

    2. Pressure: place hands firmly on or around the area where client feels pain; can provide relief of discomfort, decrease bleeding, and prevent swelling

    3. Massage: gently or briskly stimulate client's subcutaneous tissues by kneading, pulling or pressing with hands; thought to initiate gate closure; promotes relaxation and sedation

        a. Use warm lubricant, such as lotion

      b. Use long, smooth strokes to achieve relaxation; maintain continuous hand contact with skin

      c. Use rapid strokes, circular motions, and gentle squeezing of tissues to stimulate increase in the client's level of alertness or stimulate circulation

    4. Vibration: use an electrical or battery-operated vibrator to stimulate the client's subcutaneous tissues; thought to initiate gate closure

Table 8-2	Opioid Equianalgesic Chart				
Drug	**IM Route (mg)**	**PO Route (mg)**	**IM/PO Peak (hr)**	**IM/PO Duration (hr)**	**Comments**
Morphine	10	30–60	½–1 IM	3–5 IM	Morphine 10 mg IM is the analgesic dose all other drugs in this table are compared to; PO dose varies from 3–6 times the IM dose depending on drug used; also comes in suppository form, time-released oral form, and for spinal injection
Butorphanol (Stadol)	2	NA	½–1 IM	4–5 IM	Agonist-antagonist; can produce withdrawal from opioids, more likely to produce nausea and vomiting; respiratory depression rare but severe and not easily reversed by naloxone (Narcan)
Codeine	130	200	½–1 IM 2 PO	4–5 IM 3–4 PO	More toxic in higher doses than morphine; causes more nausea and vomiting and is extremely constipating; adding 650 mg of acetaminophen or aspirin will significantly increase analgesic effect
Fentanyl (Sublimaze)	0.05	NA	7–8 min IM	1–2 IM	Commonly used for anesthetic; IV substituted for high-dose morphine in terminally ill clients
Hydromorphone (Dilaudid)	1.5	7.5	½–1 IM ½–2 PO	3 IM 3–4 PO	Shorter-acting than morphine; also available as rectal suppository or high-potency injection 10 mg/mL; may be used for PCA or epidural
Levorphanol (Levo-Dromoran)	2	4	½–1 SC ½–2 PO	6–8 SC 6–8 PO	Longer-acting than morphine when given in repeated, regular doses; good alternative to methadone; drug accumulates so analgesic effect may increase with repeated doses; subcutaneous route better than IM
Meperidine (Demerol)	75	300	½–1 IM ½–2 PO	2–4 IM 2–4 PO	Oral dose of 300 mg not recommended; shorter-acting than morphine; transformed to normeperidine, a toxic metabolite that stimulates the CNS and causes seizures; effects of normeperidine not reversed by naloxone
Methadone (Dolophine)	10	20	10–20 IM ½–1 PO	4–6 IM 4–12 PO	Long plasma half-life, so regular doses lead to accumulation of drug and increased analgesia; dosage must be carefully titrated over days to weeks; use with caution in elderly or in clients with liver or kidney failure
Nalbuphine (Nubain)	10	NA	½–1 PO	4–5 PO	Agonist-antagonist; similar to butorphanol; may cause withdrawal if used in clients receiving opioids; longer-acting and less likely to cause hypotension than morphine; less respiratory depression
Oxycodone	NA	30	1 PO	3–4 PO	Faster onset and higher peak effect than most oral opioids; available as single agent and in combination with acetaminophen
Pentazocine (Talwin)	60	180	½–1 IM ½–2 PO	3–4 IM 2–4 PO	Agonist-antagonist; similar to butorphanol but much higher incidence of psychomimetic effects; may cause withdrawal if used in clients receiving opioids
Propoxyphene (Darvon)	NA	500	½–2 PO	3–4 PO	Never give in 500 mg dose; may be used for mild to moderate pain; doses of 65–130 mg are usual

Source: Agency for Healthcare Policy and Research (AHCPR). *Acute pain management: Operations or medical procedures and trauma. Clinical practice guideline.* AHCPR Publication No. 92-0032.

     5. Heat/cold applications: are better labeled as "warm" and "cool"

        a. Indications: either heat or cold may be used as preferred for muscle aches or spasms, joint pain, or itching; heat may be used for rectal pain, while cool applications may be used for headaches or surgical incisions

        b. Equipment: heat sources typically include warm moist compresses, heating pads or bottles, immersion in water, or use of plastic wraps (to retain body heat); cold sources include ice bags, gel packs, bags of frozen vegetables that are small and fairly smooth, plastic zip-lock bags with ice/water/slush (combination of ⅓ alcohol with ⅔ water, or soaked towels

        c. Cautionary notes

           1) Heat or cold therapy should not be continued if pain increases

           2) Use moderation with temperature (neither too hot nor too cold)

           3) Cover heat or cold source with a towel for insulation and to protect skin surfaces

           4) Moisture increases the effect or intensity of heat or cold therapy

           5) Do not use heat on areas that are bleeding, have sustained recent injury, or that have menthol or oil on them

           6) Do not use cold on areas that have poor circulation; remove cold from an area if it becomes numb

        d. Apply heat or cold source for 10 to 20 minutes at a time, but it may be used for longer periods at the discretion of the client if it remains comfortable and does not cause skin irritation; do not use at temperatures less than 70°F or greater than 110°F

        e. If it is not possible to apply heat or cold therapy directly to a painful area, try placing it to the same point on the opposite side of the body, or above or below the painful site

B. Trancutaneous electrical nerve stimulation (TENS)

     1. A battery-operated unit with electrodes applied to skin to produce tingling, vibration, or buzzing sensation

     2. Can be used for acute or chronic pain, but is most frequently used for chronic pain (such as with arthritis)

     3. Based on gate control theory; thought to decrease pain through stimulation of nonpain receptors in the same area as the fibers that transmit pain

     4. The client adjusts placement of electrodes, and the timing and intensity of stimuli to obtain best pain relief

     5. TENS is most effective in clients who understand and are motivated to learn the device

     6. A client may need help with electrode placement, so it is helpful and generally beneficial to include family or other support people in client teaching sessions

     7. TENS units can be attached to battery packs so the unit is portable

C. Distraction

     1. The client focuses on something other than pain to decrease number of painful stimuli being transmitted to brain

     2. Examples include watching television, listening to music, visiting with friends/family, playing games

     3. Stimulation of several senses (sight, sound and touch) are generally more effective in reducing pain than a single sense

D. Relaxation

1. Involves learning activities or techniques that deeply relax the body and mind; provides distraction, lessens effects of stress from pain, increases effectiveness of other pain relief measures, and increases perception of pain control

2. Diaphragmatic breathing can relax muscles, improve oxygen levels, and provide a feeling of release from tension
   a. Is more effective when client sits or lies down
   b. The client should have quiet environment, closed eyes
   c. The client should inhale and exhale slowly and regularly

3. Progressive muscle relaxation may be used alone or with deep breathing to manage pain
   a. Teach the client to tighten one group of muscles, hold tension for a few seconds, then relax the muscle group completely
   b. The client should repeat this action for all parts of body
   c. Audio tapes may be helpful to assist with the relaxation process

4. Guided imagery: uses the imaginative power of the mind with the assistance of the nurse to create a scene or sensory experience that relaxes muscles and moves the client's focus away from the pain experience
   a. The client must be able to concentrate, use imagination, and follow directions
   b. Facilitate this process by using a calm, soothing voice to reinforce the pleasant places or situations imagined
   c. Audio tapes may be helpful to assist with the imagery process

5. Meditation: is a process whereby the client empties the mind of all sensory data and concentrates on a single object, word, or idea
   a. Produces a deeply relaxed state
   b. Oxygen consumption decreases, muscles relax, and endorphins are produced

Practice to Pass

A client is interested in exploring nonpharmacological methods of pain relief. What methods should the nurse discuss with the client?

E. Acupuncture

1. Ancient Chinese technique involving stimulation of certain points on the body to enhance the flow of vital energy (*chi*) along pathways called meridians

2. Points can be stimulated with needles, application of heat, massage, laser or electrical stimulation

F. Biofeedback

1. Is an electronic method of measuring physiologic responses with intent to condition or control the responses

2. The client goal is to exercise voluntary control over sensations to promote relaxation, lessen anxiety, and decrease pain

3. It requires trained facilitator to assist client and monitor physiologic data such as skin temperature, brain waves, and muscle contractions

4. The client eventually learns to independently repeat actions to produce desired effect (e.g., slowing circulation to reduce heart rate and warmth of skin)

G. Nursing considerations for nonpharmaceutical pain relief techniques

1. Assess the following client variables that will affect the method selected
   a. Concurrent use of analgesics (should complement, not replace their use)
   b. Attitude toward nonpharmaceutical methods in general or toward the method being contemplated for use (based on success or lack of success in past, and on cultural practices of an individual)

        c. Energy level (degree of fatigue) and ability to understand and/or follow directions

    2. Offer opportunities for family/friends/significant others to be involved with therapy

    3. Provide client and any helping individuals with adequate instruction and support materials (written instructions, audiotapes, films)

IX. COMMON NURSING DIAGNOSES FOR THE CLIENT WITH PAIN

A. Pain

    1. Applies when a client experiences discomfort or pain (either constant or intermittent) that is time-bound in that it has lasted from 1 second to less than 6 months (NANDA–I)

    2. A nursing diagnostic statement for *Pain* must include the location and any etiological/precipitating factors

B. Chronic pain

    1. Applies when the client has discomfort or pain (either constant or intermittent) that has lasted for more than 6 months (NANDA–I)

    2. A nursing diagnostic statement for *Chronic pain* must include the location and any etiological/precipitating factors

C. Altered comfort: applies when the client experiences some type of discomfort in response to a specific stimulus that is noxious in nature (NANDA–I)

D. Other pertinent nursing diagnoses

    1. Ineffective coping (individual and/or family) related to persistent pain that may add stress that affects the client's and/or family's ability to cope

    2. Deficient knowledge related to lack of information or misinformation regarding pain treatment strategies

    3. Impaired physical mobility related to movement limited by pain

    4. Disturbed sleep pattern related to persistent pain

    5. Anxiety related to loss of control

    6. Fear related to pain

    7. Powerlessness related to illness-related regimen

    8. Ineffective role performance related to a change in health status and impaired coping

    9. Ineffective sexuality patterns related to illness and pain

    10. Activity intolerance related to pain and/or depression

    11. Self-care deficit (total or partial) related to pain

Case Study

A 75-year-old woman has been admitted to an orthopedic unit following a right fractured hip repair. She lives alone and fell while hanging curtains in her bedroom. Her postoperative orders include a PCA pump prescribed as morphine 1 mg every 10 minutes. She is currently alert and tells the nurse, "I am in so much pain, I'd rather be dead." Vital signs are as follows: oral temperature 99.2˚F, pulse 102, respirations 20 and BP 142/92.

1. What common physiologic responses are expected for a client in acute pain?

2. What are several nonopioid medications that could be used to manage pain in addition to the PCA pump?

3. What are the nursing priorities for a client using a PCA pump?

4. What additional comfort measures could be used for this client?

5. What nursing diagnoses related to pain are anticipated for this client?

For suggested responses, see page 337–338.

POSTTEST

❶ An anxious-appearing client with acquired immunodeficiency syndrome (AIDS) tells the nurse that he has a burning sensation with shooting pain to both feet that is excruciating in nature. The nurse should interpret this client's report as indicating:

1. The client is experiencing neuropathic pain to the distal lower extremities.
2. Psychogenic pain to both feet is accompanied by an anxious appearance.
3. There is referred pain described as excruciating to the bilateral feet.
4. Severe phantom pain is present to the feet and is resulting in anxiety.

❷ A male client is very anxious about the pain he may experience postoperatively. Which interventions would be most effective in helping him deal with this fear? Select all that apply.

1. Teach him relaxation techniques such as deep breathing and guided imagery.
2. Explain the availability of pain medications after surgery.
3. Demonstrate various positioning techniques that promote postop comfort.
4. Distract the client from discussing pain by focusing on surgical preparation.
5. Encourage the client to verbalize his concerns.

❸ When caring for a client receiving epidural morphine (Duramorph), the nurse would develop a care plan using which nursing diagnosis?

1. Impaired urinary elimination related to polyuria
2. Ineffective breathing pattern related to tachypnea
3. Imbalanced nutrition: less than body requirements related to nausea
4. Risk for impaired skin integrity related to pruritis

POSTTEST

4 A nurse asks a client to describe the quality of pain currently experienced. The nurse would anticipate documenting which of the following client symptoms?

1. Severe
2. Aching
3. Intermittent
4. Chronic

5 The nurse would evaluate successful client teaching with regard to morphine administration via patient-controlled analgesia (PCA) when the client makes which statement?

1. "I will probably use less morphine this way than with taking injections in my hip."
2. "I will get a dose of morphine every time I push the button."
3. "Using this device will keep me comfortable at all times."
4. "If I push the control button too often, I may get more medicine than needed."

6 A hospital discharge planning nurse is making arrangements for a client (who has an epidural catheter for continuous infusion of opioids) to be placed in a long-term care facility in the client's neighborhood to encourage family visiting. The facility has never cared for a client with this type of need. What would be the discharge planning nurse's best action?

1. Ask the physician for an extension of hospitalization until epidural catheter is discontinued to allow for placement at neighborhood facility.
2. Arrange for staff at the long-term-care facility to receive immediate in-services on pain management using epidural catheters.
3. Explain the situation to client and family and seek another long-term-care facility for discharge from the hospital.
4. Encourage family to hire private-duty nurses skilled in epidural catheter pain management to allow for client transfer to neighborhood facility.

7 Which of the following would be the most appropriate goal statement for teaching a client with chronic pain how to use visual imagery?

1. Exercises will decrease the need for analgesia.
2. Exercises will actively involve the client in his or her own pain management.
3. Exercises will decrease pain sensation.
4. Exercises will allow for better rest periods.

8 Which of the following clients would require the most frequent reassessment of pain after the administration of an analgesic?

1. An elderly client taking over-the-counter (OTC) medication for osteoarthritis
2. A client taking oral narcotics regularly for chronic low back pain
3. A young adult taking medication for frequent migraine headaches
4. A child with sickle cell anemia receiving IV analgesia for his or her first painful crisis

9 A student nurse is caring for a hospitalized client who is requesting medication for pain rated as "severe." The client is watching television with visitors and is eating. Which statement indicates to the nurse that the student understands principles of pain management?

1. "His distractions must not be very effective."
2. "He's probably anxious being in the hospital."
3. "If he says he hurts, then he must hurt."
4. "Social stimulation can increase one's pain."

10 A home health nurse is preparing to apply a fentanyl (Duragesic) transdermal patch for pain management. The nurse would not apply the patch to the client's upper arm if the client:

1. Had bilateral mastectomies performed a year ago.
2. Has minimal hair distribution to this area.
3. Has intravenous catheters placed in the hands.
4. Uses an overhead trapeze bar for bed mobility.

➤ *See pages 229–231 for Answers & Rationales.*

POSTTEST

ANSWERS & RATIONALES

Pretest

1 **Answer: 3** Chronic pain may be difficult to treat. It persists for 6 months or longer and can affect adults of all age groups. The etiology is often difficult to determine. Nerve damage may be one of numerous causes.
Cognitive Level: Application **Client Need:** Physiological Integrity: Basic Care and Comfort **Integrated Process:** Teaching/Learning **Content Area:** Fundamentals **Strategy:** The core issue of the question is knowledge of the characteristics of chronic pain. Recall the challenges in chronic pain management to choose correctly among the various options. **Reference:** Kozier, B., Erb, G., Berman, A., & Snyder, S. J. (2004). *Fundamentals of nursing: Concepts, process, and practice* (7th ed.). Upper Saddle River, NJ: Pearson Education, p. 1133.

2 **Answer: 1** Unless the client is cognitively impaired, the best technique for validation of pain is to use a scale to rate the intensity. Behavioral and physiologic responses are not as reliable; however, they can be used to support the quantitative method of validation.
Cognitive Level: Application **Client Need:** Physiological Integrity: Basic Care and Comfort **Integrated Process:** Nursing Process: Assessment **Content Area:** Fundamentals **Strategy:** The critical term is *most effective method.* Recall that pain assessment tools and instruments are key to effective pain assessment. **Reference:** Kozier, B., Erb, G., Berman, A., & Snyder, S. J. (2004). *Fundamentals of nursing: Concepts, process, and practice* (7th ed.). Upper Saddle River, NJ: Pearson Education, pp. 1140–1142.

3 **Answer: 4** When one medication is used alone, the dose must be higher to be effective. Using the opioid with the NSAID decreases the opioid dose required for adequate pain relief. This method reduces, although does not eliminate, the potential side effects of the opioid. NSAIDs target more than muscle pain.
Cognitive Level: Application **Client Need:** Physiological Integrity: Pharmacological and Parenteral Therapies **Integrated Process:** Teaching/Learning **Content Area:** Fundamentals **Strategy:** Knowledge of the pharmacologic effect of common analgesics is needed to select an answer. Recall general pharmacological principles of the two types of analgesics and use the process of elimination to make a selection. **Reference:** Kozier, B., Erb, G., Berman, A., & Snyder, S. J. (2004). *Fundamentals of nursing: Concepts, process, and practice* (7th ed.). Upper Saddle River, NJ: Pearson Education, pp. 1151–1153.

4 **Answer: 1** TENS is thought to be effective for chronic pain clients as a result of stimulating the non-nocicep-

tors. This device does not provide a distraction, reduce cell damage, or alter cell function.
Cognitive Level: Application **Client Need:** Physiological Integrity: Basic Care and Comfort **Integrated Process:** Teaching/Learning **Content Area:** Fundamentals **Strategy:** The critical word in the question is *rationale.* Use knowledge of the purposes of nonpharmacologic techniques for promoting comfort to choose the response that is appropriate for client education. **Reference:** Kozier, B., Erb, G., Berman, A., & Snyder, S. J. (2004). *Fundamentals of nursing: Concepts, process, and practice* (7th ed.). Upper Saddle River, NJ: Pearson Education, p. 1161.

5 **Answer: 2** Respiratory compromise is rare with opioid administration yet feared by many healthcare workers (option 4). Sedation precedes a fall in respiratory rate and/or depth and therefore should be noted and recorded. It may not be feasible to allow the surgical client to rest uninterrupted for a several-hour period (option 1). The infusion pump continuously records the amount of medication infused (option 3).
Cognitive Level: Application **Client Need:** Physiological Integrity: Pharmacological and Parenteral Therapies **Integrated Process:** Nursing Process: Implementation **Content Area:** Fundamentals **Strategy:** The critical words are *highest priority.* Recall information about common side effects of patient-controlled analgesia to assist you in assuring client safety during its use. **Reference:** Kozier, B., Erb, G., Berman, A., & Snyder, S. J. (2004). *Fundamentals of nursing: Concepts, process, and practice* (7th ed.). Upper Saddle River, NJ: Pearson Education, p. 1160.

6 **Answer: 3** A client who is breathing 8 breaths per minute is experiencing a potentially life-threatening side effect of the analgesia. This is the highest priority for the nurse. A respiratory rate of 24 may indicate pain, and this client may need additional teaching about PCA use, but this is a lesser priority than the decreased respiratory rate. It is anticipated that postoperative discomfort may be experienced when ambulating but not at rest. A state of sleeping but arousable indicates effective pain control.
Cognitive Level: Application **Client Need:** Physiological Integrity: Pharmacological and Parenteral Therapies **Integrated Process:** Nursing Process: Implementation **Content Area:** Fundamentals **Strategy:** To answer this question accurately, it is necessary to understand the adverse effects of PCA. Use knowledge that PCA utilizes opioid or narcotic analgesics and recall their major adverse ef-

fects to make a selection. **Reference:** Kozier, B., Erb, G., Berman, A., & Snyder, S. J. (2004). *Fundamentals of nursing: concepts, process, and practice* (7th ed.). Upper Saddle River, NJ: Pearson Education, pp. 1158–1160.

7 Answer: 2 Prior to administering opioid analgesics through an epidural catheter, gently aspirate to ensure there is no return of cerebrospinal fluid or blood. Obtaining a pulse oximetry reading and changing the client's position would be important actions regardless of epidural catheter placement (options 1 and 3). The catheter insertion site does not require an hourly assessment; rather it is done once a shift or each time medication is administered (option 4).
Cognitive Level: Application **Client Need:** Physiological Integrity: Pharmacological and Parenteral Therapies **Integrated Process:** Nursing Process: Implementation **Content Area:** Fundamentals **Strategy:** The critical term is *safe care.* Recall care measures for clients receiving spinal analgesics that are essential to client safety and use the process of elimination to make a selection. **Reference:** Kozier, B., Erb, G., Berman, A., & Snyder, S. J. (2004). *Fundamentals of nursing: Concepts, process, and practice* (7th ed.). Upper Saddle River, NJ: Pearson Education, p. 1157

8 Answer: 4 The purpose of biofeedback in pain management is to teach the client self-control over physiologic variables that relate to the pain, such as muscle contraction and circulation. The therapy requires working with a trained counselor; therefore, financial obligations are present in the early phases of training. This is a self-control treatment that does not include group therapy.
Cognitive Level: Application **Client Need:** Physiological Integrity: Basic Care and Comfort **Integrated Process:** Teaching/Learning **Content Area:** Fundamentals **Strategy:** The critical words are *biofeedback* and *understand.* Familiarity with nonpharmacological techniques for promoting comfort will allow you to assess client understanding of this treatment measure. **Reference:** Kozier, B., Erb, G., Berman, A., & Snyder, S. J. (2004). *Fundamentals of nursing: Concepts, process, and practice* (7th ed.). Upper Saddle River, NJ: Pearson Education, p. 230.

9 Answer: 4 A client's statement about pain intensity and pain relief should be what guides the nurse in determining medication route, dosage, and frequency. The other responses are generalizations that may not be accurate for the client's condition.
Cognitive Level: Application **Client Need:** Physiological Integrity: Pharmacological and Parenteral Therapies **Integrated Process:** Communication and Documentation **Content Area:** Fundamentals **Strategy:** The critical term is *best reply.* Recall principles regarding the use of anal-

gesics to assist you in assessing medication effectiveness and communicating these criteria to clients and families. **Reference:** Kozier, B., Erb, G., Berman, A., & Snyder, S. J. (2004). *Fundamentals of nursing: Concepts, process, and practice* (7th ed.). Upper Saddle River, NJ: Pearson Education, p. 1138.

10 Answers: 1, 5 Reaction to pain is very individualized and varies based on many subjective factors such as the meaning of pain and the environment of the client. The tolerance to pain reflects the amount of pain the client is willing to endure. The client may not request pain medication and may need frequent assessment (option 5). This does not mean the client will not experience pain (option 3), but may need less medication than other people in the same age group with a similar injury. Options 2 and 4 are more consistent with a low tolerance for pain.
Cognitive Level: Application **Client Need:** Physiological Integrity: Pharmacological and Parenteral Therapies **Integrated Process:** Nursing Process: Planning **Content Area:** Fundamentals **Strategy:** The critical phrase is *unbelievable tolerance for pain.* Being able to identify clients that are at risk for poor pain assessment and treatment will ultimately result in more effective pain management strategies for all clients. **Reference:** Kozier, B., Erb, G., Berman, A., & Snyder, S. J. (2004). *Fundamentals of nursing: Concepts, process, and practice* (7th ed.). Upper Saddle River, NJ: Pearson Education, p. 1139.

Posttest

1 Answer: 1 Neuropathic pain is the result of a disturbance of the peripheral or central nervous system that results in pain not necessarily associated with an ongoing tissue damage process. It is usually described as shooting, stabbing, burning, or pins and needles. It is severe in nature and is frequently seen in clients with AIDS. Psychogenic pain is emotionally based; referred pain is felt from a distant site than the actual tissue damage; and phantom pain occurs after the loss of an extremity.
Cognitive Level: Application **Client Need:** Physiological Integrity: Basic Care and Comfort **Integrated Process:** Nursing Process: Analysis **Content Area:** Fundamentals **Strategy:** The critical words are *AIDS, shooting pain,* and *excruciating.* Recall typical client descriptions of pain quality, which can provide to valuable data on the source of the client's pain. **Reference:** Kozier, B., Erb, G., Berman, A., & Snyder, S. J. (2004). *Fundamentals of nursing: Concepts, process, and practice* (7th ed.). Upper Saddle River, NJ: Pearson Education, p. 1134.

2 Answers: 2, 5 The client is most likely experiencing anxiety because of fears related to the postoperative pain.

The best interventions are to encourage him to verbalize his concerns and reassure him that pain medication will be available to provide relief from discomfort. Teaching relaxation techniques and discussing positioning requires concentration from the client that may not be possible because of anxiety. Promoting distraction does not address his fears and thereby may lead to increased anxiety.

Cognitive Level: Analysis **Client Need:** Physiological Integrity: Basic Care and Comfort **Integrated Process:** Nursing Process: Implementation **Content Area:** Fundamentals **Strategy:** The critical phrase is *most effective;* note that multiple answers may be selected. Recall basic communication techniques and information about available pharmacologic analgesics to provide reassurance and education to the concerned client. **Reference:** Kozier, B., Erb, G., Berman, A., & Snyder, S. J. (2004). *Fundamentals of nursing: Concepts, process, and practice* (7th ed.). Upper Saddle River, NJ: Pearson Education, p. 1140.

3 Answer: 4 Pruritis and/or development of a skin rash are commonly associated with the administration of epidural opiates. This may be due in part to histamine release. The other potential physiologic problems to be anticipated include hypotension, headache, and urinary retention. Options 1, 2, and 3 do not apply.

Cognitive Level: Application **Client Need:** Physiologic Integrity: Pharmacological and Parenteral Therapies **Integrated Process:** Nursing Process: Analysis **Content Area:** Fundamentals **Strategy:** The critical words are *epidural morphine* and *greatest likelihood.* Recall the common side effects of various analgesics to assist you to recognizing the etiology of the stated client problem.

Reference: Kozier, B., Erb, G., Berman, A., & Snyder, S. J. (2004). *Fundamentals of nursing: Concepts, process, and practice* (7th ed.). Upper Saddle River, NJ: Pearson Education, p. 1153.

4 Answer: 2 Using the PQRST technique, aching would describe the quality (Q) of pain the client is experiencing. Severe would fall under the category of severity (S), intermittent indicates the timing (T) of the pain, and chronic reflects the type of pain.

Cognitive Level: Application **Client Need:** Physiological Integrity: Basic Care and Comfort **Integrated Process:** Nursing Process: Assessment **Content Area:** Fundamentals **Strategy:** The critical term is *quality of pain.* Use nursing knowledge of the range of characteristics that are part of pain assessment to choose correctly from the available options. **Reference:** Kozier, B., Erb, G., Berman, A., & Snyder, S. J. (2004). *Fundamentals of nursing: Concepts, process, and practice* (7th ed.). Upper Saddle River, NJ: Pearson Education, p. 1142.

5 Answer: 1 Research has shown that small, frequent doses of an opioid as administered through PCA provide better pain relief and less total medication than with traditional intramuscular (IM) injections used every 3 to 4 hours PRN. Only the client should push the control button. The goal of PCA is to provide relief of discomfort; however, with movement, stress, procedures, and so on, the client may still experience periods of pain. The pump device is regulated to avoid overdosing and will limit the amount of medication the client can receive within a given timeframe. Pushing the button after a maximum dose has been infused will not result in the client receiving more medication.

Cognitive Level: Application **Client Need:** Physiological Integrity: Pharmacological and Parenteral Therapies **Integrated Process:** Teaching/Learning **Content Area:** Fundamentals **Strategy:** Nursing knowledge of routes of analgesia administration is needed to answer this question. Recall specific information about PCA and use the process of elimination to make a selection. **Reference:** Kozier, B., Erb, G., Berman, A., & Snyder, S. J. (2004). *Fundamentals of nursing: Concepts, process, and practice* (7th ed.). Upper Saddle River, NJ: Pearson Education, pp. 1159–1160.

6 Answer: 3 According to JCAHO pain standards, if a facility cannot treat a client for pain, the individual must be referred to a facility that can provide the skill. The physician may not be able to extend hospitalization because of insurance limitations (option 1). It is the long-term care facility's decision and responsibility to become prepared to provide a new service (option 2). Private-duty nurses may be cost prohibitive for the family, and the long-term care facility may not have the resources needed to provide safe care for this client (option 4).

Cognitive Level: Application **Client Need:** Safe, Effective Care Environment: Management of Care **Integrated Process:** Nursing Process: Planning **Content Area:** Fundamentals **Strategy:** Recall accreditation agencies standards on pain control to allow you to plan acceptable care measures. **Reference:** Kozier, B., Erb, G., Berman, A., & Snyder, S. J. (2004). *Fundamentals of nursing: Concepts, process, and practice* (7th ed.). Upper Saddle River, NJ: Pearson Education, p. 1148.

7 Answer: 2 Relaxation exercises such as guided imagery enhance other pain-relief measures to promote comfort of the client. They offer the client the opportunity to participate actively in pain control. Complementary therapies for pain control should not be used as substitutes for analgesia as these measures do not decrease pain sensation.

Cognitive Level: Application **Client Need:** Physiological Integrity: Basic Care and Comfort **Integrated Process:** Nursing Process: Planning **Content Area:** Fundamentals **Strategy:** Recall knowledge of nonpharmacological techniques for managing pain to guide you in setting appropriate client outcomes. **Reference:** Kozier, B., Erb, G., Berman, A., & Snyder, S. J. (2004). *Fundamentals of nursing: Concepts, process, and practice* (7th ed.). Upper Saddle River, NJ: Pearson Education, pp. 231–232.

8 **Answer: 4** The regularity of pain assessment depends on the degree to which the client's condition and/or pain status is changing. More rapidly progressive disease requires more frequent client assessment. Options 1, 2, and 3 all reflect clients with recurrent, long-standing problems. Their pain should be thoroughly assessed and documented, but option 4 reflects the client with the most rapidly changing condition that would require the most frequent reassessment.

Cognitive Level: Analysis **Client Need:** Physiological Integrity: Pharmacological and Parenteral Therapies **Integrated Process:** Nursing Process: Evaluation **Content Area:** Fundamentals **Strategy:** The critical term is *most frequent.* Awareness of criteria for the reassessment of pain following analgesic administration is necessary to evaluate the safety and efficacy of pain-control medications. **Reference:** Kozier, B., Erb, G., Berman, A., & Snyder, S. J. (2004). *Fundamentals of nursing: Concepts, process, and practice* (7th ed.). Upper Saddle River, NJ: Pearson Education, pp. 1151–1152.

9 **Answer: 3** Although options 1, 2, and 4 may be accurate for this particular client, the best choice for the nurse is to act based directly on the client's verbal report. According to McCaffery and Pasero (1999), "Pain is whatever the person says it is, experienced whenever they say they are experiencing it." Nurses must realize that individuals react very uniquely when in pain and there are no defining characteristics that are applicable to the majority of clients.

Cognitive Level: Application **Client Need:** Physiological Integrity: Basic Care and Comfort **Integrated Process:** Nursing Process: Assessment **Content Area:** Fundamentals **Strategy:** The core issue of the question is knowledge of fundamental pain assessments as they relate to the body of knowledge about the pain experience. Use knowledge of pain theory to guide you to make an accurate assessment of the client's pain. **Reference:** Kozier, B., Erb, G., Berman, A., & Snyder, S. J. (2004). *Fundamentals of nursing: Concepts, process, and practice* (7th ed.). Upper Saddle River, NJ: Pearson Education, p. 1133.

10 **Answer: 1** The patch is placed every 72 hours over nonhairy, nonedematous skin with good capillary flow (often over the torso, shoulders, or upper arms). Following mastectomy, the potential for lymphedema would contraindicate using the upper arms because circulation would be compromised; thus distribution of the medication would be impaired. The presence of an IV catheter or use of a trapeze bar should not affect the site.

Cognitive Level: Application **Client Need:** Physiological Integrity: Pharmacological and Parenteral Therapies **Integrated Process:** Nursing Process: Implementation **Content Area:** Fundamentals **Strategy:** Recall various routes of administration and principles of safe transdermal medication administration to make a selection. **Reference:** Kozier, B., Erb, G., Berman, A., & Snyder, S. J. (2004). *Fundamentals of nursing: Concepts, process, and practice* (7th ed.). Upper Saddle River, NJ: Pearson Education, p. 1155.

References

Berman, A., Snyder, S., Kozier, B., & Erb, G. (2008). *Fundamentals of nursing: Concepts, process, and practice* (8th ed.). Upper Saddle River, NJ: Pearson Education, pp. 1186–1230.

Harkreader, H. & Hogan, M. (2007). *Fundamentals of nursing: Caring and clinical judgment.* (3rd ed.). St. Louis, MO: Elsevier Science, pp. 1000–1035.

Jacox, A. & Carr, D. B. (1992). *Acute pain management: Operations or medical procedures and trauma. Clinical practice guidelines.* AHCPR Publication No. 92-0032. Rockville, MD: Agency for Healthcare Policy and Research, U.S. Department of Health and Human Services, Public Health Service.

Jacox, A., Carr, D. B., & Payne, R. (1994). *Management of cancer pain: Clinical practice guideline,* No. 9. AHCPR Publication No. 94-0592. Rockville, MD: Agency for Health Care Policy and Research, U.S. Department of Health and Human Services, Public Health Service.

LeMone, P. & Burke, K. (2008). *Medical-surgical nursing: Critical thinking in client care* (4th ed.). Upper Saddle River, NJ: Pearson Education.

McCaffery, M. & Pasero, C. (1999). *Pain: Clinical manual* (2nd ed.). St. Louis, MO: Mosby, pp. 177–270, 404, 410.

Potter, P. & Perry, A. (2005). *Fundamentals of nursing* (6th ed.). St. Louis, MO: Mosby, pp. 1229–1268.

Smeltzer, S. & Bare, B. (2006). *Brunner and Suddarth's textbook of medical-surgical nursing* (11th ed.). Philadelphia: Lippincott Williams & Wilkins.

World Health Organization. (1990). *Cancer pain relief and palliative care.* Technical Report Series 804. Geneva, Switzerland.

ANSWERS & RATIONALES

9

Meeting the Needs of the Perioperative Client

Chapter Outline

Overview of Perioperative Nursing

Purposes and Types of Surgery and Anesthesia

Components of the Preoperative Assessment

Informed Consent

Developmental Considerations of Individuals Having Surgery

Physical Preparation of Individuals Having Surgery

Intraoperative Factors Affecting the Postoperative Phase

Postoperative Nursing Care

Nursing Process Related to Perioperative Nursing

 NCLEX-RN® Test Prep

Use the CD-ROM enclosed with this book to access additional practice opportunities.

Objectives

➤ Explain the concept of perioperative nursing.

➤ Describe the purposes and types of surgical procedures and anesthesia.

➤ Identify the components of a comprehensive preoperative assessment.

➤ Explain the nurse's role in informed consent.

➤ Review the developmental needs and physical preparation of individuals undergoing surgery.

➤ Describe intraoperative factors that can affect a client's psychophysiologic functioning postoperatively.

➤ Identify assessment parameters and nursing interventions necessary to prevent and detect postoperative complications.

➤ Discuss the nursing process in the preoperative, intraoperative, and postoperative phases of care.

Review at a Glance

anesthesia partial or complete loss of sensation

conscious sedation a form of anesthesia that raises the pain threshold and provides some amnesia but allows the client to respond to verbal and physical stimuli; intravenous narcotics and antianxiety agents are used; the client can maintain a patent airway; also called moderate sedation

dehiscence partial or total rupture of a sutured wound

drain tube inserted into wound during surgery and designed to allow the removal of excessive fluids

exudate fluid and cells that accumulate in a wound

informed consent a formal process, the responsibility of the physician, whose purpose is to gain permis-

sion from the client for an invasive procedure and involves an explanation of the procedure as well as the risks, benefits, and alternatives to the procedure

intraoperative phase the period of surgery; during surgery

moderate sedation a newer term for conscious sedation

palliative relieves or reduces pain or symptoms of a disease without curing the disease

preoperative phase begins with a determination that surgical intervention is necessary and ends with client transport to the operating room

postoperative phase begins with the admission to the postanesthesia care unit (PACU) and ends with a follow-up evaluation in the clinical setting or home

purulent pus-containing

regional anesthesia loss of sensation in one part of the body as a result of an anesthetic agent

sanguineous bloody, refers to body fluid

serosanguineous refers to fluid composed of serum and blood

serous appearing like serum

surgical asepsis activities designed to keep operative or other sites free from the presence of microorganisms

surgical scrub a specific handwashing technique used by operating room personnel that is designed to reduce microorganisms, particularly on the hands

sterile field a microorganism-free area

PRETEST

1 Which of the following activities would the nurse carry out in the preoperative period for a client scheduled for surgery?

1. Identify potential or actual health problems.
2. Perform specialized procedures to maintain safety.
3. Assess client's response to interventions.
4. Intervene to prevent complications.

2 The nurse interprets that which client would be most likely to undergo an ablative procedure?

1. A client scheduled for breast reconstruction following a mastectomy 2 years ago
2. A client scheduled for biopsy of a lung tumor
3. A child awaiting an adenoidectomy
4. A client undergoing a nerve root resection

3 A client having surgery has a degree of risk associated with the surgery. The nurse would evaluate which of the following client-related factors as contributing to a high degree of risk associated with surgery? Select all that apply.

1. Type of institution where surgery is performed
2. Involvement of vital organs
3. Average nutritional status
4. Little likelihood of complications
5. A history of respiratory disease and diabetes

4 An infant who is having surgery has a higher risk than an adult. The nurse would interpret that which of the following is a reason for the increased risk?

1. Decline in functioning
2. Immaturity of vital organs
3. Increased possibility of hyperthermia
4. Fluctuation in volume of blood

5 A 4-year-old boy is facing surgery and may have fears related to the surgery. The type of fears the nurse would anticipate in this child would be which of the following?

1. That the surgical procedure is punishment for being bad
2. Looking drastically different after surgery
3. Not being able to do the things he used to do after the surgery
4. Of medical personnel not being competent to perform procedures correctly

6 A client has just entered the postanesthesia care unit (PACU) from surgery. The postoperative client's immediate needs include initial monitoring of which of the following items by the nurse?

1. Vital signs, level of consciousness, and presence of pain
2. Skin coloring, surgical incision, limb movements
3. Skin temperature, blood pressure, mental status
4. Temperature, emotional status, social support

7 The nurse in the postanesthesia care unit (PACU) is assessing a postoperative client. Which of the following indicators suggest to the nurse an alteration in tissue perfusion?

1. Pallor
2. Difficulty with mobility
3. Pain in the incisional area
4. Fluid loss

8 After surgery, the nurse encourages the client to move from side to side at least every 2 hours. The client questions this activity. The nurse explains that which of the following is the purpose of this intervention?

1. Assist peristalsis to return more quickly.
2. Lessen muscle weakness.
3. Increase client's ability to sleep.
4. Let the lungs alternately achieve maximum expansion.

9 The nurse is assessing the client's surgical wound in the postoperative period. Which finding indicates to the nurse that the first stage of healing is taking place?

1. Inflammation in the wound edges
2. Bleeding around the incision
3. Clot binding the wound edges
4. Collagen synthesis

10 The nurse is creating a care plan for a postoperative client. The nursing diagnosis is *Pain*. Which of the following would be an appropriate outcome for this client?

1. Balanced fluid intake and output
2. Seeks help as needed
3. Absence of nonverbal signs of discomfort
4. Performs leg exercises as instructed

➤ *See pages 252–254 for Answers & Rationales.*

I. OVERVIEW OF PERIOPERATIVE NURSING

A. Definitions

1. Perioperative nursing is defined as "those nursing activities performed by the professional nurse in the preoperative, intraoperative, and postoperative phases of the patient's surgical experience" (AORN, 2006)

   a. The Association of Operating Room Nurses (AORN) is the professional organization of perioperative registered nurses, whose mission is to "promote quality patient care by providing its members with education, standards, services, and representation" (AORN, 2006)

   b. Practice settings of perioperative nurses include hospitals, physician offices, and free-standing surgical settings

2. Perioperative phases

   a. **Preoperative phase** begins with a determination that surgical intervention is necessary and ends with the transport of client to operating room (OR); nursing activities include:

   1) Identification of the client

   2) Assessment of the client

   3) Identifying potential or actual health problems

   4) Beginning postoperative teaching about self-care

   b. Intraoperative phase (the surgical period) begins when the client is transferred to the operating table and ends when the client is admitted to the postanesthesia care unit (PACU); nursing activities include:

   1) Preparing the client for induction of anesthesia

   2) Maintaining homeostasis and asepsis throughout the procedure

   3) Assisting surgeon and team as needed by providing an aseptic environment, a hazard-free environment, and needed supplies in a timely manner

   c. Postoperative phase begins with the client's admission to PACU and ends with a follow-up evaluation in the clinical setting or home; nursing activities include:

   1) Assessment for physical adaptation following anesthesia and surgical intervention

   2) Assisting in orienting the client back to consciousness

   3) Providing continuity of information between nursing units about client progress and adaptation following the procedure

B. Nursing roles/responsibilities during the perioperative phases

   1. Preoperative

   a. Interview: current health status, allergies, current medications, previous surgical experiences, mental status, understanding of the surgical procedure and anesthesia, smoking habit, alcohol and drug use, coping strategies, social resources, and cultural considerations

   b. Arranging for pre-admission testing, consultations and education related to management of recovery from surgery and anesthesia

   1) Ordering appropriate tests, etc.

   2) Ensuring reports are available on chart

   3) Reporting to surgeon or anesthesiologist any pertinent abnormalities

   c. Day of surgery: after appropriate identification of the client, the nurse verifies the completion of paperwork and secures valuables; if the procedure is being performed as an outpatient, transportation home is verified; the nurse then proceeds with:

   1) Determining the client's cognitive understanding of procedure

   2) Performing a physical assessment

   3) Planning nursing diagnoses

   4) Reinforcing preoperative teaching for postoperative care

   5) Physical preparation: skin preparation, vital signs, antiembolism stockings, catheterization, and starting an IV infusion

   6) Ensure client has been NPO (if ordered)

   7) Ensure that there is a signed consent form and it is placed in client record

   2. Intraoperative

   a. Administer IV infusions and medications as needed

   b. Provide safe, effective care

   1) Position client to ensure functional alignment and exposure of surgical site

   2) Apply grounding device

   3) Provide emotional and physical support if awake

    4) Account for all equipment and supplies

    5) Maintain aseptic environment

    6) Perform physiologic monitoring

    7) Assess fluid loss/gain

    8) Monitor cardiac, respiratory, and neurological status

    9) Monitor the client response to preoperative medications

    10) Prepare the surgical site according to policy

  c. Nursing roles during the intraoperative period (the period of surgery)

    1) Circulating nurse

      a) Assist scrub nurses and surgeons

      b) Sterile scrubbing and gloving not necessary

    2) Scrub nurses

      a) Assist the surgeons

      b) Maintain sterile gowns, gloves, caps

      c) Account for used sponges, needles and instruments

3. Postoperative

  a. Immediate care

    1) Assess the effects of anesthetic agents/surgical procedure

    2) Monitor vital functions

    3) Provide pain relief measures to promote comfort

  b. Ongoing care

    1) Assess for client adaptation to surgery

    2) Provide pain management

    3) Position the client appropriately and reposition every 2 hours to prevent atelectasis and pneumonia

    4) Promote the use of the incentive spirometer, and deep breathing and coughing exercises

    5) Assist with postoperative exercises, such as ankle circles, calf pumps

    6) Maintain hydration and monitor fluid balance

    7) Promote urinary elimination

    8) Maintain suction to devices as needed; monitor all catheters, tubes, and drains

    9) Provide wound care and assess surgical site

    10) Continue client teaching and discharge planning

    11) Provide for safety

II. PURPOSES AND TYPES OF SURGERY AND ANESTHESIA

A. Purposes

  1. Diagnostic or exploratory: confirms or establishes a diagnosis (e.g., breast biopsy)

  2. Curative: removes pathological cause (e.g., removal of cancer)

  3. Ablative: removes a diseased body part (e.g., tonsils for tonsillitis)

  4. Reconstructive: restores function or appearance (e.g., cleft lip repair)

  5. Palliative: relieves or reduces pain or symptoms (e.g., removal of sensory nerves for intractable pain)

B. General classification of surgery

1. According to degree of risk

   a. Major: high degree of risk; may include a prolonged intraoperative period, large loss of blood, involvement of a vital organ, or postoperative complications (e.g., liver biopsy, colectomy)

   b. Minor: lesser degree of risk to the client; usually associated with few complications, may be described as "one-day surgery" or outpatient surgery (e.g., cyst removal, ingrown toenails)

2. Urgency classification

   a. Emergent: performed immediately to save a person's life, limb, or organ (e.g., testicular torsion)

   b. Urgent: requires prompt attention, usually within 24 hours (e.g., reduction of a broken bone)

   c. Required: necessary for client's well-being, usually within weeks to months (e.g., cholecystectomy, if not acute)

   d. Elective: surgery is necessary but not imminently life-threatening; will improve the client's life (e.g., some types of plastic surgery)

   e. Optional: personal preference on part of client (e.g., gastric stapling)

C. Administration of *anesthesia* (partial or complete loss of sensation)

1. Anesthetic agents are drugs used to effect a partial or complete loss of pain sensation; the client may be conscious or unconscious

2. Three major classifications of anesthesia

   a. Moderate sedation (also called **conscious sedation**)

   1) An anesthesia state that involves minimal depression of level of consciousness allowing the client the ability to respond to verbal and physical stimuli; the client can still maintain a patent airway while the pain threshold is raised

   2) Uses IV narcotics and antianxiety agents to maintain moderate sedation

   3) Examples: endoscopy, balloon angioplasty

   b. Regional anesthesia: the loss of sensation in one part of the body as a result of an anesthetic agent

   1) Local

      a) Injected in a specific area for minor surgical procedures

      b) Example of use: lidocaine for suturing a small wound

   2) Nerve block

      a) Anesthetic agent injected into and around a nerve or group of nerves

      b) Example: pudendal block used to numb the perineum for an episiotomy in childbirth

   3) Epidural block

      a) Anesthetic agent injected into the epidural space to anesthetize larger areas

      b) The client is awake and aware of surroundings but feels no pain

      c) Example of use: vaginal childbirth

   4) Spinal anesthesia

      a) Anesthesia is injected through a lumbar puncture into the subarachnoid space

        b) The client is conscious but has no sensation or movement of the lower extremities up to a specific area

        c) Example: used for hernia repairs or cesarean section deliveries

    c. General anesthesia

        1) Anesthesia that involves the loss of all sensation and consciousness

        2) It is usually administered by intravenous (IV) infusion or by inhalation of gases

        3) Examples of use: major surgery, exploratory laparotomy

  3. Stages of general anesthesia

    a. Stage I

        1) Beginning anesthesia

        2) The client is drowsy and dizzy

        3) Pain sensation is depressed

    b. Stage II

        1) Excitement

        2) The client demonstrates irregular breathing and involuntary motor movements

        3) It is important to avoid stimulating the client, which can trigger vomiting, holding the breath, and increased activity

        4) Ensure the client's safety by the proper use of safety straps

    c. Stage III

        1) The stage of anesthesia appropriate for surgical procedures

        2) The client demonstrates skeletal muscle relaxation, constricted pupils, and the absence of eyelid reflex

    d. Stage IV

        1) Medullary depression

        2) Pupils are fixed and dilated, respirations are weak and pulse is rapid and thready

        3) The client is near death

  4. Preanesthesia classifications of client's physical condition: the anesthesiologist reviews the client's medical history as well as current findings related to diagnosis, medication use, allergies, and drug reactions (see Table 9-1 for an

Table 9-1	Physical Status	Findings	Examples of Accompanying Disease
American Society of Anesthesiology Physical Status Classification System	I	Healthy client with no systemic disease	None
	II	Mild systemic disease	Moderate obesity, mild hypertension
	III	Severe systemic disease	Morbid obesity, pulmonary insufficiency
	IV	Severe systemic disease that presents as a constant threat to survival	Advanced renal disease, hepatic insufficiency
	V	Client who is not expected to survive without surgical procedure	Ruptured abdominal aneurysm
	VI	Brain-dead client whose organs are being donated	
	E	Emergency operation of a client with a poorer physical status	

Table 9-2	Anesthetic Agent	Route	Advantages	Disadvantages	Complications
Brief Overview of Anesthetic Agents	Xylocaine	Topical, injected	Quick acting	May be absorbed through mucosal surfaces and open wounds	Cardiac side effects if absorbed
	EMLA (Lidocaine and Prilocaine)	Topical	Very little absorption through skin	Must be done 60 min. prior to procedure	Blanching or erythema at application site
	Fentanyl (Sublimaze)	Parenteral	Moderate sedation	Prolonged use may cause myoclonus and/or tremors	Rapid infusion will cause chest wall tightening
	Midazolam (Versed)	Parenteral	Promotes sedation	Pain at injection site	
	Nitrous oxide	Inhalation	Quick acting	May lead to vomiting postprocedure	

example of the American Society of Anesthesiology physical status classification system)

5. Anesthetic agents may be administered either by inhalation or IV (see Table 9-2 for a brief overview of some anesthetic agents)

   a. Inhalation anesthetic agents are inhaled in gaseous forms

      1) Administered by mask or by endotracheal tube

      2) Induction is usually rapid

      3) Drugs are eliminated by the respiratory system

      4) With normal lung function, recovery rate is predictable

   b. IV anesthesia

      1) Administered alone or in combination with inhalation anesthesia

      2) Rapid onset of unconsciousness

      3) Metabolized primarily by the liver and excreted by kidneys

      4) Reversal agents may be required to stop the drug's effects

► **Practice to Pass**

Describe five purposes of surgery and include examples of each.

III. COMPONENTS OF THE PREOPERATIVE ASSESSMENT

   A. Client's history

      1. Medical history: current and past

         a. Current health status including any chronic disease that might affect the client's response to surgery and anesthesia

         b. Past medical illnesses and treatments; previous surgical experiences including complications that occurred with any previous surgical or anesthesia experience

         c. Report of severe anxiety associated with surgery

      2. Medication use: all current medications, including prescription, over-the-counter (OTC), and herbal products

      3. Allergies: food, medication, and environmental (latex, tape, soap, and antiseptic agents)

4. Tobacco use: may indicate potential problems of the respiratory tract
   a. Type of product and amount/frequency used
   b. When possible, urge client to stop smoking 6 to 8 weeks prior to major surgery
5. Alcohol and controlled substance use
   a. Type of product and amount/frequency
   b. Potential for problems with withdrawal
6. Psychosocial/economic factors
   a. Occupation
   b. Financial concerns
   c. Support systems
   d. Spiritual needs
   e. Cultural beliefs
   f. Coping mechanisms used in the past
   g. Fear/anxieties related to procedure (such as body image, pain, or grieving a loss of body part)

▶ Practice to Pass

Discuss six issues to assess preoperatively regarding a client's history.

B. Physical assessment

1. Assessment of factors that will affect the client's response to surgery or anesthesia
2. General assessments
   a. Overall appearance, gestures, facial expression
   b. Height/weight (obesity increases risk)
   c. Vital signs (hypertension increases risk)
3. Head and neck
   a. Oral mucous membranes reveal hydration status
   b. Identify loose teeth, dentures, and orthodontic work
   c. Inspect soft palate, nasal sinuses, cervical lymph nodes
   d. Note presence of jugular venous distention
4. Integumentary
   a. Evaluate skin over entire body
   b. Note any areas where skin is thin, dry, or has poor turgor
5. Chest and lungs
   a. Auscultate for adventitious breath sounds
   b. Note degree of chest expansion, presence of cough, upper airway congestion, and/or obstructed nasal passages
6. Cardiovascular system
   a. Assess apical rate and rhythm
   b. Check color and temperature of extremities
   c. Note presence of pacemaker, arteriovenous (AV) shunts
7. Gastrointestinal (GI) system
   a. Distinguish between obesity and distention of abdomen
   b. Assess baseline bowel sounds and elimination patterns
   c. Note gag reflex and history of nausea/vomiting postoperatively

d. Validate NPO (nothing by mouth) status when applicable; anesthetics are known to depress GI functioning; clients are usually NPO for 6 to 8 hours prior to surgery to reduce the risk of vomiting and aspiration

8. Genitourinary/reproductive system

a. Determine alterations in urinary elimination, color, appearance, and usual amount of urine output

b. Note presence of abnormal vaginal discharge, uterine bleeding in women

9. Neurological/mobility status

a. Determine baseline level of consciousness (LOC)

b. Note presence of sensory/perceptual deficits

c. Assess range of motion (ROM) and ability to perform activities of daily living (ADLs)

C. Diagnostic screening

1. Laboratory tests are done prior to surgery to screen for existing abnormalities and to use as a baseline for future assessments

2. Additional tests may be ordered related to specific condition

3. Verify that test results are present prior to surgery

4. Abnormal findings may need to be corrected prior to surgery

5. See Table 9-3 for routine preoperative screening tests

> **Practice to Pass**
>
> Describe one abnormal assessment finding for each body system the nurse may note while completing a physical assessment that could affect the outcome of the surgical procedure.

Table 9-3	**Test**	**Rationale**
Routine Preoperative Screening Tests	Complete blood count (CBC)	RBCs, hemoglobin (Hgb), and hematocrit (Hct) are important to the oxygen-carrying capacity of the blood; WBCs are an indicator of immune function
	Blood grouping and cross-matching	Determined in case blood transfusion is required during or after surgery
	Serum electrolytes (Na^+, K^+, Ca^{2+}, Mg^{2+}, Cl^-, HCO_3^-)	To evaluate fluid and electrolyte status
	Fasting blood glucose	High levels may indicate undiagnosed diabetes mellitus
	Blood urea nitrogen (BUN) and creatinine	To evaluate renal function
	ALT, AST, LDH, and bilirubin	To evaluate liver function
	Serum albumin and total protein	To evaluate nutritional status
	Urinalysis	To determine urine composition and possible abnormal components (eg, protein or glucose) or infection
	Chest x-ray	To evaluate respiratory status and heart size
	Electrocardiogram (ECG) (in all clients over 40 years of age and/or clients with preexisting cardiac conditions)	To identify preexisting cardiac problems or disease
	Pregnancy test	To identify if the client is pregnant

Source: Berman, A., Snyder, S., Kozier, B. & Erb, G.. (2008). *Fundamentals of nursing: Concepts, process, and practice* (8th ed.). Upper Saddle River, NJ: Pearson Education, p. 943.

IV. INFORMED CONSENT

A. Definition

1. Written permission obtained from the client by the practitioner performing the procedure or surgery prior to any invasive procedure or one that has potentially serious side effects or complications

2. The client has the right to accept or reject the procedure after an explanation has been provided

3. Informed consent is the process which includes providing the client with information about:

   a. Nature and purpose of a treatment or procedure

   b. Expected outcomes and probabilities of success, material risks, benefits and consequences of treatment

   c. Alternatives to the procedure and supporting information

   d. Effect of doing without the procedure/treatment including the effect on prognosis

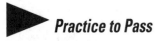

Practice to Pass

Describe four factors the nurse must consider while obtaining informed consent from a client.

B. Three elements of informed consent

1. The consent is given voluntarily

2. The consent is given by an individual with the capacity and competence to understand what the procedure involves

   a. Adults have the legal authority to make decisions for themselves

   b. If the client is a minor, the parent or legal guardian has the right to provide consent

   c. Many states recognize emancipated minors who can provide consent for themselves

   d. Many states allow minors to provide consent for treatment in cases related to sexually transmitted disease, pregnancy, abortion, and contraception

   e. Legal power of attorney for health care allows another individual to make decisions should the client become incapacitated

3. Sufficient information must be provided to the client to allow for an informed decision

   a. This requires that the health care worker must communicate in a means the client can understand

   b. An interpreter may be needed to ensure adequate communication

4. In emergencies when informed consent cannot be obtained from the client or the next of kin, consent is implied by law; the specific information about the emergency situation and the reason informed consent was not obtained must be documented in the medical record

C. Legal standards for informed consent

1. Professional standard: what the physician believes the consumer should know

2. Subjective standard: what the particular consumer believes the consumer should know

3. Objective standard: what a reasonable person believes the consumer should know

D. Nurse's role with informed consent

1. The informed consent is part of the physician–client relationship

2. Because the nurse does not perform surgery or procedures, informed consent is not part of the nursing responsibility

3. The physician has obligation to acquire consent

4. The nurse's role is to serve as witness to the following:

   a. Authority on consent form is authentic

   b. The client has the capacity to make informed consent

   c. The client has the authority to consent

   d. Consent is being given voluntarily

V. DEVELOPMENTAL CONSIDERATIONS OF INDIVIDUALS HAVING SURGERY

A. Children and adolescents

1. Take care with all children and adolescents while explaining procedures as they may misinterpret the meaning

2. Infancy: surgery and separation from parents may interfere with bonding; children of this age have no understanding of the process but are aware of adult emotions; no explanations about procedures are required for the child, but the parents will need complete preparation

3. Toddler: children of this age may suffer from separation anxiety; their security lies in the presence of their caregivers; when the caregivers are not present, the child may suffer; immediately prior to a procedure, give the toddler a brief, simple explanation

4. Preschoolers: often view illness as a punishment for bad behavior; they have an inadequate understanding of cause–effect and thus misinterpret relationships; explanations continue to be simple and near to the time of the procedure; play therapy may be beneficial in aiding the child to express his or her feelings

5. School-age children: are better able to withstand separation from parents and are accustomed to dealing with adults other than family; children of this age fear pain and mutilation; give more complete, yet age-appropriate instructions and consider using pictures, dolls, and videos

6. Adolescents: concerns are separation from peers and body image/physical attractiveness; protect the adolescent's privacy

B. Adults

1. Fear of the unknown/separation from support systems

2. Dependence and loss of control

3. Disruption in career goals, family living patterns, and financial worries

4. Concern over cancer and/or death

VI. PHYSICAL PREPARATION OF INDIVIDUALS HAVING SURGERY

A. Preparing for anesthesia

1. Anesthetic needs and risks are assessed by anesthesiologist

2. The type of anesthetic along with method of administration, risks, and recovery is explained

B. Preparing the skin

1. Purpose: cleansing and removing transient microbes from the skin
2. Includes the following components:
   a. Cleansing: begins with morning shower or bath; the surgical site is then cleansed with an antimicrobial agent immediately prior to surgery
   b. Hair removal: removing hair from the surgical site may be ordered to further reduce microbial growth; care must be taken to maintain an intact skin

C. Preparing the GI tract

1. NPO prior to OR in order to:
   a. Reduce risk of vomiting/aspiration
   b. Prevent contamination of operative site from fecal material
   c. Reduce post-op nausea, vomiting, gastric distention, or bowel obstruction
2. Colon cleansing may be ordered for surgical procedures involving the GI tract; colon cleansing reduces contamination of the surgical field; postoperative constipation may be prevented; cleansing may occur using:
   a. Enemas
   b. Laxatives
   c. Oral antibiotics

D. Preparation on the day of surgery

1. Routine care for most outpatient/ hospitalized clients
   a. Ensure consent form is signed
   b. Administer any preoperative medications
   c. Provide emotional support to client/family
   d. Complete preoperative teaching, including information about postoperative care
2. General care
   a. Record vital signs for baseline information
   b. Remove dentures/bridgework; note loose teeth on chart
   c. Assist client to put on hospital gown without undergarments in most cases (for children and minor procedures, there may be exceptions)
   d. Have client void to empty the bladder
   e. Remove cosmetics/nail polish
   f. Remove jewelry per agency policy and place in secure area for safekeeping; if client does not want to remove wedding band, tape it in place; in certain situations, this would also require removal because of the risk of postoperative edema
   g. Leave hearing aids in place and note their presence on the preoperative checklist
   h. Remove eyeglasses, contact lenses, and other prostheses
   i. Antiembolism stockings may be ordered; these stockings promote return circulation from the legs

E. Preoperative medications

1. May be ordered at a scheduled time or "on call" to the operating room
2. Purposes
   a. Sedate/tranquilize

       b. Decrease respiratory tract secretions

       c. Provide analgesia

       d. Reduce nausea and prevent vomiting

       e. Reduce gastric acid

   3. Classifications of preoperative medication

       a. Barbiturates

          1) Use: sedation, narcotic enhancer

          2) Major side effects: central nervous system (CNS) depression, respiratory depression

       b. Tranquilizers

          1) Use: sedation, medication enhancer

          2) Major side effect: CNS depression

       c. Narcotic/opioid analgesics

          1) Use: reduce dosages needed of anesthetics

          2) Major side effect: CNS depression

       d. Anticholinergics

          1) Use: reduce secretion of body fluids such as saliva

          2) Major side effect: GI system depression

       e. Antinausea agents

          1) Use: reduce probability of emesis and aspiration

          2) Major side effect: respiratory depression

       f. Antacid, H_2-receptor blockers

          1) Use: reduce gastric acidity and reflux

          2) Major side effect: rebound acidity

       g. Prophylactic anti-infectives

          1) Use: reduce risk of infection

          2) Major side effect: tolerance to antibiotics

VII. INTRAOPERATIVE FACTORS AFFECTING POSTOPERATIVE PHASE

A. Principles of perioperative asepsis

   1. General

       a. Keep sterile supplies dry and unopened

       b. Check package sterilization expiration date to verify sterility

       c. Maintain general cleanliness in surgical suite

       d. Maintain **surgical asepsis** (activities designed to keep sites free from the presence of microorganisms) throughout the procedure (refer back to Chapter 6, Table 6-2, pp. 143–144, for principles and practices for surgical asepsis)

   2. Personnel

       a. Personnel with signs of illness should not report to work

       b. **Surgical scrub,** a specific handwashing technique used by operating room personnel designed to reduce microorganisms on the hands and arms, is done for the length of time designated by hospital policy

1) A sensor-controlled or knee- or foot-operated faucet allows the water to be turned on and off without the use of the hands

2) Remove all rings and watches

3) Use liquid soaps to prevent the spread of microorganisms

4) Keep the fingernails short and well-trimmed; clean fingernails with a nail stick under running water

5) Hold the hands higher than the elbows throughout the handwashing procedure so that run-off goes to the elbows; this allows the cleanest part of the arms to be the hands

6) A scrub brush facilitates the removal of microorganisms; clean all areas of skin on the hands and arms in sequence starting at the hands and ending at the elbows

7) After rinsing, dry the hands with paper towels, drying first one arm from hand to elbow, then using a second towel to dry the second hand

3. Maintaining a **sterile field** (a microoganism-free area)

   a. Create a sterile field using sterile drapes

   b. Use the sterile field to place sterile supplies where they will be available during the procedure

   c. Drape equipment prior to use

   d. Keep drapes dry and out of contact with nonsterile objects

   e. Utilize sterile technique while adding or removing supplies from sterile fields

4. Sterile supplies and solutions

   a. Check expiration dates for sterility

   b. Don't use solutions that were opened prior to current use

   c. "Lip" the solutions after initial use by pouring a small amount of liquid out of the bottle into a waste container to cleanse the bottle lip

B. **Potential environmental health hazards during the intraoperative period**

   1. Injuries caused by equipment

      a. Laser tools used for a surgical procedure can cause burns

      b. Improperly grounded cautery devices can cause burns

      c. Prevent by ensuring proper grounding for electrical equipment and checking equipment prior to beginning surgical procedure

      d. Latex allergy affects many people, both clients and hospital personnel

         1) Clients with spina bifida and those who have had multiple surgical procedures are at greatest risk

         2) Exposure can occur percutaneously, mucosally, parenterally, and via inhalation

         3) Symptoms can vary from contact dermatitis to anaphylaxis

         4) Symptoms in the anesthetized client would include flushing, facial swelling, urticaria, bronchospasm, hypotension, and cardiac arrest

         5) Be aware of equipment that contains latex, including tourniquets, ambu bags, balloon catheters, surgical gowns, boots, and drapes among other items

   2. Exposure to blood and body fluids

      a. Is a concern for client and staff alike

      b. Use goggles and fluid-protectant shields; gloves worn for extended period can leak and should be changed periodically

      c. Use caution with sharps

C. Potential intraoperative complications

Practice to Pass

What nursing interventions will the OR nurse carry out to prevent hypothermia in the surgical client?

1. Nausea and vomiting: ensure that the client is NPO for the prescribed time period

2. Hypoxia/respiratory complications

   a. Complications

   1) Aspiration of secretions or vomitus may be caused by loss of pharyngeal and cough reflexes

   2) Respiratory depression can occur from anesthetic agents

   3) Respiratory muscles become weakened or paralyzed by neuromuscular agents

   4) Positioning can negatively affect lung expansion

   b. Tissue perfusion is monitored by anesthesiologist

   c. Use of a pulse oximeter assists with the monitoring of oxygenation

3. Hypothermia

   a. Is related to room temperature of OR and exposure of internal organs

   b. Is minimized by preventing exposure of nonsurgical body parts, use of head covering and blankets, warmed IV fluids and anesthetic agents

4. Malignant hyperthermia

   a. Is defined as excessive heat production related to stress, trauma, infection; may be attributed to anesthetic agent; seen more commonly in males; there is a tendency towards development if inherited as an autosomal dominant trait

   b. Symptoms include rapid rise in body temperature, tachycardia and tachypnea, and respiratory and metabolic acidosis

   c. Skin initially appears flushed then becomes mottled and cyanotic

   d. Treatment includes administering 100% oxygen, cooling blankets and cold packs, cool IV fluids and stomach irrigation

   e. Can be fatal

5. Paresthesia related to positioning: use padding and proper position

6. Excessive fluid/blood loss: monitor bleeding and intake and output

VIII. POSTOPERATIVE NURSING CARE

A. Assessments in immediate period following surgery (PACU—postanesthesia care unit) (see Box 9-1)

1. The client is admitted from the surgical unit into the PACU; upon admission, the PACU nurse will:

   a. Confirm the client's identity

   b. Receive report from the OR/surgical nurse, which includes surgical procedure, anesthesia, drugs and IV fluids administered, and estimated blood loss

   c. Note location, types, and conditions of catheters, **drains,** or packs; drains are tubes inserted into wounds to allow the removal of excessive **serosanguineous** (fluid composed of serum and blood) or **purulent** (containing pus) material from the wound

2. The nurse in the PACU will:

   a. Maintain a patent airway

   1) This is a priority nursing concern

   2) The airway may be affected by the continued effects of anesthesic drugs, relaxtion of the tongue, oropharyngeal secretions, or by vomitus

Box 9-1	➤ Adequacy of airway
Clinical Assessment in the Immediate Postanesthetic Phase	➤ Oxygen saturation

➤ Adequacy of airway

➤ Oxygen saturation

➤ Adequacy of ventilation

  ➤Respiratory rate, rhythm, and depth

  ➤Use of accessory muscles

  ➤Breath sounds

➤ Cardiovascular status

  ➤Heart rate and rhythm

  ➤Peripheral pulse amplitude and equality

  ➤Blood pressure

  ➤Capillary filling

➤ Level of consciousness

  ➤Not responding

  ➤Arousable with verbal simuli

  ➤Fully awake

  ➤Oriented to time, person, and place

➤ Presence of protective reflexes (e.g., gag, cough)

➤ Activity, ability to move extremities

➤ Skin color (pink, pale, dusky, blotchy, cyanotic, jaundiced)

➤ Fluid status

  ➤Intake and output

  ➤Status of IV infusions (type of fluid, rate, amount in container, patency of tubing)

  ➤Signs of dehydration or fluid overload

➤ Condition of operative site

  ➤Status of dressing

  ➤Drainage (amount, type, and color)

➤ Patency of and character and amount of drainage from catheters, tubes, and drains

➤ Discomfort (i.e., pain) (type, location, and severity), nausea, vomiting

➤ Safety (e.g., necessity for side rails, call bell within reach)

Source: Berman, A., Snyder, S. Kozier, B., Erb, G., (2008). *Fundamentals of nursing: Concepts, process, and practice* (8th ed.). Upper Saddle River, NJ: Pearson Education, p. 957.

    3) Position the client on his/her side unless contraindicated

    4) Monitor respiratory rate, breath sounds, and suction as necessary

  b. Maintain cardiovascular stability

    1) The client is typically on a cardiac and respiratory monitor

    2) Vital signs are monitored according to hospital policy (often every 15 minutes) until stable and then every 30 minutes

    3) Changes in vital signs should be reported immediately

    4) Antiembolism stockings or pneumatic compression boots may be utilized to promote circulation in the lower extremities

  c. Assess for hypotension/shock

    1) May be related to fluid/blood loss or as a reaction to drugs

      2) Monitor dressings and drains for amount and type of drainage

      3) Symptoms include restlessness, cool moist skin, pallor followed by cyanosis, and decreased urine output

      4) Monitor and maintain IV infusion flow rates

    d. Assess for hemorrhage

      1) Monitor dressings and drains for amount of discharge; observe appearance of urine; observe for distention of body tissues

      2) A client with excessive blood loss may require a transfusion; ensure the blood product and type are appropriate

    e. Assess for hypertension/dysrhythmias

    f. Relieve pain and anxiety

      1) Pain can negatively affect vital signs and recovery

      2) Assess location and cause of pain

      3) Administer analgesics as ordered

      4) Observe effectiveness of analgesics

3. The client will be discharged from the PACU when:

    a. Vital signs are stable and spontaneous respirations have returned

    b. Gag reflex is present

    c. Client is easily arousable

B. Nursing management on the surgical nursing unit

  1. Immediate nursing interventions

    a. Assess breathing and apply oxygen if prescribed

    b. Check vital signs and skin warmth, moisture, color

    c. Assess surgical site/wound drains; the partial or total rupture of a sutured wound is termed **dehiscence,** which may be preceded by sudden straining as during coughing; when dehiscence occurs, cover the wound with sterile dressings soaked in normal saline; place the client in bed with the knees bent to reduce tension on the wound and notify the surgeon; note and record any wound **exudate** (fluid and cells that accumulate in a wound); exudate varies in appearance

      1) **Serous** (appearing like serum) exudate looks watery and clear

      2) **Purulent** exudate is thick and contains pus; purulent exudate varies in color and may be blue, green, or yellow tinged

      3) **Sanguineous** exudate is bloody and may be dark red or bright red depending on the freshness of the blood

    d. Connect tubes to drain devices or suction

    e. Perform pain assessment and utilize appropriate pain relief interventions

    f. Position the client properly using support devices as necessary

    g. Monitor IV fluids and infusion pumps

    h. Monitor urine output hourly or less frequently as ordered

      1) Kidney function may have been impaired from poor perfusion during surgery; output indicates the kidney response; hourly urine output should be 30 mL or more in an adult (0.5 mL/kg/hour)

      2) Bladder distention is possible for up to 24 hours following spinal anesthesia; spontaneous voiding should occur within 6 to 8 hours postoperatively

      3) If client is unable to void, catheterization may be ordered and repeated as necessary

2. Ongoing nursing interventions
   a. Encourage deep breathing and coughing exercises
      1) Helps remove mucus that accumulates in the lungs during surgery
      2) Aids in the prevention of postoperative complications such as atelectasis and pneumonia

      3) Should be performed every 2 hours while awake
      4) Deep breathing frequently initiates coughing; encourage the client to sit up in bed and place hands one on top of the other directly on the wound dressing to reduce the discomfort of coughing
      5) When increased intracranial pressure is a risk, client may deep breathe but not cough
   b. Teach and encourage leg exercises, use of support stockings, or sequential compression device
   c. Keep the call light, emesis basin, ice chips, bedpan, urinal within reach
   d. Communicate with family/significant others
   e. Monitor for infection by noting wound characteristics, temperature, and WBC test results
   f. Teach self-care according to surgical procedure and client/family needs
   g. Encourage activity as tolerated
   h. Promote GI/GU function by providing diet/fluids once bowel sounds return; encourage early ambulation to promote bowel function; monitor voiding
   i. Provide wound care as ordered (monitor incision, change dressing as ordered); document findings
   j. Participate in discharge planning according to individual client needs

IX. NURSING PROCESS RELATED TO PERIOPERATIVE NURSING

A. **Nursing diagnoses and expected outcomes for the preoperative period**

1. Diagnosis: *Deficient knowledge:* operative procedure, postoperative complications, postoperative exercises, etc. (no etiology is required to explain a knowledge deficit)
2. Client outcomes: client describes operative procedure and potential complications; client demonstrates postoperative exercises
3. Diagnosis: *Anxiety* related to unknown outcome of surgery
4. Client outcomes: client expresses fears and identifies two activities that will reduce his/her fear

B. **Nursing diagnoses and expected outcomes for the intraoperative period**

1. Diagnosis: *Risk for impaired gas exchange* related to depressant effect of anesthestic agents
2. Client outcome: client's repiratory rate remains between 16 and 20
3. Diagnosis: *Risk for ineffective airway clearance* related to impaired gag reflex and unconscious state
4. Client outcome: client's breath sounds remain clear
5. Diagnosis: *Risk for ineffective peripheral tissue perfusion*
6. Client outcome: oxygen saturation measured by pulse oximeter remains 95–100%

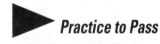

Practice to Pass

For the diagnosis *Risk for impaired gas exchange related to accumulation of secretions during surgery,* list one client goal and three nursing interventions that will aid achievement of that goal.

C. Nursing diagnoses and expected outcomes for the postoperative period

1. Nursing diagnoses related to gas exchange/airway clearance and tissue perfusion continue to be important for this period

2. Diagnosis: *Risk for infection* related to loss of skin integrity

3. Client outcome: the client remains free of infection as evidenced by temperature within normal range, normal WBC count, and lack of wound redness

4. Diagnosis: *Impaired skin integrity* related to surgical procedure

5. Client outcome: the client's skin heals within two weeks

6. Diagnosis: *Pain* related to trauma to tissue secondary to surgical procedure

7. Client outcome: the client remains pain free as evidenced by verbalization, relaxed facial expression, and participation in postoperative activities

Case Study

A 14-year-old female is admitted for an abdominal exploratory laparotomy. She has been complaining of abdominal pain intermittently for several months.

1. What ethical issues surround obtaining informed consent?

2. Discuss pertinent questions the nurse needs to ask about her history.

3. List two preoperative nursing diagnoses that might be appropriate for her.

4. Discuss what she needs to be taught about her postoperative care.

5. The client will have general anesthesia. Discuss what the nurse should tell her about the anesthesia.

For suggested responses, see page 338.

POSTTEST

1 A client is being admitted to the hospital on the day before a scheduled surgery. Which of the following is the most appropriate initial question to ask this preoperative client?

1. "Has your doctor talked to you about the type of surgery you are having? What did the doctor say?"
2. "What questions do you have about your surgery?"
3. "What type of surgery are you having and why are you having it done?"
4. "What do you know about what will be done to you?"

2 A presurgical client asks the nurse for more information about the advantages of a general anesthetic. Which of the following would be appropriate for the nurse to include in a response to the client?

1. Respiratory and circulatory functions are depressed.
2. Client loses consciousness and does not perceive pain.
3. Anesthetic agent is not rapidly excreted so that the timing of surgery can be adjusted.
4. General anesthesia reduces the chance that the client suffers from amnesia.

3 A benzodiazepine has been administered to a client preoperatively. After the drug has been administered, the nurse plans to monitor the client for which side effects? Select all that apply.

1. Anxiety
2. Hypotension
3. Hypocalcemia
4. Extrapyramidal reactions
5. Sedation

4 A preoperative client has an elevated hemoglobin and hematocrit. What would the nurse suspect regarding the significance of this increased value?

1. Immune deficiency
2. Kidney dysfunction
3. Malignancy
4. Dehydration

5 The nurse has completed preoperative teaching with a pregnant woman. During the discussion, the nurse describes the different types of anesthesia available. Which statement by the client indicates to the nurse an understanding of regional anesthesia?

1. "In spinal anesthesia, the anesthetic is injected into the subarachnoid space."
2. "The anesthetic is injected into the dura mater of the spinal cord for epidural anesthesia."
3. "I will be sedated and have some awareness of the event."
4. "Regional anesthesia produces analgesia and amnesia."

6 The client arrives in the postanesthesia care unit (PACU) in an unconscious state. In what position would the nurse place the unconscious client in the immediate postanesthesia stage?

1. Side lying with the face slightly down
2. Side lying with a pillow under the client's head
3. Semiprone position with the head tilted to the side
4. Dorsal recumbent with head turned to the side

7 The client has been in the postanesthesia care unit (PACU) for 1 hour. The client is now groggy but able to respond to voice commands. While assessing the client, the nurse checks the bedclothes underneath the client to detect which of the following?

1. Drainage from the tubes or drains
2. Fluid balance
3. Possible hemorrhage
4. Perspiration

8 A client is in the postoperative stage and the physician has ordered ambulation. The client has difficulty understanding the necessity for early ambulation. The nurse would formulate which appropriate nursing diagnosis for this client?

1. Self-care deficit
2. Deficient knowledge
3. Ineffective coping
4. Risk for injury

9 The nurse is assessing the client upon return to the nursing unit from the postanesthesia care unit (PACU) and notes the presence of a drain in the surgical wound. A family member sees the drain and asks why the tube was left in the wound. The nurse explains that drains:

1. Allow drainage of excessive fluids such as blood, edema, or pus from the surgical site.
2. Allow healing to occur at a very rapid rate.
3. Have to be shortened to allow healing to occur from the inside out.
4. Have to be connected to suction tubes.

10 A client is being discharged following outpatient surgery. The nurse who is providing the caregiver with instructions for wound care would instruct the caregiver to report which finding to the surgeon?

1. Scar formation
2. Increased redness or drainage
3. No odor of the wound drainage
4. Slight serous color of the drainage

➤ *See pages 254–256 for Answers & Rationales.*

ANSWERS & RATIONALES

Pretest

1 **Answer: 1** Assessment in the preoperative phase includes anticipating any health problems that may occur during and after surgery. Option 2 is applicable during the intraoperative phase, where specific specialized activities are carried out in the operating room. Option 3 is a very general activity that should occur at any time.

Prevention of complications (option 4) occurs in the postoperative stage.
Cognitive Level: Application **Client Need:** Physiological Integrity: Reduction of Risk Potential **Integrated Process:** Nursing Process: Implementation **Content Area:** Fundamentals **Strategy:** The critical term is *preoperative period*. Recall activities associated with each phase of the perioperative period to direct you to provide care to

clients in each phase. **Reference:** Kozier, B., Erb, G., Berman, A., & Snyder, S. J. (2004). *Fundamentals of nursing: Concepts, process, and practice* (7th ed.). Upper Saddle River, NJ: Pearson Education, p. 902.

2 **Answer: 3** Ablative surgery involves removal of diseased body parts. Option 1 involves reconstructive surgery, option 2 is carried out for a diagnostic purpose, and option 4 is completed for palliation.
Cognitive Level: Application **Client Need:** Physiological Integrity: Reduction of Risk Potential **Integrated Process:** Nursing Process: Analysis **Content Area:** Fundamentals **Strategy:** Knowledge of terminology related to purposes and types of surgery will enable you to recognize the accurate option and make a correct selection. **Reference:** Kozier, B., Erb, G., Berman, A., & Snyder, S. J. (2004). *Fundamentals of nursing: Concepts, process, and practice* (7th ed.). Upper Saddle River, NJ: Pearson Education, p. 897.

3 **Answers: 2, 5** When surgery is performed on vital organs (option 2) and when there is a greater likelihood for complications due to client age and condition (option 5), there is a greater likelihood for complications and therefore the risk is higher. Risk is not associated with the place where surgery is performed (option 1); also, this is not a client-related factor. Risk is associated with poor nutritional status, so option 3 is incorrect. The higher the likelihood of complications, the greater the risk making option 4 incorrect.
Cognitive Level: Analysis **Client Need:** Physiological Integrity: Reduction of Risk Potential **Integrated Process:** Nursing Process: Assessment **Content Area:** Fundamentals **Strategy:** The critical terms are *client-related factors* and *high degree of risk*. Being able to recall surgical risks is vital to care and client education and is the core issue of the question. Use nursing knowledge and the process of elimination to make a selection. **Reference:** Kozier, B., Erb, G., Berman, A., & Snyder, S. J. (2004). *Fundamentals of nursing: Concepts, process, and practice* (7th ed.). Upper Saddle River, NJ: Pearson Education, pp. 898–899.

4 **Answer: 2** The infant has immature vital organs that affect the infant's ability to metabolize medications such as the anesthetic and the ability to resist infection (option 2). Infants do not suffer from declines in functioning (option 1). Hypothermia is more likely to occur than hyperthermia since the infant has an immature temperature regulation and large body surface area (option 3). The volume of blood in an infant is limited and does not fluctuate (option 4).
Cognitive Level: Application **Client Need:** Physiological Integrity: Reduction of Risk Potential **Integrated Process:** Nursing Process: Analysis **Content Area:** Fundamentals

Strategy: To answer the question correctly, it is necessary to have knowledge of surgical risk factors, which will then enable you to make an accurate selection.
Reference: Kozier, B., Erb, G., Berman, A., & Snyder, S. J. (2004). *Fundamentals of nursing: Concepts, process, and practice* (7th ed.). Upper Saddle River, NJ: Pearson Education, p. 898.

5 **Answer: 1** Option 1 is correct. Since preschool children have a very limited understanding of cause and effect, they often interpret illness and related procedures such as surgery as punishment for bad behavior. The other options are incorrect. Appearance is not a primary concern at this age (option 2), anticipating inability to do certain things is not a concern at this developmental level (option 3), and children at this age are unaware of competency issues of medical personnel (option 4).
Cognitive Level: Analysis **Client Need:** Health Promotion and Maintenance **Integrated Process:** Nursing Process: Analysis **Content Area:** Fundamentals **Strategy:** The critical words are *preschool child*. Understanding developmental stages and tasks will enable you to make the best selection using the process of elimination. **Reference:** Kozier, B., Erb, G., Berman, A., & Snyder, S. J. (2004). *Fundamentals of nursing: Concepts, process, and practice* (7th ed.). Upper Saddle River, NJ: Pearson Education, p. 898.

6 **Answer: 1** Although all the options contain aspects that need assessment, initially all of the parameters in option 1 are the most important to assess because they relate to both physiological needs and are more global indicators of overall functioning than the other options.
Cognitive Level: Analysis **Client Need:** Physiological Integrity: Reduction of Risk Potential **Integrated Process:** Nursing Process: Assessment **Content Area:** Fundamentals **Strategy:** The critical term is *immediate needs*. Recall the necessary nursing responsibilities for the postoperative client and their relative importance to enable you to set priorities for care. **Reference:** Kozier, B., Erb, G., Berman, A., & Snyder, S. J. (2004). *Fundamentals of nursing: Concepts, process and practice* (7th ed.). Upper Saddle River, NJ: Pearson Education, p. 913.

7 **Answer: 1** The color of the skin, nails, and lips are indicators of tissue perfusion, and pallor and cyanosis indicate an alteration. Mobility, pain, and fluid loss are incorrect as they are not signs of tissue perfusion, although fluid loss could ultimately contribute to reduced tissue perfusion.
Cognitive Level: Analysis **Client Need:** Physiological Integrity: Reduction of Risk Potential **Integrated Process:** Nursing Process: Assessment **Content Area:** Fundamentals **Strategy:** The critical phrase is *alteration in tissue perfusion*. Recall manifestations of common postoperative

complications to assist you in making accurate nursing diagnoses. **Reference:** Kozier, B., Erb, G., Berman, A., & Snyder, S. J. (2004). *Fundamentals of nursing: Concepts, process, and practice* (7th ed.). Upper Saddle River, NJ: Pearson Education, p. 913.

8 Answer: 4 Turning side to side allows the lungs alternatively to expand properly. Peristalsis increases with movement even if it is not turning, and muscle weakness can be lessened with movement. Turning does not necessarily induce sleep.
Cognitive Level: Application **Client Need:** Physiological Integrity: Reduction of Risk Potential **Integrated Process:** Teaching/Learning **Content Area:** Fundamentals **Strategy:** Knowledge of potential postoperative complications will enable you to use client education as a tool to prevent their occurrence. Recall that promoting lung expansion prevents complications. **Reference:** Kozier, B., Erb, G., Berman, A., & Snyder, S. J. (2004). *Fundamentals of nursing: Concepts, process, and practice* (7th ed.). Upper Saddle River, NJ: Pearson Education, p. 915.

9 Answer: 3 The first sign of healing is absence of bleeding and wound edges bound by fibrin in the clot. Inflammation at the wound edges follows the first sign, and then when the clot diminishes, inflammation decreases and collagen forms a scar.
Cognitive Level: Analysis **Client Need:** Physiological Integrity: Reduction of Risk Potential **Integrated Process:** Nursing Process: Evaluation **Content Area:** Fundamentals **Strategy:** The critical term is *first stage of healing.* Recall the differences among the various stages of healing to make an appropriate selection. **Reference:** Kozier, B., Erb, G., Berman, A., & Snyder, S. J. (2004). *Fundamentals of nursing: Concepts, process, and practice* (7th ed.). Upper Saddle River, NJ: Pearson Education, p.924.

10 Answer: 3 Absence of nonverbal signs of discomfort indicates that the client is likely meeting the goal. The other options may be useful in the overall client management but are not directly related to the stated problem (pain).
Cognitive Level: Application **Client Need:** Physiological Integrity: Basic Care and Comfort **Integrated Process:** Nursing Process: Planning **Content Area:** Fundamentals **Strategy:** The critical word is *Pain.* Recall that client outcome statements must always be directly related to the problem. **Reference:** Kozier, B., Erb, G., Berman, A., & Snyder, S. J. (2004). *Fundamentals of nursing: Concepts, process, and practice* (7th ed.). Upper Saddle River, NJ: Pearson Education, p. 918.

Posttest

1 Answer: 3 Option 1 is not the best question initially as it focuses not on the client but on the doctor. Option 2 is

not an appropriate initial question. Option 4 is challenging and not appropriate as an initial question. Option 3 is correct as it is exploratory in nature and will provide a basis for further communication with the client.
Cognitive Level: Application **Client Need:** Physiological Integrity: Reduction of Risk Potential **Integrated Process:** Communication and Documentation **Content Area:** Fundamentals **Strategy:** The critical term is *most appropriate.* Recall that preoperative care responsibilities to include assessment of client knowledge of the impending procedure, which will then enable client teaching that enhances postoperative outcomes. **Reference:** Kozier, B., Erb, G., Berman, A., & Snyder, S. J. (2004). *Fundamentals of nursing: Concepts, process, and practice* (7th ed.). Upper Saddle River, NJ: Pearson Education, p. 899.

2 Answer: 2 General anesthetics produce central nervous system depression so clients do not feel the pain of surgery. Respiratory and circulatory depression is a disadvantage of general anesthetics because there is a greater risk for complications, especially for clients with chronic illnesses. General anesthetic agents are rapidly excreted and produce amnesia.
Cognitive Level: Application **Client Need:** Physiological Integrity: Pharmacological and Parenteral Therapies **Integrated Process:** Teaching/Learning **Content Area:** Fundamentals **Strategy:** Recall the major classifications of anesthesia and their advantages and disadvantages and use the process of elimination to make a selection. **Reference:** Kozier, B., Erb, G., Berman, A., & Snyder, S. J. (2004). *Fundamentals of nursing: Concepts, process, and practice* (7th ed.). Upper Saddle River, NJ: Pearson Education, p. 910.

3 Answers: 2, 5 Benzodiazepines such as lorazepam and diazepam decrease anxiety and produce side effects such as hypotension and sedation. Major tranquilizers such as chlorpromazine produce extrapyramidal symptoms, but benzodiazepines do not. Hypocalcemia is not an adverse effect of this class of drugs.
Cognitive Level: Application **Client Need:** Physiological Integrity: Pharmacological and Parenteral Therapies **Integrated Process:** Nursing Process: Evaluation **Content Area:** Fundamentals **Strategy:** The critical words are *benzodiazepine* and *side effects.* Recall common side effects of frequently used perioperative medications and use the process of elimination to make a selection. **Reference:** Kozier, B., Erb, G., Berman, A., & Snyder, S. J. (2004). *Fundamentals of nursing: Concepts, process, and practice* (7th ed.). Upper Saddle River, NJ: Pearson Education, p. 907.

4 Answer: 4 An increased hemoglobin and hematocrit may be a result of dehydration. Immune deficiency is

an indication of decreased white blood cell count (option 1), while an increase in electrolytes such as potassium, sodium, or chloride indicate kidney dysfunction (option 2). Malignancy may be suspected in increased platelet count (option 3).
Cognitive Level: Analysis **Client Need:** Physiological Integrity: Reduction of Risk Potential **Integrated Process:** Nursing Process: Analysis **Content Area:** Fundamentals **Strategy:** The critical phrase is *elevated hemoglobin and hematocrit*. Recall the usual causes of common lab abnormalities and use the process of elimination to identify conditions that need to be corrected prior to surgery. **Reference:** Kozier, B., Erb, G., Berman, A., & Snyder, S. J. (2004). *Fundamentals of nursing: Concepts, process, and practice* (7th ed.). Upper Saddle River, NJ: Pearson Education, p. 906.

5 **Answer: 1** The anesthetic agent is injected into the subarachnoid space for spinal anesthesia and into the epidural space (which is outside the dura mater) in epidural anesthesia. Regional anesthesia can include local or topical anesthesia or nerve blocks and do not require clients to have sedation or produce amnesia.
Cognitive Level: Application **Client Need:** Physiological Integrity: Pharmacological and Parenteral Therapies **Integrated Process:** Teaching/Learning **Content Area:** Fundamentals **Strategy:** Recall information about the basic types of regional anesthesia and use the process of elimination to make a selection. **Reference:** Kozier, B., Erb, G., Berman, A., & Snyder, S. J. (2004). *Fundamentals of nursing: Concepts, process, and practice* (7th ed.). Upper Saddle River, NJ: Pearson Education, p. 910.

6 **Answer: 1** Option 1 is the correct answer as in this position, gravity keeps the tongue forward, which prevents aspiration. A pillow would elevate the head (option 2); the semiprone position is unsafe in most cases as it may interfere with breathing (option 3). A dorsal recumbent position (option 4) does not protect the client from risk of aspiration because secretions could pool at the back of the throat.
Cognitive Level: Application **Client Need:** Physiological Integrity: Reduction of Risk Potential **Integrated Process:** Nursing Process: Implementation **Content Area:** Fundamentals **Strategy:** The critical words are *immediate postanesthesia stage*. Recall interventions for airway maintenance in the postanesthesia period to enable you to provide safe care for this client. **Reference:** Kozier, B., Erb, G., Berman, A., & Snyder, S. J. (2004). *Fundamentals of nursing: Concepts, process, and practice* (7th ed.). Upper Saddle River, NJ: Pearson Education, p. 912.

7 **Answer: 3** Excessive bloody drainage on dressings or the bedclothes often underneath (because of gravity) the client indicates hemorrhage. This technique would not be useful in determining tube drainage, fluid balance in the general sense, or perspiration.
Cognitive Level: Application **Client Need:** Physiological Integrity: Reduction of Risk Potential **Integrated Process:** Nursing Process: Assessment **Content Area:** Fundamentals **Strategy:** The critical phrase is *underneath the client*. Recall that gravity will cause blood from a wound to travel to the lowest point, which is generally beneath the client. **Reference:** Kozier, B., Erb, G., Berman, A., & Snyder, S. J. (2004). *Fundamentals of nursing: Concepts, process, and practice* (7th ed.). Upper Saddle River, NJ: Pearson Education, p. 913.

8 **Answer: 2** Option 2 is the correct answer as the client is unable to retain the information and therefore has a deficiency in knowledge base. Self-care deficit is incorrect as there is no indication of inability to perform self-care activities such as bathing and eating. Options 3 and 4 (coping and injury) are definitely incorrect.
Cognitive Level: Application **Client Need:** Physiological Integrity: Reduction of Risk Potential **Integrated Process:** Teaching/Learning **Content Area:** Fundamentals **Strategy:** The critical term is *difficulty understanding*. Select the nursing diagnosis that focuses on a learning need. **Reference:** Kozier, B., Erb, G., Berman, A., & Snyder, S. J. (2004). *Fundamentals of nursing: Concepts, process, and practice* (7th ed.). Upper Saddle River, NJ: Pearson Education, pp. 914., 920

9 **Answer: 1** Placement of surgical drains will allow for drainage of excessive fluid or possibly purulent material that may have accumulated during the surgery. Healing is promoted, but not necessarily at a rapid rate (option 2), and not all drains have to be shortened (option 3) or connected to suction (option 4).
Cognitive Level: Analysis **Client Need:** Physiological Integrity: Reduction of Risk Potential **Integrated Process:** Teaching/Learning **Strategy:** The critical phrase is *explains drains*. Recall the uses of surgical site wound drains and use the process of elimination to make a selection. **Reference:** Kozier, B., Erb, G., Berman, A., & Snyder, S. J. (2004). *Fundamentals of nursing: Concepts, process, and practice* (7th ed.). Upper Saddle River, NJ: Pearson Education, p. 928.

10 **Answer: 2** Option 2 could indicate wound infection. All other options indicate normal wound healing or characteristics.
Cognitive Level: Analysis **Client Need:** Physiological Integrity: Reduction of Risk Potential **Integrated Process:** Teaching/Learning **Content Area:** Fundamentals **Strategy:** The core issue of the question is knowledge of which

postoperative findings warrant notification of the surgeon. Recall basic nursing knowledge about postoperative care and teaching and use the process of elimination to make a selection. **Reference:** Kozier, B., Erb, G., Berman, A., & Snyder, S. J. (2004). *Fundamentals of nursing: Concepts, process, and practice* (7th ed.). Upper Saddle River, NJ: Pearson Education, p. 930.)

References

Association of PeriOperative Registered Nurses (AORN) (2006). *Standards, recommended practices and guidelines.* Denver: AORN, Inc.

Ball, J. & Bindler, R. (2006). *Child health nursing: Caring for children* and families (3rd ed.). Upper Saddle River, NJ: Pearson Education.

Berman, A. J., Snyder, S., Kozier, B. & Erb, G. (2008). *Fundamentals of nursing: Concepts, process, and practice* (8th ed.). Upper Saddler River, NJ: Pearson Education, pp. 939–977.

Harkreader, H. & Hogan, M. (2007). *Fundamentals of nursing: Caring and Clinical Judgment* (3rd ed.). St. Louis, MO: Elsevier Science, pp. 1271–1312.

LeMone, P. & Burke, K. (2008). *Medical surgical nursing: Critical thinking in client care* (4th ed.). Upper Saddle River, NJ: Pearson Education.

Potter, P. & Perry, A. (2005). *Fundamentals of Nursing* (6th ed.). St. Louis, MO: Mosby., pp. 1593–1644.

ANSWERS & RATIONALES

Meeting the Needs of the Client with Altered Skin Integrity, Sensory Perception, or Mobility

10

Chapter Outline
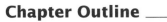

Skin Integrity and Wound Care

Alterations in Sensory/Perceptual Ability

Altered Mobility

Objectives

➤ Classify types of wounds and the products used to promote skin integrity.

➤ Define the elements associated with alterations in sensory perception.

➤ Identify methods the nurse can use to promote self-care and safety for clients with sensory perception deficits.

➤ List common causes and complications of immobility.

➤ Discuss the purpose and types of exercise for individuals with mobility problems.

➤ Describe the correct and safe use of assistive devices that facilitate ambulation.

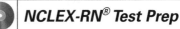

NCLEX-RN® Test Prep

Use the CD-ROM enclosed with this book to access additional practice opportunities.

Review at a Glance

conductive hearing loss interrupted transmission of sound through ear

debridement removal of dead necrotic tissue from a wound

dehiscence an unintentional opening of a wound

evisceration bursting open of a suture line with protrusion of organs

hyperopia farsightedness

keloid scar tissue

myopia nearsightedness

orthostatic intolerance also called postural hypotension, a drop in blood pressure caused by a change in position that may be accompanied by dizziness or vertigo; the client should change positions slowly

presbycusis loss of hearing related to aging process

presbyopia loss of elasticity of the lens of the eye

primary intention healing of a wound without infection or scarring; wound edges are well approximated

pressure ulcers lesions involving the skin and underlying tissues caused by inadequate blood supply secondary to unrelieved pressure

purulent exudate wound drainage containing pus

secondary intention wound healing by granulation or indirect union; edges are widely separated and granulation tissue fills in between the edges

sensory deprivation lack of stimuli that is meaningful

sensory overload bombardment of an individual by stimuli that have no meaning to that person

wound a break in the skin or mucous membrane resulting from physical means

PRETEST

1 The nurse assessing a bedridden client notes a large erythemic area on the client's buttocks. In addition, the center of the area looks like an abrasion with a shallow crater. The nurse would document this ulcer as being at which stage?

1. Stage I
2. Stage II
3. Stage III
4. Stage IV

2 A client was assessed to have a Stage I pressure ulcer on his hip despite every 2-hour turning and positioning. The nurse formulates which of the following as the appropriate nursing diagnosis for this client?

1. Impaired skin integrity related to infrequent turning and positioning
2. Impaired skin integrity related to the effects of pressure
3. High risk for impaired skin integrity related to redness
4. Risk for pressure ulcer

3 The client is postoperative for an abdominal surgical procedure. In assessing the abdominal suture line, which characteristics would indicate to the nurse a possible delay in wound healing?

1. Suture line clean and dry
2. Incision healing by primary intention
3. Purulent drainage on dressing
4. Sanguineous drainage in the wound collection device

4 A nurse is working in a geriatric screening clinic. The nurse expects that the skin of a normal elderly client will have which of the following characteristics? Select all that apply.

1. Appearance of being tight and shiny with edema in distal legs
2. Moist with elastic skin turgor
3. Skin turgor showing a loss of elasticity
4. Overhydration causing the skin to wrinkle
5. Fragile skin that is wrinkled

5 A hospitalized client exhibits all of the following symptoms: excessive yawning, drowsiness, impaired memory, crying, and depression. The nurse would suspect which of the following problems?

1. Sensory deprivation
2. Sensory overload
3. Visual deficit
4. Auditory deficit

6 In planning nursing care to prevent pressure ulcers in the bedridden client, the nurse should include which of the following interventions?

1. Slide the client when turning.
2. Turn and position the client b.i.d.
3. Vigorously massage bony prominences.
4. Post a turning schedule at the client's bedside.

7 A nurse preceptor overhears a group of student nurses discussing techniques for dressing changes. The nurse concludes that the student who needs to review the skill is the one who makes which of the following statements?

1. "I will clean the wound from the center out."
2. "To remove the used dressing, I should wear sterile gloves."
3. "After I clean the wound, I should do my assessments."
4. "While irrigating the wound, I can use a catheter, which is placed close to the open area."

8 A client with a hearing impairment is admitted to a busy hospital unit. Which intervention is most important for the nurse to employ to meet the client's needs while preventing sensory overload?

1. Allow all of the client's family members to stay with the client as much as possible.
2. Address the client directly and face the client during the conversation.
3. Keep the television or radio on for the client continuously.
4. Keep the overhead light on at all times.

9 A 78-year-old visually impaired client is admitted to the nursing unit. Which of the following interventions selected by the nurse would be most appropriate in reducing sensory deprivation?

1. Partially close window shades to reduce glare.
2. Keep doors open to provide bright light in the room.
3. Keep curtains or shades open to allow the sun to shine brightly in the room.
4. Keep lights in the room dimmed.

10 A client uses a cane to assist with ambulation. After teaching the client how to use a cane, the client makes the following statements. Which one indicates to the nurse the need for additional teaching?

1. "My elbow should be slightly flexed while using the cane."
2. "I should hold the cane on my weaker side."
3. "A walker would be more difficult to use than a cane."
4. "While walking here in the hospital, socks alone may cause me to slip."

➤ *See pages 280–281 for Answers & Rationales.*

I. SKIN INTEGRITY AND WOUND CARE

A. Normal skin integrity

1. The skin is the largest organ in the body

2. Five functions of skin

   a. It is the body's first line of defense against microorganisms; as such, it serves as a barrier preventing invasion by microorganisms; this function is interrupted if the skin is not intact

   b. It regulates the body temperature

   c. It is a sense organ transmitting the sensations of pain, temperature, touch, and pressure

   d. It produces and absorbs vitamin D

   e. It secretes sebum that has several functions, including softening and lubricating the skin and hair

3. Layers of skin vary in thickness but in places can be as thick as ¼ inch; the skin can be divided into the layers of epidermis and dermis; beneath the dermis is a subcutaneous layer of tissue

    a. Epidermis: the outermost layer of skin made of stratified squamous epithelial cells; the epidermis can be further divided into five layers, the innermost of which is the basal-cell layer, the cells responsible for replacing sloughed and damaged cells

    b. Dermis: the second layer of skin composed of connective tissue; is the layer that gives elasticity to the skin; blood vessels, nerve fibers, glands, and hair follicles are embedded in this layer of skin

    c. Subcutaneous tissue: consists of adipose tissue and provides support and blood flow to the dermis

4. Skin glands: the skin has three kinds of glands, sebaceous glands, soporiferous glands, and cerumenous glands

    a. Sebaceous glands are within the dermis; they secrete an oily substance called sebum, made up of fats, cholesterol, proteins, and salts; sebum protects hair from drying, forms a protective film on the skin that prevents excessive evaporation of water, and inhibits the growth of certain bacteria on the skin

    b. Sudoriferous glands (sweat glands) produce a watery secretion; the body has up to 5 million sweat glands which are present at birth; there are two types: apocrine and eccrine

        1) Apocrine glands are primarily in the axilla and pubic regions and begin functioning at puberty; the secretions are odorous because, when decomposed by bacteria, they produce an unpleasant odor

        2) Eccrine glands are distributed throughout the skin; they are chiefly found on the palms of the hands, soles of the feet, and forehead; they produce a watery discharge to help cool the body through evaporation

    c. Ceruminous glands secrete a thick, oily substance called cerumen, a waxy secretion of the external ear (also known as earwax)

5. Skin alterations related to aging: overall health status, age, nutritional status, and energy/activity level play a role in maintaining a client's skin condition; problems associated with skin alterations in the elderly include:

    a. The epidermis thins and has a lower water content, leading to dry skin

    b. Elasticity and some of the fatty cushion is lost, resulting in wrinkles and fragile skin

    c. Blood vessels in the skin also become more fragile with aging, leading to easy bruising

B. Classification of wounds: a wound is a break in the skin or mucous membrane resulting from physical means; a wound may be superficial (affecting only the surface of the skin) or deep (involving blood vessels, nerves, muscle, fascia, tendons, ligaments, and bones)

1. Open versus closed: is a classification of wounds according to the continuity of the surface it covers (tissue involved)

    a. An open wound is characterized by a break in the skin and could be superficial or deep; examples are an abrasion, laceration, or puncture

    b. A closed wound is one in which there is no break in the skin; examples are a contusion and ecchymosis; these injuries may be caused by a blow or another type of blunt force or trauma

2. Superficial and full and partial thickness refer to depth of the injury and are used most frequently to refer to burns

    a. Superficial thickness involves only the epidermis

      b. Partial thickness involves the entire epidermis and part of the dermis; sweat glands and hair follicles are intact

      c. Full thickness involves epidermis and dermis extending to the subcutaneous tissue, possibly even muscle and bone

  3. Noninfected versus infected wounds

      a. A noninfected or clean wound has not been invaded by pathogenic microorganisms; a clean wound heals without infection

      b. An infected wound or septic wound is one in which pathogenic microorganisms have invaded the wound and clinical signs and symptoms of infection develop

  4. Surgical wound: an intentional wound made by a surgeon for therapeutic purposes using a sharp cutting instrument; it is a clean wound that heals without infection

  5. **Pressure ulcers:** lesions caused by unrelieved pressure; this in turn damages underlying tissues

      a. Contributing factors

        1) Pressure ulcers occur mainly in people who are chair-bound, bed-bound, or have an altered level of consciousness (LOC) that causes them to be immobile

        2) Older adults are at greater risk for developing pressure ulcers because of the fragility of the skin

        3) Moisture on the skin from sweating or incontinence can lead to skin breakdown

        4) Malnutrition contributes because of reduced nutrient stores including protein for tissue repair

        5) Shearing pressures cause injury by contributing to tissue hypoxia; this often occurs when the head of the bed is elevated, when the skin remains stationary while the underlying tissues shift with the pull of gravity

        6) Friction that occurs when a client is moved in the bed contributes to tissue damage and can be a precursor to a pressure ulcer

        7) Contributing factors can be assessed to determine an individual client's relative risk using scales such as the Braden Scale or the Norton Scale (see Table 10-1)

      b. Four stages of pressure ulcers

        1) Stage I: the skin is intact, although nonblanching erythema will be noted; blanching is done by applying and quickly releasing pressure to an area to determine color changes of the skin; nonblanching erythema shows no color change, while blanching erythema is a reddened area that turns white or pale when blanched; the client may report tingling or burning; darker-skinned clients may have skin discoloration, warmth, edema, and induration or hardness as indicators

        2) Stage II: involves superficial or partial-thickness skin loss with blister or abrasion-like appearance; it may also look like a shallow crater

        3) Stage III: full-thickness skin loss; necrotic tissue will be seen in the subcutaneous layer that extends down to (but not through) underlying fascia; the ulcer will appear as a deeper crater with or without undermining of surrounding tissue

        4) Stage IV: continuation of Stage III with damage to muscle, bone, and supporting structures such as tendons or joint capsule; undermining of tissue and sinus tracts may also be present

Table 10-1	Pressure Ulcer Risk Assessment Scales

Norton Scale

Physical Condition		Mental Condition		Activity		Mobility		Continence	
Good	4	Alert	4	Walks	4	Full	4	Good	4
Fair	3	Apathetic	3	Walks with help	3	Slightly limited	3	Occasional incontinence	3
Poor	2	Confused	2	Sits in chair	2	Very limited	2	Frequent incontinence	2
Very poor	1	Stuporous	1	Remains in bed	1	Immobile	1	Urine and fecal incontinence	1
Total ____		Total ____		Total ____		Total ____		Total ____	

Grand total = _____

A score of 14 or less indicates risk of pressure ulcer; a score under 12 indicates high risk.

Braden Scale

Sensory Perception		Moisture		Activity		Mobility		Nutrition		Friction and Shear	
No impairment	4	Rarely moist	4	Walks frequently	4	No limitations	4	Excellent	4		
Slightly limited	3	Occasionally moist	3	Walks occasionally	3	Slightly limited	3	Adequate	3	No apparent problems	3
Very limited	2	Moist	2	Chairfast	2	Very limited	2	Probably inadequate	2	Potential problem	2
Completely limited	1	Constantly moist	1	Bedfast	1	Immobile	1	Very poor	1	Problem	1
Total ____		Total ____		Total ____		Total ____		Total ____		Total ____	

Grand total = _____

Assign a score of 1 to 4 in each category. Total the score; no risk: 19–23; at risk: 15–18; moderate risk: 13–14; high risk: 10–12; very high risk: 9 or below.

Source: Smith, S., Duell, D., & Martin, B. (2004). *Clinical nursing skills: Basic to advanced skills* (6th ed.). Upper Saddle River, NJ: Prentice Hall, p. 853.

C. Wound healing

1. The process of wound healing can be divided into three phases

   a. Inflammatory phase: occurs immediately after injury and lasts 3 to 4 days; a blood clot forms a fibrin matrix, which becomes the framework for cell repair; the wound surface dries out, forming a scab that seals the skin; blood flow increases to the area, bringing oxygen and nutrients for healing; phagocytosis occurs to remove microorganisms and cellular debris

   b. Proliferative phase: fibroblasts synthesize collagen to add tensile strength to the wound and deposit fibrin as this phase occurs (4 to 21 days), granulation tissue forms and is very friable, soft, and pinkish red in color because of the new capillaries in the area; next epithelial cells grow from the edges to cover the wound; connective tissue then fills the area and becomes a scar that is stronger than granulation tissue; when the wound is extensive and cannot close by epithelialization, the area becomes covered with eschar, consisting of dead cells and dried plasma proteins

    c. Maturation or remodeling phase is the healing of the scar; this phase often occurs by day 21, but can extend for 1 to 2 years after the injury; this phase is characterized by reorganization of collagen fibers, wound remodeling and contraction, and tissue maturation; a fully healed wound has tensile strength that still will not exceed 80% of the preinjury state, making it more susceptible to injury in the future; in some clients (particularly those with dark skin), an abnormal amount of collagen is laid down, forming a hypertrophic scar called a **keloid**

2. Factors affecting wound healing include age, nutrition, condition of the tissue, efficiency of circulation, medication, and the relationship between rest and anxiety or stress

    a. Age: healthy children and adults heal faster than the older client; see Box 10-1 for factors that inhibit healing in older adults

    b. Nutrition: good physiological functioning is essential for wound healing; protein is needed to build new tissue and vitamin C for the maturation of fibrous tissue; vitamin C also enhances protein synthesis; overall nutrition also affects healing; undernourished clients may lack adequate body stores to utilize as nutrients, while obese clients tend to have decreased blood flow to the tissue and have a greater risk of developing infection

    c. Condition of the tissues: wound contamination and infection will slow down the healing process; organisms present in the wound will compete with body cells for oxygen and nutrition

    d. Efficiency of circulation: any factor that restricts blood supply to a wound will interfere with healing; the blood transports the products used in healing; therefore factors such as damaged arteries, tissue edema, and dehydration impede healing; anemia and blood dyscrasias may interfere with oxygen reaching the tissue; conditions such as diabetes and liver dysfunction can also delay healing; individuals who participate in regular exercise tend to have better circulation and thus tend to heal faster; smoking is a risk factor that may limit the amount of oxygen the blood can supply to tissues

Box 10-1	
Factors Inhibiting Wound Healing in Older Adults	➤ Vascular changes associated with aging, such as atherosclerosis and atrophy of capillaries in the skin, can impair blood flow to the wound.
	➤ Collagen tissue is less flexible, which increases the risk of damage from pressure, friction, and shearing.
	➤ Scar tissue is less elastic.
	➤ Changes in the immune system may reduce the formation of antibodies and monocytes necessary for wound healing.
	➤ Nutritional deficiencies may reduce the numbers of red blood cells and leukocytes, thus impeding the delivery of oxygen and the inflammatory response essential for wound healing. Oxygen is needed for the synthesis of collagen and the formation of new epithelial cells.
	➤ Having diabetes or cardiovascular disease increases the risk of delayed healing due to impaired oxygen delivery to these tissues.
	➤ Cell renewal is slower, leading to delayed healing.

Source: Berman, A., Snyder, S., Kozier, B. & Erb, G., (2008). *Fundamentals of nursing: Concepts, process, and practice* (8th ed.). Upper Saddle River, NJ: Pearson Education, p. 912.

    e. Rest, anxiety, and stress: adequate rest of the injured part will affect the wound closure; anxiety and stress can stimulate the release of hormones that will slow down healing; it is important that the client with a wound take measures to ensure adequate rest and reduce stress whenever possible

    f. Medications: anti-inflammatory drugs such as steroids or hormones slow down the formation of fibrous tissue and therefore impair healing

3. Wound closures: wound healing can be a natural function as occurs with primary and secondary union or as the result of surgical intervention in the nature of sutures and clips

    a. The first type of healing is **primary intention,** characterized by the return of the tissues to normal with minimal inflammation and little if any scarring; wound edges are well approximated and the wound heals without infection

    b. **Secondary intention** healing occurs when the wound is extensive, and wound edges cannot or should not be approximated; there is greater injury and more granulation tissue is needed to close the wound; healing by secondary intention is different from primary intention in a variety of ways: the healing time is more prolonged, there is a deeper, more extensive scar, and the risk for infection is greater since the first line of defense is broken for an extended period

    c. Surgical interventions: sutures, staples, and clips are devices used to help approximate the edges of the wound; sutures are threads used to sew tissues together; a variety of materials may be utilized, some that absorb and others that have to be removed; staples and clips are alternatives to suturing and are usually made of silver; these require removal in approximately 7 to 10 days

4. Complications that affect wound healing

    a. Hemorrhage: after tissue damage occurs (from pressure, surgery, or trauma) bleeding usually results; this may result from rupture of small blood vessels or from trauma; internal hemorrhage may be noted by distention in the area of the wound; external hemorrhage is noted by blood on the dressing or leaking from the dressing; if bleeding is severe the client may exhibit signs and symptoms of shock; the risk of hemorrhage is greater within the first 48 hours; if pressure dressings do not successfully stop the bleeding, surgical intervention may be necessary

    b. Infection results from pathogenic microorganisms invading the wound; local clinical signs and symptoms of infection include redness, swelling, heat, and pain at the site; **purulent exudate** (consisting of leukocytes, liquefied dead tissue debris, and dead and living bacteria) may be noted; the client may be anorexic, nauseous, febrile, and have chills (systemic signs of infection); the physician will order a wound culture and antibiotics will be administered after the culture is obtained

    c. **Dehiscence** occurs when a wound's suture line accidently reopens; it usually involves an abdominal wound, but any wound could have this complication; layers of tissue under the wound separate; this may occur because of an infected suture line or if the client has any factor previously discussed that impedes wound healing; clients often state they "feel something giving way;" when dehiscence occurs, place the client in bed with head of bed low to eliminate gravity and with the knees bent to decrease pull on the suture line; cover the wound bed with large sterile dressings moistened with normal saline; notify the surgeon immediately since surgical repair is necessary

       d. Eviceration occurs when the edges of a suture line separate and the internal organs (viscera) protrude through the incision; a number of factors contribute to this complication including infection, poor nutrition, failure of suture material, dehydration, and excessive coughing; evisceration is treated in a manner similar to dehiscence

Practice to Pass

The nurse is caring for a client who is 1 week postop from abdominal surgery. What would the nurse expect assessment of this wound to reveal?

D. Wound management therapies

1. Physicians and certified wound care nurse consultants may choose a variety of therapies to treat wounds

2. The decision to apply or not to apply a dressing is based on several factors including the location, size, and type of wound along with the amount of exudate and the presence or absence of infection; dressed and undressed wounds may require cleansing and irrigation to aid healing

E. Wound assessment

1. Inspect the wound and gently palpate the surrounding area regularly

2. Note whether wound edges are approximated; as an incision heals, a healing ridge may be noted

3. Note the presence and characteristics of any drainage from the wound

4. Observe for signs of infection: redness, swelling, increased tenderness, or disruption of wound edges; note body temperature and white blood cell count as other indicators

5. Purposes for dressing a wound

    a. Absorb drainage

    b. Splint or immobilize the wound to provide rest

    c. Protect the wound from mechanical injury

    d. Promote hemostasis

    e. Prevent contamination

    f. For the mental and physical comfort of the client

6. Purposes for maintaining a wound undressed

    a. Eliminate darkness and moisture that favor growth of microorganisms

    b. Allow for better observation and assessment of the wound

    c. Facilitate bathing and hygiene

    d. Avoid adhesive tape reaction

    e. Avoid the friction and irritation that destroy new epithelial cells

7. Wound irrigation: may be needed to cleanse or flush the wound to enhance healing; normal saline and antibiotic solutions are the solutions frequently used (see Box 10-2 for information on irrigating a wound)

F. Wound management products

1. Wound cleansers: all wounds need to be cleansed appropriately; in clean wounds where the tissue is granulating, minimize any disruption of the wound bed; the method used to clean the wound should be gentle cleansing and rinsing away of debris with normal saline (see Box 10-3 for wound cleaning clinical guidelines)

2. Dressings: a variety of dressing materials are available, each with different purposes; some are designed to provide barrier protection from contamination;

Box 10-2	**Irrigating a Wound**

Purposes

➤ To clean the area

➤ To apply heat and hasten the healing process

➤ To apply an antimicrobial solution

Assessment

Appearance and size of the wound; the character of the exudate; presence of pain and the time of the last pain medication; clinical signs of systemic infection; allergies to the wound irrigation agent or tape

Planning

Before irrigating a wound, determine (a) the type of irrigating solution to be used, (b) the frequency of irrigations, and (c) the temperature of the solution

Equipment

☐ Sterile dressing eqiupment and dressing materials

☐ Sterile irrigating syringes (e.g., a 30- to 60-mL piston syringe) with a catheter of an appropriate size (e.g., #18 or #19) or an irrigating (catheter) tip syringe

☐ Sterile graduated cylinder for the irrigating solution

☐ Moistureproof bag

☐ Sterile basin to receive the irrigation returns

☐ Irrigating solution, usually 200 mL (6.5 oz) of solution warmed to body temperature, according to the agency's

or primary care provider's choice

☐ Clean disposable gloves

☐ Sterile gloves

☐ Moistureproof sterile drape

Intervention

1. General preparation

➤ Verify physician order and client identity.

➤ Explain procedure to client.

➤ Perform hand hygiene.

➤ Ensure irrigating fluid is at correct temperature.

2. Prepare the client

➤ Assist the client to a position in which the irrigating solution will flow by gravity from the upper end of the wound to the lower end and then into the basin.

➤ Place the waterproof drape over the client and the bed.

➤ Put on clean gloves and remove and discard the old dressing.

➤ If indicated, clean from the center of the wound outward, using circular strokes.

➤ Use a separate swab for each stroke, and discard each swab after use.

➤ Assess the wound and drainage.

➤ Remove and discard clean gloves.

3. Prepare the equipment

➤ Open the sterile dressing set and supplies.

➤ Pour the ordered solution into the solution container.

➤ Put on sterile gloves.

➤ Position the sterile basin below the wound to receive the irrigating fluid.

4. Irrigate the wound

➤ Instill a steady stream of irrigating solution into the wound; make sure all areas of the wound are irrigated.

➤ Use either a syringe with a catheter attached or with an irrigating tip to flush the wound.

➤ If you are using a catheter, insert the catheter into the wound until resistence is met; do not force the catheter.

➤ Continue irrigating until the solution becomes clear (no exudate is present).

➤ Dry the area around the wound.

5. Assess and dress the wound

➤ Assess the appearance of the wound, noting in particular the type and amount of exudate and the presence and extent of granulation tissue.

➤ Using sterile technique, apply a dressing to the wound based on the amount of drainage expected.

6. Document all relevant information

➤ Document the irrigation and client response in the client record using forms or checklists supplemented by narrative notes any when appropriate.

Evaluation

Perform followup based on findings that deviate from expected or normal for client. Relate findings to previous assessment if available. Report significant findings to primary care provider.

Condensed from Berman, A., Snyder, S. Kozier, B., Erb, G., (2008). *Fundamentals of nursing: Concepts, process, and practice* (8th ed.). Upper Saddle River, NJ: Prentice Hall, pp. 925–926.

some may be impregnated with antibiotics; others are moist and aid in liquefying necrotic tissue; dressing types include:

a. Gauze dressing: plain or impregnated with an anti-microbial; this dressing packs and fills the wound; it absorbs drainage; gauze dressings are used for full- and partial-thickness wounds with drainage; may be applied dry to cover wound or as damp–to–damp dressing to pack a wound requiring debridement

b. Transparent dressing: adhesive membrane that is occlusive to liquids and bacteria; protects the wound and promotes autolytic **debridement** (the removal of dead tissue from a wound); Op-site™ and Tegaderm™ are examples; transparent dressings are impermeable to bacteria

c. Composite dressing: contains an absorbent pad and an adhesive covering; purpose is to absorb drainage; the advantage of this type of wound coverage is that it only has to be changed three times per week

d. Hydrocolloids: adhesive made of gelatin; Duoderm™ and Tegasorb™ are examples; this dressing is occlusive to microorganisms and liquids and promotes absorption of wound exudates; autolysis of necrotic tissue within the wound bed is enhanced

e. Hydrogel: water or glycerin is the primary component of this nonadherent dressing; the hydrogel maintains a moist wound surface and provides some absorption; these products are permeable to oxygen and can fill dead spaces in a wound; a secondary nonadhesive dressing may be required

---

Box 10-3	➤ Follow standard precautions for personal protection. Wear gloves, gown, goggles, and mask as indicated.
Clinical Guidelines for Cleaning Wounds	➤ Use solutions such as isotonic saline or wound cleansers, to clean or irrigate wounds. If antimicrobial solutions are used, make sure they are well diluted.

➤ Microwave heating is not recommended. When possible, warm the solution to body temperature before use. This prevents lowering of the wound temperature, which slows the healing process. Microwave heating could cause the solution to be too hot.

➤ If a wound is grossly contaminated by foreign material, bacteria, slough, or necrotic tissue, clean the wound at every dressing change. Foreign bodies and devitalized tissue act as a focus for infection and can delay healing.

➤ If a wound is clean, has little exudate, and reveals healthy granulation tissue, avoid repeated cleaning. Unnecessary cleaning can delay wound healing by traumatizing newly produced, delicate tissues, reducing the surface temperature of the wound, and removing exudate which itself may have bactericidal properties.

➤ Use gauze squares. Avoid using cotton balls and other products that shed fibers onto the wound surface. The fibers become embedded in granulation tissue and can act as foci for infection. They may also stimulate "foreign body" reactions, prolonging the inflammatory phase of healing and delaying the healing process.

➤ Clean superficial noninfected wounds by irrigating them with normal saline. The hydraulic pressure of an irrigating stream of fluid dislodges contaminating debris and reduces bacterial colonization.

➤ To retain wound moisture, avoid drying a wound after cleaning it.

➤ Hold cleaning sponges with forceps or with a sterile gloved hand.

➤ Clean from the center of the wound in an outward direction to avoid transferring organisms from the surrounding skin into the wound.

➤ Consider not cleaning the wound at all if it appears to be clean.

Source: Berman, A., Snyder, S. Kozier, B., & Erb, G., (2008). *Fundamentals of nursing: Concepts, process, and practice* (8th ed.). Upper Saddle River, NJ: Prentice Hall, p. 925.

    f. Calcium alginates: a pad made of seaweed fibers; the purpose of this dressing is to absorb larger amounts of drainage

    g. Exudate absorbers, also called polyurethane foam: semipermeable polyurethane foam dressings that absorb large amounts of exudate while keeping the wound moist; these dressings are nonadherent

    h. Absorptive or filler dressings: have the ability to absorb moderate amounts of drainage; Duo-Derm™ paste is an example

3. Bandages are strips of cloth used to wrap a body part

    a. Bandages are made of gauze, which is light and porous, or of an elasticized material, which provides pressure to the area

    b. Widths of bandages vary from 1 to 4 inches and are determined by the part of body to be wrapped

    c. Purposes include to anchor dressings, provide support to a body part, immobilize a body part, or to promote circulatory return

    d. Guidelines for bandaging

        1) Bandage with the body part in a normal or functional position

        2) Pad bony prominences

        3) Bandage from distal to proximal area to support blood return

        4) Use even pressure while applying bandage; this is especially important when using elastic bandages that could impair circulation

        5) Inspect and palpate the area regularly; assess a fresher wound more frequently and an older wound less frequently; note the presence of drainage from the wound; assess neurovascular status of the extremity including temperature, blanching, and sensation; assess for pain and evaluate its cause

4. Enzymatic debriding agents: an enzyme paste or solution that is applied to necrotic tissue; the enzyme digests necrotic tissue; e.g., Elase

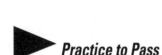

Practice to Pass

A 72-year-old client is admitted with a Stage I pressure ulcer on his sacrum. What wound care should the nurse provide for this client?

II. ALTERATIONS IN SENSORY PERCEPTUAL NEEDS

A. Factors affecting sensation/perception

1. Numerous factors affect sensory function; these include illness, developmental stage, medications, stress, and lifestyle

2. Illness may result in hospitalization; this change of environment may have an effect on mentation, especially for the older client; this could be the result of the underlying disease process or simply a change in the physical environment

3. Developmental stage affects sensory perception; infants have adequate sensory organs but have no mental concepts to understand sensory input; as development occurs, the individual develops understanding of sensory input; adults have many learned responses to sensory cues; with aging, sensory input diminishes because of decreased sense organ functioning

4. Medications can affect both sensory function and sensory awareness; many drugs are known to decrease the LOC; others contribute to mental confusion; in the older adult, polypharmacy may lead to drug interactions that result in decreased sensory functioning

5. Stress can be described as eustress or distress

    a. Eustress is the stress that stimulates the individual functioning; an example is a student who wants to do well on an exam, and stress encourages the student to study and score well on the exam

      b. Distress is the presence of more stress that depresses the individual functioning; anxiety tends to limit the amount of sensory input a client can deal with effectively; if the student in the above scenario had test anxiety, the student may be unable to score well on the exam

      c. Illness and hospitalization can both cause distress; today, hospitals have made great efforts to create an aesthetic environment more conducive to healing, such as bright and cheerful walls that are hung with beautiful pictures, floors that may be carpeted, and an overall attempt to create a pleasant "home-like" environment

  6. Lifestyle influences sensory perception; one individual may thrive in a stimulating environment that may overwhelm others

B. Sensory perceptual alterations

  1. Identified factors that contribute to alterations in the client's behavior include, but are not limited to, sensory deprivation, sensory overload, and sensory deficits

  2. **Sensory deprivation** is defined as a lack of meaningful stimuli; the actual amount of incoming stimuli is reduced because of either a decrease of environmental stimuli or impairment in one or more of the client's senses; decreased sensory input can lead to disorientation over a period of time

      a. If the client cannot derive meaning from the environment, this can lead to sensory deprivation; an example is a blind client who is admitted to the hospital; the environment for this client has changed drastically because landmarks that were present at home are gone

      b. Changes in any kind of sensory input could lead to deprivation; an example is a person who has a visual impairment and loss of tactile perception as a result of a neurological illness; sensory deprivation can then lead to distortions in perception, which may then affect the client's ability to perceive his environment correctly

      c. Risk factors that may lead to sensory deprivation include dysfunction of the senses; medications, immobility, isolation, and language barriers can also contribute

      d. See Box 10-4 for clinical signs and symptoms of sensory deprivation

      e. Hospital rooms now have clocks, calendars, and possibly boards that identify the names of caregivers on that shift, all of which provide meaningful stimuli to the hospitalized client and promote orientation to surroundings

Box 10-4	➤ Excessive yawning, drowsiness, sleeping
Clinical Signs of Sensory Deprivation	➤ Decreased attention span, difficulty concentrating, decreased problem solving
	➤ Impaired memory
	➤ Periodic disorientation, general confusion, or nocturnal confusion
	➤ Preoccupation with somatic complaints, such as palpitations
	➤ Hallucinations or delusions
	➤ Crying, annoyance over small matters, depression
	➤ Apathy, emotional liability

Source: Berman, A., Snyder, S., Kozier, B. & Erb, G. (2008). *Fundamentals of nursing: Concepts, process, and practice* (8th ed.). Upper Saddle River, NJ: Prentice Hall, p. 982.

3. **Sensory overload** is defined as an increase in the intensity of stimuli to levels beyond normal; it generally occurs when a person is unable to process the amount or intensity of stimuli and with exposure to numerous stimuli that are not meaningful

   a. Two factors contribute to sensory overload

      1) Increased quantity of internal stimuli as in anxiety

      2) Increased quantity of external stimuli in the environment such as noise, equipment, multiple healthcare personnel

   b. Sensory overload leads to sleep deprivation, which adds to the deterioration of the individual's coping abilities; when overloaded with sensory stimuli, the client may feel that he or she is not in control; assess the environment and recognize that sights and sounds familiar to the healthcare worker may add to the overload for the client

   c. Contributing factors that add to overload could be pain, anxiety, and lack of sleep

   d. Clinical signs and symptoms of sensory overload include increased muscle tension, fatigue and inability to sleep, irritability and restlessness, inability to concentrate, and decreased problem-solving performance

   e. Sensory overload is frequently experienced by the client in the intensive care unit (ICU)

      1) This syndrome was recognized in the 1960s and was named ICU psychosis

      2) It was noted that clients in the ICU experienced confusion, disorientation, and memory loss after 2 to 3 days in the ICU

      3) ICU syndrome served as the motivation behind changes in the hospital environment; ICU and other units now have calendars, clocks, windows, and television; ICU rooms are now private rooms, and to help maintain client orientation, timing of care activities may be arranged to allow for a more natural sleep cycle (see Chapter 7)

4. **Sensory deficit:** is impairment of both reception and perception of one or more of the senses; when the loss of sensory function is gradual, the individual compensates for the loss; for instance, someone with impaired vision may decrease the area in which he or she travels alone

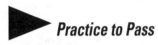

Practice to Pass

An elderly client is admitted to the nursing unit. What are some of the factors that will contribute to the sensory overload the client may experience?

C. **Common sensory deficits**

1. Visual: vision is an important sense because it allows people to interact with their environment

   a. People with visual impairment may wear glasses or contact lens to correct refraction errors of the lens of the eye

   b. Some of these refraction errors include

      1) **Myopia,** commonly called nearsightedness

      2) **Hyperopia,** or farsightedness

      3) **Presbyopia,** the loss of elasticity of the lens of the eye; as a result, there is a loss of ability to see objects that are close; presbyopia is the visual disturbance that occurs with aging, often beginning around the age of 45; bifocal glasses are often used to correct this problem

   c. Cataracts are another problem that occur with aging; they are often seen in clients over 65 years of age and occur when the lens of the eye becomes opaque; lens opacity blocks light rays and distorts and impairs the visual field; surgical removal is often required as the cataract progresses

d. Glaucoma: is a painless blockage in the circulation of aqueous fluid in the eye that leads to an increase in intraocular pressure and possibly blindness

        1) Signs of glaucoma can include blurry or foggy vision, loss of peripheral vision, difficulty adjusting to dark rooms

        2) This disease of the eye can be controlled using ophthalmic medications if diagnosed and treated early; therefore, screening is important

        3) Diabetic retinopathy: is the leading cause of blindness among adults from 20 to 70 years old; proliferative retinopathy or neurovascular disease occurs when ischemic retinal blood vessels bleed, causing vitreous hemorrhage; this hemorrhage can be repetitive and may lead to permanent visual loss

        4) Macular degeneration: refers to the degenerative changes in the layer of blood vessels that arise in the retina; macular blood vessels then leak and damage the macula; scarring occurs and visual loss results; signs and symptoms are blurring and distortion of visual images

2. Hearing: difficulty with hearing may make the client feel isolated; it can interfere with health teaching and even increase the risk of injury for a client

    a. **Conductive hearing loss** is the result of interrupted transmission of sound waves through the outer and middle ear; possible causes are a tear in the eardrum (tympanic membrane), obstruction in the auditory canal caused by swelling or other factors, degeneration of the hammer, anvil, and stirrup from infection, or continuous low sensory input

    b. Sensorineural hearing loss is the result of damage to the inner ear, the auditory nerve, or the hearing center in the brain from viral infection or ototoxic medications (whose names often end with *mycin*)

    c. **Presbycusis** is the loss of hearing ability related to aging; gradual loss of hearing is more common in men than women

3. Balance: with aging comes a gradual reduction of power and contraction of muscles; after age 50, there is a steady decrease in muscle fibers; often balance is impaired with this process as well; there may be degenerative joint changes making movement more restricted

4. Taste: the reduction in the ability to taste can affect appetite and contribute to poor nutrition; if a corresponding loss of the sense of smell occurs, the client's appetite will also not be stimulated by the aroma of the food

5. Smell: in addition to its effect on the client's appetite, loss of the sense of smell can be a safety issue; with the decrease in smell, the client will not be aware of a gas leak, for example, from the stove at home

6. Touch: tactile deprivation can occur from a disease or an injury that leads to destruction of or damage to nerve cells

    a. Children born with myelomeningocele have damage to the nerves below the level of the pathology; injuries that destroy the nerves will have the same effect; the loss of tactile ability may contribute to safety issues; a client who has suffered loss of sensation of a part of the body could easily be burned because the client cannot feel pain

    b. Peripheral neuropathy is a disease process that interferes with innervation of the peripheral nerves; with aging, diabetes, or arteriosclerosis, the overall effectiveness of blood vessels decreases; the body compensates by constricting superficial blood vessels to divert blood to larger blood vessels; with constriction of peripheral blood vessels, peripheral nerve endings in the area that are supplied by these blood vessels suffer the effects of decreased blood flow; as a result, neuropathy develops

c. Multisensory deficit conditions: some conditions lead to damage to more than one of the senses, such as strokes or "brain attack" resulting from either thrombus, embolus, or hemorrhage into an area of the brain; this process leads to ischemia in the area of the brain affected; the results may be decreased mobility, decreased sensation, and/or paresis or paralysis of the extremities, as well as aphasia, blindness, or other visual impairment, or impaired swallowing

D. Promoting self-care

1. Screening/prevention: early detection of sensory deprivation is an important health screening function

   a. Routine auditory testing is done at birth

   b. Periodic vision screening of all school-aged children is done

   c. Health fairs often provide a means to screen a large number of healthy people

   d. Be aware of disease processes that can lead to sensory deprivation and screen for symptoms; this can lead to early recognition of sensory problems

   e. Health measures should be taught to protect sensory organs; encourage protective eyewear and ear gear; emphasize, especially to teenagers, the risk of damage to the ears from loud noises or music

   f. Teach clients general health measures such as regular eye and ear exams

   g. The Occupational Safety and Health Administration (OSHA) provides regulations and guidelines to limit hazards affecting the senses to those in the workplace; OSHA guidelines are carefully followed in healthcare settings also

2. Assistive aids: assist clients who have a sensory deficit by encouraging the use of specific aids to support their sensory function; promote the use of the other senses and communicating effectively; and work to ensure the client's safety

   a. Visual and hearing aids are available to the client with visual and hearing deficits; these aids can be used in the hospital and home setting

   b. For clients with smell and taste deficits, supply diets that include a variety of flavors, temperatures, and textures that may then stimulate taste buds

   c. Each client with a sensory deficit should be evaluated to determine the appropriate assistive device

   d. Encourage clients to utilize the aids available and promote their use; for example, if a client who has limited mobility also wears glasses offer the client his or her eyeglasses upon awakening; see Box 10-5 for information on possible visual and auditory aids

3. Communication

   a. Communication is the exchange of information; the client with a sensory deficit is at risk for not accurately interpreting communication

   b. It is important to convey respect to the client and enhance his or her self-esteem

   c. A person with a hearing deficit needs to concentrate at all times during a conversation

   d. When speaking to a client with a hearing deficit, face the client and speak directly to him or her without large numbers of people around; too many people in the environment will be a distraction

   e. The client with visual deficits might misinterpret nonverbal clues during conversation

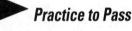

Practice to Pass

An 80-year-old client has a hearing impairment (presbycusis). What would be the nurse's best approach when communicating with this client to ensure client understanding?

Box 10-5	The nurse can help a client select aids that are appropriate for that client.	
Aids for Clients with Visual and Auditory Deficits	**For Clients with Visual Deficits**	**For Clients with Auditory Deficits**

For Clients with Visual Deficits

➤ Prescription eyeglasses

➤ Proper lighting in rooms and use of nightlights

➤ Shades on windows to reduce glare

➤ Large-print books

➤ Color-code or textured appliances and medicine containers

➤ Books on tape

➤ Seeing-eye dog

➤ Red-tipped cane or laser cane

➤ Magnifying glass

➤ Phone and clock with large numbers

For Clients with Auditory Deficits

➤ Hearing aids

➤ Closed caption for television

➤ Telephone with amplifiers

➤ Flashing alarms in the home for smoke detectors, doorbells, etc.

➤ Telecommunication device for the deaf (TDD) phone

➤ Telephone with light that flashes when ringing

➤ Vibrating or flashing alarm clock

➤ Wireless page, phone, and email service

f. See Box 10-6 for further information about communicating with clients who have visual or hearing deficits

III. ALTERED MOBILITY

A. Activity develops and maintains the proper functioning of the body

1. Inactivity can lead to physical deterioration; clients can have impaired mobility because of paralysis, hemiplegia, muscle weakness, poor balance or poor coordination, spinal cord injuries, or because they wear a cast

2. In general, any client who is weakened by illness or surgery will have some degree of impaired mobility

3. The musculoskeletal system is one of the body's largest systems and accounts for 50% of body weight; muscle strength peaks at age 25 to 30 and is maintained through the fifth decade; after the fifth decade the system decreases in its strength and becomes noticeably weaker after the seventies

B. Common causes of immobility

1. Common causes that place a client at risk for immobility are pain, motor function impairment, structural problems, generalized inactivity, psychological problems, and medically induced problems such as surgery (especially orthopedic surgery)

2. Pain: clients who are in pain will reduce spontaneous movement in an attempt to decrease the painful stimuli; pain will also cause the client to refuse to participate in rehabilitative activities including coughing and deep breathing

3. Motor and nervous system impairment: disorders of the musculoskeletal and nervous system can limit mobility; certain neurological diseases can cause muscles to become stiff or lose function

   a. Arthritis and amputations are obvious examples of musculoskeletal conditions that would impair mobility

Box 10-6	
Communicating with Clients Who Have a Visual or Hearing Deficit	**Visual Deficit**

Visual Deficit

➤ Always announce your presence when entering the client's room and identify yourself by name.

➤ Stay in the client's field of vision if the client has a partial vision loss.

➤ Speak in a warm and pleasant tone of voice; some people tend to speak louder than necessary when talking to a blind person.

➤ Always explain what you are about to do before touching the person.

➤ Explain the sounds in the environment.

➤ Indicate when the conversation has ended and when you are leaving the room.

Hearing Deficit

➤ Before initiating a conversation, convey your presence by moving to a position where you can be seen or by gently touching the person.

➤ Decrease background noises (e.g., radio) before speaking.

➤ Talk at a moderate rate and in a normal tone of voice; shouting does not make your voice more distinct and in some instances makes understanding more difficult.

➤ Address the person directly; do not turn away in the middle of a remark or story; make sure the person can see your face easily and that it is well lighted.

➤ Avoid talking when you have something in your mouth, such as chewing gum; avoid covering your mouth with your hand.

➤ Keep your voice at about the same volume throughout each sentence, without dropping the voice at the end of each sentence.

➤ Always speak as clearly and accurately as possible; articulate consonants with particular care.

➤ Do not "overarticulate"; mouthing or overdoing articulation is just as troublesome as mumbling; pantomime or write ideas, or use sign language or finger spelling where appropriate.

➤ Use longer phrases, which tend to be easier to understand than short ones; for example, "Will you get me a drink of water?" presents much less difficulty than "Will you get me a drink?"; word choice is important: "Fifteen cents" and "fifty cents" may be confused, but "half a dollar" is clear.

➤ Pronounce every name with care; make a reference to the name for easier understanding, for example, "Joan, the girl from the office" or "Sears, the big downtown store."

➤ Change to a new subject at a slower rate, making sure that the person follows the change to the new subject; a key word or two at the beginning of a new topic is a good indicator.

Source: Berman, A., Snyder, S. Kozier, B. & Erb, G., (2008). *Fundamentals of nursing: Concepts, process, and practice* (8th ed.). Upper Saddle River, NJ: Prentice Hall, p. 990.

  b. Multiple sclerosis and Parkinson's disease are neurological conditions that may render the muscles unable to function normally

  c. Alterations in LOC and stroke or cerebrovascular accident (CVA) could also leave the client immobile

 4. Functional problems: some chronic conditions that limit the supply of oxygen and nutrients to the body will affect activity tolerance, such as chronic obstructive lung disease (COPD), congestive heart failure (CHF), angina, and obesity; these conditions increase the heart's workload and thus restrict or impair the client's activity

5. Generalized weakness

a. A client's age affects body strength; as a client ages, muscle tone and bone density decreases; flexibility and reaction time slows; osteoporosis (demineralization of the bone) begins to wear away the bone; the changes associated with aging will affect posture, balance and gait

b. Chronic illness may also cause bodily changes that affect the client's energy level and ability to be active; for an example, anemia and low hemoglobin, which lowers the oxygen-carrying capacity of the blood, will cause the person to experience fatigue; this, in turn, will reduce mobility

6. Psychological problems: emotional disorders such as depression or stress can reduce a client's desire to be active

a. Depression may cause the client to lack the motivation and energy to participate in the activities of daily living

b. A client who is under prolonged stress can also be depleted of energy

c. Fear may also prevent the client from going outside or leaving the home

7. Medically induced immobility

a. Healthcare providers may place clients on bedrest or restricted activity to facilitate healing

b. Orthopedic devices can also restrict mobility; traction, casts, splints, and braces can all lead to inactivity of some part(s) of the body

C. Major effects of immobility

1. Psychological effects: powerlessness and loss of self-concept

2. Atrophy and contractures

3. Disuse osteoporosis

4. Pressure ulcers

5. **Orthostatic intolerance** (also known as postural or orthostatic hypotension)

6. Deep vein thrombosis

7. Pneumonia

8. Decrease in peristalsis (paralytic ileus)

9. Kidney stones

D. Nursing interventions for impaired mobility

1. Exercise: a repetitive, planned body movement performed to either improve or maintain physical movement; activity is essential in preventing complications of immobility

2. Exercise is necessary for the healthy functioning of the body

3. The American Heart Association recommends that for a healthy heart and cardiovascular system, exercise should be performed most days of the week for 30 minutes

4. Benefits of exercise

a. Exercise improves the tone and strength of muscles; it also improves joint flexibility and range of motion

b. Exercise promotes good pulmonary ventilation; this, in turn, prevents pooling of secretions in the lungs and reduces the risk of pneumonia

c. Gastrointestinal motility and tone is improved, thereby improving digestion and elimination

d. Since exercise decreases bone loss of calcium, the urine maintains acidity and thus decreases the risk for renal calculi

5. Types of exercise

a. Isometric: produces tension or restistance in a muscle without a change in muscle length; are helpful for the immobilized client because they strengthen muscle groups that will be used later in ambulation; teach the client to push or pull against a stationary object as a form of isometric exercise; the muscles exercised here are the abdominal, gluteus, and quadriceps

b. Isotonic: shortens the muscle to produce contraction and active movement; there is no significant change in resistance during movement, so the force of the contraction stays stable; increases muscle tone and maintains joint flexibility; using a trapeze to lift the body or pushing the body into a sitting position are examples of isotonic exercises for the bedridden client

c. Passive range of motion: are exercises accomplished with the assistance of another individual who will support the client's body part while moving it

d. Active range of motion: are exercises performed independently; these are isotonic exercises of each joint in the body and can maintain or improve muscle strength; they prevent deterioration of joint movement and subsequent contractures

E. Assistive ambulation devices

1. There are many devices available to assist the client in mobility; these devices include crutches, canes, and walkers

2. Crutches: are devices used to assist the client in moving and ambulating unassisted; all crutches require rubber tips to prevent slipping on slippery floors

a. There are various types of crutches (see Figure 10-1)

1) An axillary crutch is the most frequently used type of crutch

2) A Lofstrand or forearm crutch is used as a substitute for a cane; it consists of a single tube of aluminum with a handle and a cuff for the forearm; it allows the user to release the hand bar because the metal cuff maintains crutch placement and prevents it from falling

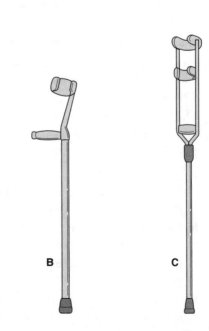

Figure 10-1

Three types of crutches.
A. Axillary crutch;
B. Lofstrand crutch;
C. Canadian or elbow extension crutch.

A   B   C

            3) The Canadian or elbow extensor crutch is used for the client whose forearm extensor muscles are weak; it allows the upper arm to provide stability to the crutch

        b. Proper fit: it is critical that the client be fitted correctly for the chosen crutch

            1) Measure the client who is lying supine from the anterior fold of the axilla to the heel of the foot and add 1 inch (2.5 cm)

            2) Also measure the placement of the hand on the crutch while the client stands and adjust the crutch so that it maintains the elbow at a 30-degree angle

            3) With the client standing erect, ensure that the shoulder rest of the crutch is 3 fingerwidths (2.5 to 5 cm, or 1 to 2 inches) below the axilla

        c. Safety: in addition to the rubber tip on the end of the crutch, the client needs to know the appropriate gait; prior to gait training, assist the client in preparing for crutch walking by encouraging the client to push the body off the bed with the hands and arms; while utilizing crutches, the client's weight is borne by the arms, not the axillae, as continued pressure in this area can cause nerve damage

        d. Gaits used: there are five crutch-walking gaits; the choice depends upon the client's ability to bear weight and maintain balance on both legs or one leg; while using a crutch, the client alternates body weight between one or both legs and the crutches; the five gaits and their uses include:

            1) Four-point gait: partial weight-bearing

                a) The client must be able to bear weight on both legs

                b) It is the safest gait and provides three points of support at all times

                c) It requires constant shifting of weight and coordination of movement of legs and crutches

            2) Three-point gait: requires one leg to be able to bear weight of entire body

                a) Non-weight-bearing on affected leg

                b) Alternates between good leg and affected leg with both crutches

            3) Two-point gait: requires partial weight-bearing on both feet

                a) Client can move at a faster gait than with the four-point gait

                b) Two points are used to support the body at all times

                c) Crutch movement is similar to the swinging of the arms while walking

            4) Swing-through gait: weight-bearing gait that requires strength and coordination

                a) Client moves both crutches forward together

                b) Then the client lifts his or her body weight and swings through

            5) Swing-to gait: weight-bearing on both feet

                a) Similar to swing-through gait except body motion is only to level of crutches

                b) Useful for clients with paralysis of legs and hips

    3. Cane: assists a client to walk with greater balance and support

        a. Three types of canes are available depending on the number of feet

            1) Quad cane: four feet

            2) Tri-pod: three feet

            3) Straight cane

      b. Canes are adjustable; the length should allow the elbow to bend slightly

      c. Canes allow clients to ambulate with faster speed, and they do not get fatigued as quickly

      d. Clients may use one or two canes; a single cane is used on the unaffected side

      e. A rubber cap is fitted at the tips of the foot (feet) to prevent slipping

4. Walker: device that provides the client with more support than a cane

      a. A walker is useful for clients who have poor balance, cardiac problems, or who cannot use crutches

      b. The standard walker has four legs with rubber tips on the legs and plastic grips for the hands

          1) The client needs to be partial weight-bearing and have strength in his or her wrists and arms

          2) The client uses his or her upper body to propel the walker forward

      c. Another type of walker is the two- or four-wheeled walker

          1) Clients who are too weak or not stable enough to move a walker by lifting it use these walkers

          2) They may contain a seat at the back to allow the client to sit and rest while walking

      d. Walkers can have their height adjusted

F. Hydraulic lift

    1. This apparatus is used for clients who are not able to stand and are too heavy for the healthcare workers to lift safely; e.g., Hoyer Lift

    2. The lift has three parts: the sling, the arm, and the base; a pressure release valve is on the base

    3. The sling is placed under the client: the arm of the device has a hook that hooks into the sling; the lift is raised to elevate the client

    4. The lift is then moved and aligned with the chair; the pressure release valve is released, and the client is lowered to the chair

    5. The sling can be removed from the hooks but left under the client to facilitate returning the client to bed

> ► **Practice to Pass**
>
> The nurse wants to assist the client in strengthening his arm muscles in preparation for crutch walking. Describe the exercises the nurse would teach.

Case Study

A 30-year-old client came to the Emergency Department with a swollen ankle. The nurse notes swelling over the ankle extending down to the toes. X-rays are negative for a fracture. A sprained ankle is diagnosed. The doctor orders a compression (Ace™) bandage for the ankle and the use of crutches with no weight bearing on the right ankle.

1. Describe how to apply the compression bandage and give a rationale.

2. Describe how the nurse will teach the client to use the crutches without bearing weight on the right foot.

3. Describe the process for measuring the client for crutches.

4. What type of wound did this client have? How long will it take to heal?

5. What safety concerns would you include in discussions about crutch use?

For suggested responses, see page 338.

POSTTEST

1 A client has been on bed rest with cervical traction for 2 weeks. The traction is discontinued and the client is to ambulate. Prior to getting the client out of bed, it is important for the nurse to take which of the following initial actions? Select all that apply.

1. Raise the head of the bed slowly.
2. Assess lower leg muscle strength.
3. Provide the client with a cane.
4. Get a neck brace for the client.
5. Take the client's blood pressure prior to ambulation.

2 A 76-year-old client is admitted to the hospital. In planning for client teaching, the nurse would assess for which condition that is often associated with aging and that is most likely to interfere with the client's ability to participate in education activities?

1. Presbyopia
2. Conductive hearing loss
3. Presbycusis
4. Tinnitus

3 A client who visits the optometrist for an eye exam is told that he has myopia. The client asks the nurse what the treatment will be. The nurse's reply would include information about which of the following standard treatments?

1. Surgical removal
2. Eye drops or ointment
3. Glasses or contact lenses
4. Oral antibiotics

4 The nurse is performing wound care on a pressure ulcer. The doctor orders a wet-to-damp dressing. A family member asks why the dressing is put on wet. The nurse explains that the purpose of this type of dressing is to:

1. Protect the wound.
2. Dilute thick exudate.
3. Promote collagen deposit.
4. Debride the wound.

5 The nurse assesses a wound of a client and finds that a scab has formed. The nurse concludes that this wound is at what point in the phases wound healing?

1. End of the inflammatory phase
2. End of the proliferative phase
3. Midpoint of the reparative phase
4. Beginning of the maturation phase

6 A client has a large pressure ulcer on his lower extremity. The nurse instructs the client about nutrients needed for healing, especially vitamin C and protein. While evaluating intake, the nurse determines that the instruction was successful after noting that the client is eating which of the following breakfasts?

1. Coffee, buttered toast with jelly, and bacon
2. Milk, scrambled eggs, and cantaloupe
3. Pancakes with butter and syrup and hot tea
4. Oatmeal with butter, diet soda, and bacon

7 The nurse is using the Braden scale to assess a client's risk for developing a pressure ulcer and calculates a score of 7. The nurse should interpret that this client has which level of risk for development of pressure ulcers?

1. High risk
2. Moderate risk
3. Low risk
4. Unlikely to develop pressure ulcers

8 During an exercise session with a client who had vascular surgery to the leg, the nurse dorsiflexes and then plantar flexes the foot. The client looks surprised and asks why the nurse is performing this activity. What should the nurse include in a response?

1. "Active range of motion will allow the fastest recovery for your leg."
2. "Passive range of motion will help maintain muscle tone until you can participate more actively in the exercises."
3. "Isometric exercise such as this will use muscles to push against resistance and build up the muscles in your leg."
4. "Isotonic exercise lets me do the work and your muscles get the benefit."

POSTTEST

9 Which assessment of the immobilized client would prompt the nurse to take further action?

1. Client reports fatigue
2. Urinary output of 50 mL/hour
3. White blood cell count of 9500/mm^3
4. Hypoactive bowel sounds

10 The nurse is assessing several clients with different types of injuries. The nurse would conclude that the client who is least likely to develop a wound infection would be the client with which of the following?

1. A contusion
2. A wound healing by second intention
3. A septic wound
4. A wound with purulent exudate

➤ See pages 281–283 for Answers & Rationales.

ANSWERS & RATIONALES

Pretest

1 **Answer: 2** Stage I ulcers have nonblanchable erythematous skin that is intact. Stage II is reddened by the skin is also broken, giving the appearance of a broken blister. Stage III is a deep ulcer with necrotic tissue, while Stage IV involves tissue necrosis and extends to underlying tissue such as muscle and bone. **Cognitive Level:** Analysis **Client Need:** Physiological Integrity: Physiological Adaptation **Integrated Process:** Nursing Process: Assessment **Content Area:** Fundamentals **Strategy:** The critical word in the question is *classify*. Recall the various stages of pressure ulcer, visualize each stage, and then compare them to the ulcer description in the question to make a selection. **Reference:** Kozier, B., Erb, G., Berman, A., & Snyder, S. J. (2004). *Fundamentals of nursing: Concepts, process, and practice* (7th ed.). Upper Saddle River, NJ: Pearson Education, p. 859.

2 **Answer: 2** Impaired skin integrity is a result of constant shearing force and pressure (option 2). The client was turned and positioned frequently enough, making option 1 incorrect; in addition, this type of statement is incorrectly written as it implies that the staff are to blame for the client's condition. Options 3 and 4 are incorrect because the client has an actual diagnosis, not a risk diagnosis. **Cognitive Level:** Analysis **Client Need:** Physiological Integrity: Basic Care and Comfort **Integrated Process:** Nursing Process: Analysis **Content Area:** Fundamentals **Strategy:** The critical phrase is *appropriate nursing diagnosis*. Discriminate between actual and risk diagnoses to eliminate options 3 and 4, and then use information in the question to choose option 2 over option 1. **Reference:** Kozier, B., Erb, G., Berman, A., & Snyder, S. J. (2004). *Fundamentals of nursing: Concepts, process, and practice* (7th ed.). Upper Saddle River, NJ: Pearson Education, pp. 868–869.

3 **Answer: 3** Purulent drainage is a sign of infection. The wound healing will be delayed if infection is present. Primary intention is a normal process of wound healing and a clean and dry suture line is normal. Sanguineous drainage indicates the drainage of blood that is in the tissues. **Cognitive Level:** Application **Client Need:** Physiological Integrity: Reduction of Risk Potential **Integrated Process:** Nursing Process: Assessment **Content Area:** Fundamentals **Strategy:** The core issue of the question is the ability to identify data that are consistent with a delay in wound healing. Eliminate option 4 first because it does not directly relate to healing. Choose option 3 over options 1 and 2 because it indicates abnormal data. **Reference:** Kozier, B., Erb, G., Berman, A., & Snyder, S. J. (2004). *Fundamentals of nursing: Concepts, process, and practice* (7th ed.). Upper Saddle River, NJ: Pearson Education, p. 924.

4 **Answers: 3, 5** A loss of elastic skin turgor with wrinkling and increased fragility is part of the normal process of aging of the skin. Tight shiny skin with edema and overhydration are not expected assessment findings of the elderly client's skin. **Cognitive Level:** Application **Client Need:** Health Promotion and Maintenance **Integrated Process:** Nursing Process: Assessment **Content Area:** Fundamentals **Strategy:** The core issue of the question is knowledge of age related changes in the older adult client. Use knowledge of how skin changes with aging and the process of elimination to make a selection. **Reference:** Kozier, B., Erb, G., Berman, A., & Snyder, S. J. (2004). *Fundamentals of nursing: Concepts, process, and practice* (7th ed.). Upper Saddle River, NJ: Pearson Education, p. 402.

5 **Answer: 1** Symptoms of sensory deprivation, in addition to the above, would include preoccupations with somatic complaints, hallucinations, and apathy. Sensory overload symptoms would include sleeplessness, irritability, disorientation, and reduced problem-solving

ability. Visual and hearing deficits would relate to the involved sense.
Cognitive Level: Analysis **Client Need:** Psychosocial Integrity **Integrated Process:** Nursing Process: Analysis **Content Area:** Fundamentals **Strategy:** Note that the client in the question is hospitalized and review the client's manifestations. Consider how the hospital environment could affect the client to make a selection. Eliminate options 3 and 4 first because a single sense is not affected. Compare the client's symptoms to the remaining terms to make a final selection. **Reference:** Kozier, B., Erb, G., Berman, A., & Snyder, S. J. (2004). *Fundamentals of nursing: Concepts, process, and practice* (7th ed.). Upper Saddle River, NJ: Pearson Education, p. 940.

6 **Answer: 4** Posting a turning schedule with a sign sheet will help ensure the client is turned. A client needs to be turned at least every 2 hours therefore b.i.d. is insufficient. Massaging bony prominences is a therapeutic intervention; however, doing it vigorously may damage capillaries in the area.
Cognitive Level: Application **Client Need:** Physiological Integrity: Basic Care and Comfort **Integrated Process:** Nursing Process: Planning **Content Area:** Fundamentals **Strategy:** The critical words are *bedridden* and *planning nursing care.* Recall the major complications of immobility and common nursing interventions to prevent those complications to eliminate the incorrect options. **Reference:** Kozier, B., Erb, G., Berman, A., & Snyder, S. J. (2004). *Fundamentals of nursing: Concepts, process, and practice* (7th ed.). Upper Saddle River, NJ: Pearson Education, pp. 857–858.

7 **Answer: 2** Sterile gloves are not required to remove contaminated dressings. All of the other responses indicate correct dressing change procedures.
Cognitive Level: Application **Client Need:** Safe, Effective Care Environment: Safety and Infection Control **Integrated Process:** Nursing Process: Evaluation **Content Area:** Fundamentals **Strategy:** The critical phrase is *the student who needs to review the skill.* This tells you the correct answer is the statement that contains incorrect information. Use knowledge of wound management techniques and the process of elimination to make a selection. **Reference:** Kozier, B., Erb, G., Berman, A., & Snyder, S. J. (2004). *Fundamentals of nursing: Concepts, process, and practice* (7th ed.). Upper Saddle River, NJ: Pearson Education, p. 926.

8 **Answer: 2** Having the conversation directed to the client meets the client's needs while creating fewer disturbances. This will help decrease overstimulation, especially for the client who is hearing impaired. Lights in the room should be dimmed to reduce visual overload.

Having too many family members with the client will only add to the already sensory-overloaded client.
Cognitive Level: Application **Client Need:** Physiological Integrity: Basic Care and Comfort **Integrated Process:** Nursing Process: Implementation **Content Area:** Fundamentals **Strategy:** The critical words in the question are *hearing impairment* and *preventing sensory overload.* Use knowledge of techniques for communicating with clients who have sensory deficits and the process of elimination to make a selection. **Reference:** Kozier, B., Erb, G., Berman, A., & Snyder, S. J. (2004). *Fundamentals of nursing: Concepts, process, and practice* (7th ed.). Upper Saddle River, NJ: Pearson Education, p. 949.

9 **Answer: 1** Reducing glare can help improve vision for the older client. Bright lighting can decrease the client's visual accommodation. Dim lights reduce the clients' perception of the environment.
Cognitive Level: Application **Client Need:** Physiological Integrity: Basic Care and Comfort **Integrated Process:** Nursing Process: Implementation **Content Area:** Fundamentals **Strategy:** The critical terms are *visually impaired* and *preventing sensory deprivation.* Recall basic information about aids for clients with visual deficits and use the process of elimination to make a selection. **Reference:** Kozier, B., Erb, G., Berman, A., & Snyder, S. J. (2004). *Fundamentals of nursing: Concepts, process, and practice* (7th ed.). Upper Saddle River, NJ: Pearson Education, p. 949.

10 **Answer: 2** The client should use a cane on the unaffected (stronger) side. The elbow is held in a slight degree of flexion. There are reasons to choose a walker over a cane, but neither is "better." Clients are all at greater risk when they wear socks but no shoes.
Cognitive Level: Application **Client Need:** Physiological Integrity: Basic Care and Comfort **Integrated Process:** Teaching/Learning **Content Area:** Fundamentals **Strategy:** The critical phrase is *indicates to the nurse the need for additional teaching.* This tells you that the correct answer is an incorrect statement by the client. Use nursing knowledge of assistive ambulation devices to make a selection. **Reference:** Kozier, B., Erb, G., Berman, A., & Snyder, S. J. (2004). *Fundamentals of nursing: Concepts, process, and practice* (7th ed.). Upper Saddle River, NJ: Pearson Education, p. 1102.

Posttest

1 **Answers: 1, 5** Orthostatic intolerance or hypotension may occur if the client has been on bed rest. To decrease the problem, gradually elevate the head of the bed to assist the client to a sitting position. Also check the client's blood pressure to ensure that it is stable. Assess-

ANSWERS & RATIONALES

ing the strength of the leg muscles is not something that would be done directly before getting a client up to ambulate. A cane may or may not be ordered, and there is no information in the question to support the need for a neck brace.
Cognitive Level: Application **Client Need:** Safe, Effective Care Environment: Safety and Infection Control **Integrated Process:** Nursing Process: Implementation **Content Area:** Fundamentals **Strategy:** The critical phrases are *bed rest in cervical traction for 2 weeks* and *ambulate.* Recall the major complications of immobility and related nursing actions and use the process of elimination to determine the options that will reduce the client's risk and increase client safety when getting out of bed after prolonged bed rest. **Reference:** Kozier, B., Erb, G., Berman, A., & Snyder, S. J. (2004). *Fundamentals of nursing: Concepts, process, and practice* (7th ed.). Upper Saddle River, NJ: Pearson Education, p. 1068.

2 Answers: 3 Presbycusis is the hearing loss associated with aging. Presbyopia is the inability to focus on close objects; this condition normally accompanies aging. A conductive hearing loss involves an obstruction in the ear canal. Tinnitus is ringing in the ears.
Cognitive Level: Application **Client Need:** Health Promotion and Maintenance **Integrated Process:** Nursing Process: Assessment and Analysis **Content Area:** Fundamentals **Strategy:** The critical phrase is *aging process.* Recall sensory deficits that occur with advancing age and use the process of elimination to make a selection. **Reference:** Kozier, B., Erb, G., Berman, A., & Snyder, S. J. (2004). *Fundamentals of nursing: Concepts, process, and practice* (7th ed.). Upper Saddle River, NJ: Pearson Education, p. 403.

3 Answer: 3 Myopia or nearsightedness is a condition in which light rays come into focus in front of the retina. It is treated with eyeglasses or contact lenses. The statement in option 1, surgical removal, is incorrect because there is no "removal," although the condition could be treated surgically. Eye medication and oral antibiotics are of no use in improving the vision of the client with myopia.
Cognitive Level: Application **Client Need:** Health Promotion and Maintenance **Integrated Process:** Teaching/Learning **Content Area:** Fundamentals **Strategy:** The critical term is *myopia.* Recall information about common refractory errors to discriminate among the options and make a correct selection. **Reference:** Kozier, B., Erb, G., Berman, A., & Snyder, S. J. (2004). *Fundamentals of nursing: Concepts, process and practice* (7th ed.). Upper Saddle River, NJ: Pearson Education, p. 546.

4 Answer: 4 A wet-to-damp dressing debrides the wound. As the dressing partially dries, necrotic debris will ad-

here to the dressing. When the dressing is removed, dead tissue will be removed also. Although it provides some protection of the wound, that is not its main purpose. A wet-to-wet dressing, not wet-to-damp, would dilute a thickened or viscous exudate.
Cognitive Level: Application **Client Need:** Physiological Integrity: Reduction of Risk Potential **Integrated Process:** Teaching/Learning **Content Area:** Fundamentals **Strategy:** The critical term is *wet-to-damp dressing.* Recall the uses this type of dressing to select the option that provides accurate information to the client and family. **Reference:** Kozier, B., Erb, G., Berman, A., & Snyder, S. J. (2004). *Fundamentals of nursing: Concepts, process, and practice* (7th ed.). Upper Saddle River, NJ: Pearson Education, p. 882.

5 Answer: 1 Near the end of the inflammatory phase of wound healing, protein dries out at the top of the wound, forming a scab. This scab provides safety for the wound because the first line of defense, the skin, is again covered. Options 2 and 4 are later phases of wound healing. Option 3 is not a current term associated with phases of wound healing.
Cognitive Level Application Client Need: Physiological Integrity: Basic Care and Comfort **Integrated Process:** Nursing Process: Analysis **Content Area:** Fundamentals **Strategy:** The critical word in the question is *scab.* Recall the phases of wound healing and visualize what the wound will look like in each phase to make the correct selection. **Reference:** Kozier, B., Erb, G., Berman, A., & Snyder, S. J. (2004). *Fundamentals of nursing: Concepts, process, and practice* (7th ed.). Upper Saddle River, NJ: Pearson Education, p. 860.

6 Answer: 2 To promote healing, the client should eat a diet high in protein and vitamin C. The food options in option 2 are highest in these nutrients, with milk and scrambled eggs being higher in protein and cantaloupe having vitamin C. The menus in the other options tend to be higher in fat (foods such as bacon and butter) or low in vitamin C (an absence of any fruit or vegetables).
Cognitive Level: Analysis **Client Need:** Physiological Integrity: Basic Care and Comfort **Integrated Process:** Nursing Process: Evaluation **Content Area:** Fundamentals **Strategy:** The core issue of the question is knowledge of foods that are high in vitamin C and protein for wound healing. Use information related to nutrition and the process of elimination to make a selection. **Reference:** Kozier, B., Erb, G., Berman, A., & Snyder, S. J. (2004). *Fundamentals of nursing: Concepts, process, and practice* (7th ed.). Upper Saddle River, NJ: Pearson Education, p. 862.

7 Answer: 1 The Braden scale evaluates 6 factors: sensory perception, moisture, activity, mobility, nutrition, and friction/shear. Each factor can receive a score from 1 to

4 except friction/shear, which is scored 1 to 3. Low numbers indicate factors that are likely to contribute to the development of an ulcer. Overall scores above 19 indicate that the client has a low risk of pressure ulcer development.
Cognitive Level: Analysis **Client Need:** Physiological Integrity: Reduction of Risk Potential **Integrated Process:** Nursing Process: Analysis **Content Area:** Fundamentals **Strategy:** The critical words in the question are *Braden scale* and *score of 7*. To answer this question correctly, it is necessary to be familiar with common pressure ulcer risk assessment scales (such as the Braden or Norton scales) and recall that lower numbers rather than higher ones place the client at risk. **Reference:** Kozier, B., Erb, G., Berman, A., & Snyder, S. J. (2004). *Fundamentals of nursing: Concepts, process, and practice* (7th ed.). Upper Saddle River, NJ: Pearson Education, p. 864.

8 **Answer: 2** Passive range of motion is exercise conducted with the assistance of another individual (option 2), while active range of motion (option 1) is done by the client alone. Options 3 and 4 refer to exercises that involve resistance (option 3) or no resistance (option 4) and do not apply to the current client situation.
Cognitive Level: Application **Client Need:** Physiological Integrity: Basic Care and Comfort **Integrated Process:** Teaching/Learning **Content Area:** Fundamentals **Strategy:** The core issue of the question is knowledge of the rationales and benefits for passive range of motion exercises. Use this knowledge and the process of elimination to make a selection. **Reference:** Kozier, B., Erb, G., Berman, A., & Snyder, S. J. (2004). *Fundamentals of nursing: Concepts, process, and practice* (7th ed.). Upper Saddle River, NJ: Pearson Education, p. 1096.

9 **Answer: 4** Hypoactive bowel sounds is a complication of immobility. It could be followed by constipation and other gastrointestinal problems. Fatigue (option 1) is a complaint that any client may experience in the hospital. Urinary output is within normal range as well as the white blood count (options 2 and 3, respectively).
Cognitive Level: Analysis **Client Need:** Physiological Integrity: Reduction of Risk Potential **Integrated Process:** Nursing Process: Analysis **Content Area:** Fundamentals **Strategy:** The critical words in the question are *immobilized client* and *further action*. Recall the major complications of immobility and use the process of elimination to make a selection. **Reference:** Kozier, B., Erb, G., Berman, A., & Snyder, S. J. (2004). *Fundamentals of nursing: Concepts, process, and practice* (7th ed.). Upper Saddle River, NJ: Pearson Education, pp. 1070–1071.

10 **Answer: 1** A contusion is a crushing of the tissues; there is no break in the skin. Therefore, this wound is less likely to become infected. A septic wound is one that has been invaded by pathogenic microorganisms (option 3). Purulent exudate also is an indicator of infection (option 4). A wound healing by second intention is a wound in which there is extensive injury and the edges of the wound are not well approximated. Because of this factor, this type of wound has a risk of infection.
Cognitive Level: Analysis **Client Need:** Physiological Integrity: Reduction of Risk Potential **Integrated Process:** Nursing Process: Analysis **Content Area:** Fundamentals **Strategy:** The critical words in the question are *least likely*. This tells you that the correct option is one that has the data that is the nearest to normal of the options presented. Use nursing knowledge and the process of elimination to make a selection. **Reference:** Kozier, B., Erb, G., Berman, A., & Snyder, S. J. (2004). *Fundamentals of nursing: Concepts, process, and practice* (7th ed.). Upper Saddle River, NJ: Pearson Education, p. 856.

References

Berman, A. J., Snyder, S., Kozier, B., & Erb, G., (2008). *Fundamentals of nursing* (8th ed.). Upper Saddle River, NJ: Pearson Education, pp. 902–938, 980–1001, 1104–1162.

Harkreader, H. & Hogan, M. (2004). *Fundamentals of nursing: Caring and clinical judgment* (2nd ed.). St. Louis, MO: Elsevier Science, pp. 665–698, 826–890, 1036–1057.

LeMone, P. & Burke, K. (2008). *Medical–surgical nursing: Critical thinking in client care* (4th ed.). Upper Saddle River, NJ: Pearson Education.

Smeltzer, S. & Bare, B. (2007). *Brunner and Suddarth's textbook of medical-surgical nursing* (11th ed.). Philadelphia: Lippincott Williams & Wilkins, pp. 353–369.

Potter, P. & Perry, A. (2005). *Fundamentals of nursing* (6th ed.). St. Louis, MO: Mosby pp. 1420–1592.

ANSWERS & RATIONALES

11 Administering Medications and Intravenous Fluids

Chapter Outline

Application of Pharmacology in Nursing Practice

Pharmacokinetics

Nurse's Role in Administering Medications

Intravenous Therapy

NCLEX-RN® Test Prep

Use the CD-ROM enclosed with this book to access additional practice opportunities.

Objectives

➤ Describe legal responsibilities of the nurse related to medication administration.

➤ Discuss pharmacokinetics in relation to medication administration.

➤ Apply the use of the nursing process to the skill of medication administration.

➤ Identify the procedures and techniques for safely administering medications via all routes.

➤ Describe the purpose and types of intravenous solutions and guidelines for administering them safely.

➤ Compare and contrast the various intravenous catheters and solutions available, their indications, maintenance, and methods for evaluation of potential complications.

Review at a Glance

absorption process by which a drug moves from the administration site into the bloodstream

adverse effects more severe side effects

allergic reaction an antigen/antibody or immunologic reaction to subsequent exposure to an allergen

apothecary system oldest system of measurement, uses Roman numerals; units of measure are represented by special symbols; the unit of liquid measure is the minim and the unit for weight is the grain

aseptic free from germs

biotransformation conversion of a drug by enzymatic action of the liver into a less active and harmless substance that is easily excreted; also called metabolism or detoxification

bolus direct injection of a medication intravenously

brand name name given by each manufacturer resulting in various names for the same drug; trade name

buccal pertaining to the cheek

classification grouping drugs by pharmacologic and therapeutic categories

conjunctival sac mucosal membrane that lines the eye

excretion elimination of the drug and metabolites from the body primarily through the kidneys but also through the feces, respiration, perspiration, saliva, and breast milk

generic more useful drug name that reflects the chemical family

half-life period of time after which 50% of a medication administered has lost its effectiveness

idiosyncratic effect unexpected and unpredictable individual response to a drug manifested as an under response, over response, or completely different response

inhalation administering a drug into the respiratory tract through a mist, spray, or positive pressure

intradermal into the dermal layer of skin (dermis) just under the outside layer of skin

intramuscular into a muscle

intravenous into a vein

irrigation cleansing of a body cavity by flushing with a solution or medication, also known as lavage

lavage cleansing of a body cavity by flushing with a solution or medication, also known as irrigation

lipodystrophy atrophy or hypertrophy of the subcutaneous tissue

medication a drug administered for the treatment, mitigation, diagnosis, or prevention of disease

metric a decimal system of measurement based upon units of 10 with the gram as the unit of weight and the liter as the unit of liquid volume

narcotic strong analgesic that in moderate doses depresses the central nervous system

noncompliance failure or refusal to take medications according to the instructions

ophthalmic pertaining to the eye

parenteral injection of drugs administered by any route other than the alimentary canal (intestines)

pharmacokinetics study of the metabolism and action of drugs

side effects secondary effect of a drug that is not intended; they are usually predictable and may be harmless or life-threatening

subcutaneous the third layer of skin

sublingual under the tongue

sustained release drugs manufactured in a manner to delay absorption

therapeutic effect the desired effect or the primary intended effect; the reason the drug is prescribed

topical applied externally

toxic effects harmful effects of a drug on the body, usually the result of drug overdose, improper route of administration, and cumulative effects resulting from impaired excretion or metabolism

trade name name given by each manufacturer resulting in various names for the same drug; brand name

transdermal refers to application of a medication for absorption through the skin

PRETEST

1 The nurse risk manager is reviewing a medication error involving a known diabetic client. The nurse administered 10 units NPH insulin IV stat per the physician's order. The client had an anaphylactic reaction and died. The risk manager concludes that the nurse is:

1. Not legally liable because the nurse administered the medication as ordered by the physician.
2. Not liable because it was not an insulin reaction.
3. Legally liable for the medication administered even though the order was written incorrectly.
4. Not legally liable because the nurse gave the correct medication, regardless of the route.

2 While the nurse administers a client's dose of sublingual nitroglycerin, the client asks why it is administered under the tongue instead of swallowed. Which of the following is the best response by the nurse?

1. "It is absorbed more rapidly when placed under your tongue than when swallowed."
2. "It is absorbed more rapidly when swallowed than sublingually."
3. "The absorptions are the same so it really doesn't matter."
4. "Sublingual provides a sustained release of the medication."

3 The nurse is to administer 25 mg of promethazine (Phenergan) intramuscularly (IM) to a 150-pound client. The nurse knows that this medication should be given deep into a large muscle mass. Which site should the nurse select to inject the medication?

1. Deltoid
2. Dorsogluteal
3. Vastus lateralis
4. Ventrogluteal

4 To administer 1 mL of a flu vaccine intramuscularly (IM) to an obese adult in the deltoid area, the nurse would use a needle that is which size?

1. ½ inch
2. 1 inch
3. 1½ inches
4. 2 inches

5 The nurse is preparing an intramuscular (IM) injection of hydroxyzine (Vistaril), which is especially irritating to subcutaneous tissue. To prevent "tracking" of the medication and irritation to the tissues, it would be best for the nurse to take which action?

1. Use a small-gauge needle.
2. Administer at a 45-degree angle.
3. Apply ice to the injection site.
4. Use the Z-track technique.

6 A pediatric client has been diagnosed with conjunctivitis. The nurse is to administer eye drops 4 times per day. The nurse should administer the medication by gently dropping the medication onto which of the following areas?

1. Center of the cornea
2. Sclera by the inner canthus
3. Sclera by the outer canthus
4. Lower conjunctival sac

7 A client received a severe burn in a house fire. On the second day of hospitalization, the physician orders the client to receive albumin. The nurse's best response to the client about the rationale for albumin administration is that it will:

1. Increase the level of clotting factors and prevent bleeding.
2. Provide fluid resuscitation to prevent dehydration.
3. Replace the lost red blood cells and reduce the anemia.
4. Provide proteins to increase the osmotic pressure in the blood.

8 The nurse is to administer ranitidine (Zantac) 50 mg intravenously (IV) in 50 mL of 5% dextrose in water. The nurse should set the IV infusion pump to administer _____ mL per hour to administer the dose over a 30-minute time period. Provide a numerical answer.

Answer: _____

9 The physician has ordered a hypotonic intravenous (IV) solution for a newly admitted client. The nurse obtains which of the following solutions based on the order and the likely type of dehydration?

1. 0.9% sodium chloride for hypotonic dehydration
2. 5% dextrose in normal saline for isotonic dehydration
3. Lactated Ringer's for hypovolemic dehydration
4. 0.45% sodium chloride for cellular dehydration

10 The client has been receiving total parenteral nutrition (TPN) for several days. The central venous access device became dislodged and the nurse notes that the client's IV has not been running for the last few hours. The nurse would monitor the client for which complication related to the stopped infusion?

1. Hypocalcemia
2. Hypoglycemia
3. Sepsis
4. Hyperkalemia

➤ *See pages 323–325 for Answers & Rationales.*

I. APPLICATION OF PHARMACOLOGY IN NURSING PRACTICE

A. Drug

1. A term that is sometimes used interchangeably with **medication**

2. Substance administered for the treatment, mitigation, diagnosis, or prevention of disease

B. Names of drugs

1. Each drug can have three types of names

2. Chemical

   a. Chemical derivation of the drug that describes the ingredients of the drug

   b. An example is 1-methyl-4phenyl-4 piperidinecarboxylic acid ethyl ester hydrochloride

3. **Generic**

   a. A more useful name that reflects the chemical family

   b. An example is meperidine hydrochloride (1-methyl-4phenyl-4 piperidine-carboxylic acid ethyl ester hydrochloride)

4. **Brand/trade name**

   a. A name given by each manufacturer resulting in various names for the same drug

   b. An example is Demerol (1-methyl-4phenyl-4 piperidinecarboxylic acid ethyl ester hydrochloride; meperidine hydrochloride)

C. Classification

1. The Pharmacologic-Therapeutic Classification of the American Hospital Formulary Service (AHFS) groups drugs by pharmacologic and therapeutic categories

2. Prototypes are listed under each classification that are representative of the actions and characteristics of the other drugs in that drug classification (e.g., Demerol is classified as a central nervous system [CNS] agent, narcotic [opiate] agonist analgesic)

D. Forms/preparation

1. Drugs are prepared in a variety of forms

2. See Table 11-1 for types of drug preparations

E. Federal regulations

1. In the United States and Canada, the federal government regulates the drug industry

2. This includes the production, prescription, distribution, and administration of drugs

F. State and local regulations

1. Each state legislates a Nurse Practice Act for RNs and LVN/LPNs

2. It is the responsibility of local healthcare facilities to establish and implement policies and procedures that conform to their state's regulations

3. When the laws or regulations of a community, state, or institution differ from the federal laws, the stricter law generally prevails

G. Nurse Practice Acts

1. Define nurses' boundaries and responsibilities regarding medications

2. It is a nurse's responsibility to know the state Nurse Practice Act

Table 11-1	Types of Drug Preparations		
Type	**Description**	**Type**	**Description**
Aerosol spray or foam	A liquid, powder, or foam deposited in a thin layer on the skin by air pressure	Paste	A preparation like an ointment, but thicker and stiff, that penetrates the skin less than an ointment
Aqueous solution	One or more drugs dissolved in water		
Aqueous suspension	One or more drugs finely divided in a liquid such as water	Pill	One or more drugs mixed with a cohesive material, in oval, round, or flattened shapes
Caplet	A solid form, shaped like a capsule, coated and easily swallowed	Powder	A finely ground drug or drugs; some are used internally, others externally
Capsule	A gelatinous container to hold a drug in powder, liquid, or oil form	Suppository	One or several drugs mixed with a firm base such as gelatin and shaped for insertion into the body (e.g., the rectum); the base dissolves gradually at body temperature, releasing the drug
Cream	A nongreasy, semisolid preparation used on the skin		
Elixir	A sweetened and aromatic solution of alcohol used as a vehicle for medicinal agents		
		Syrup	An aqueous solution of sugar often used to disguise unpleasant-tasting drugs
Extract	A concentrated form of a drug made from vegetables or animals	Tablet	A powdered drug compressed into a hard small disc; some are readily broken along a scored line; others are enteric-coated to prevent them from dissolving in the stomach
Gel or jelly	A clear or translucent semisolid that liquefies when applied to the skin		
Liniment	A medication mixed with alcohol, oil, or soapy emollient and applied to the skin		
Lotion	A medication in a liquid suspension applied to the skin	Tincture	An alcohol or water-and-alcohol solution prepared from drugs derived from plants
Lozenge (troche)	A flat, round, or oval preparation that dissolves and releases a drug when held in the mouth	Transdermal patch	A semipermeable membrane shaped in the form of a disc or patch that contains a drug to be absorbed through the skin over a long period of time
Ointment (salve, unction)	A semisolid preparation of one or more drugs used for application to the skin and mucous membrane		

Source: Berman, A., Snyder, S. Kozier, B., Erb, G., (2008). *Fundamentals of nursing* (8th ed.). Upper Saddle River, NJ: Pearson Education, p. 831.

▶ ***Practice to Pass***

How do Nurse Practice Acts relate to federal and state laws?

3. Under law, nurses are responsible for their own actions (e.g., if a medication order is written incorrectly, the nurse who administers the incorrect order is also responsible for the error)

4. Law also governs nursing practice involving use and management of controlled substances

H. Nontherapeutic medication use

1. Consist of chemicals that often are derived from folklore or various cultures

2. These have not passed the Federal Drug Administration (FDA) approval process (e.g., ginseng)

II. PHARMACOKINETICS

A. Study of how medications enter the body, reach their site of action, are metabolized, and exit the body

1. **Absorption:** the process by which a drug moves from the administration site into the bloodstream; drugs are absorbed through the gastrointestinal (GI) tract, respiratory tract, or skin and are dependent upon the correct form/preparation of the drug to be administered by the correct route

2. *Distribution:* the movement of the drug from the site of absorption to the site of action; it depends upon vascularity for speed of onset and upon chemical and physical drug properties to attract the drug to a certain area of the body where it will exert its effect

3. **Biotransformation:** conversion of a drug by enzymatic action of the liver into a less active substance called a metabolite; can be affected by a variety of factors including disease states; also called detoxification or metabolism; active metabolites still exert a pharmacological effect, while inactive metabolites do not

4. **Excretion:** elimination of the drug and metabolites from the body primarily through the kidneys but also through the feces, respiration, perspiration, saliva, and breast milk; the prescriber will determine the frequency of drug dosing by noting the drug's **half-life,** the time it takes the total amount of drug to be diminished by one-half; the drug's half-life provides information about the accumulation of the drug in the body with repeated doses

B. **Types of medication effects**

1. **Therapeutic effect:** the *desired effect* or the primary intended effect for which the drug is prescribed

2. **Side effect:** an unintended secondary effect of a drug; usually predictable and may be harmless or life-threatening; some side effects can have a beneficial action such as the sedative effect of morphine when used for pain management in the postoperative period

3. **Adverse effects:** more severe side effects that often require discontinuing the drug and might require reversal of the drug

4. **Toxic effects:** harmful effects of a drug on the body, usually the result of drug overdose, ingestion of a drug intended for external use, or cumulative effects resulting from impaired excretion or metabolism

5. **Idiosyncratic effect:** unexpected and unpredictable individual response to a drug manifested as an underresponse, overresponse, or completely different response

6. **Allergic reaction:** an antigen/antibody or immunologic reaction to a drug; allergic reaction can be as mild as a rash or as severe as anaphylaxis

7. Medication interactions: inhibition or enhancement of drug's action or effects as a result of interacting with foods, drugs, or other substances; results in an improved, exaggerated, or diminished response

C. **Routes of administration**

1. Refer to Table 11-2 for a summary of routes of administration and onset of action

2. Oral routes: drugs administered through the mouth

   a. Oral: drug is swallowed and drug is absorbed from the GI system; common forms of oral drugs include tablets, capsules, and liquid preparations

   b. **Sustained release** formulations (drugs manufactured in a manner to delay their absorption) are used to slow drug absorption in a controlled and planned manner; care should be taken when administering sustained release formulations to avoid breaking or opening the formulation, which alters the predictable dosage and response; most oral drugs are administered in a bolus dosing pattern

   c. **Sublingual:** drug is placed under the tongue and absorbed through the mucous membranes of the mouth into blood vessels; uncoated tablets dissolve in the mouth and are absorbed quickly

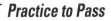

Practice to Pass

One hour ago the nurse administered 2 mg of lorazepam (Ativan) orally to a client for anxiety. The client is now reporting restlessness and increased anxiety. What response is the client experiencing and what should the nurse do?

Table 11-2	Routes	Onset and Action of Drugs
Routes of Administration and Onset of Action	*Oral Routes*	
	Oral	Slow and irregular absorption from the gastrointestinal (GI) tract
	Sublingual	Rapidly absorbed into bloodstream (systemic effect) Can be administered for local effect Bypasses the liver and is therefore more potent than oral route
	Buccal	Same as sublingual
	Parenteral Routes	
	Subcutaneous	Faster onset than oral Slower than intramuscular The abdomen has the most rapid rate of absorption of all subcutaneous sites
	Intramuscular	Rapidly absorbed: deltoid is 7% faster than vastus lateralis and 17% faster than gluteal muscles 1½-inch needle absorbs 2½ times faster than when injected through a 1-inch needle
	Intravenous	Faster onset than intramuscular, within one or more minutes
	Intradermal	Slow absorption
	Topical Routes	
	Transdermal	Prolonged systemic effect
	Inhalation	Rapid localized absorption

   d. Buccal: drug is held against the mucous membranes between the cheek and teeth and absorbed through the mucous membranes of the mouth; both buccal and sublingual administration bypass the GI tract and the liver, thus eliminating the first-pass loss when drugs are metabolized before they have reached the site of action

3. **Parenteral routes:** injection of drugs administered by any route other than the alimentary canal (intestines)

   a. Subcutaneous: injection into subcutaneous tissue, which is the third layer of tissue below skin; can be bolus or continuous infusions; volumes to be administered must be limited

   b. Intramuscular: injection into a muscle for rapid absorption into the bloodstream; some drugs may contain a substance to delay absorption (as in procaine penicillin); most intramuscular dosing patterns are bolus dosing

   c. Intravenous: injection into a vein; the onset of action is more rapid than oral or intramuscular; various dosing patterns are available such as bolus and continuous infusions; requires close monitoring due to immediacy of effect

   d. Intradermal: injection into the dermal layer of skin (dermis); just under the surface of the skin; this method is primarily used to evaluate sensitivity to different agents (e.g., PPD skin test)

4. **Topical** routes: drugs administered on the body surface that are intended for surface use only and are *not* meant for ingestion or injection; creams, lotions, ointments, powders, and patches are drug formulations used by the topical route

   a. Transdermal: surface application of a medication designed to provide a slow release of the drug; usually applied as a patch (e.g., nitroglycerine, estrogens, and nicotine)

► *Practice to Pass*

The client is experiencing a hypertensive crisis and is receiving nitroprusside (Nipride) IV drip at 0.5 micrograms/kg/min. The client weighs 160 pounds. How much nitroprusside should the client receive per minute?

   b. Inhalation: administered into the respiratory tract using a mist, spray, or positive pressure

   c. Ophthalmic: administered to the eye

   d. *Otic:* administered in the ear

   e. *Nasal:* administered in the nose for local or systemic effect

5. Medication measurement systems

   a. Metric: a decimal system of measurement based upon units of 10 with the gram as the unit of weight and the liter as the unit of liquid volume

   b. Apothecary: oldest system of measurement that uses Roman numerals and special symbols; the unit of liquid measure is the minim and the unit for weight is the grain

   c. *Household:* a less accurate system of measurement based upon drops, teaspoons, tablespoons, cups and glasses (see Table 11-3 for approximate weight equivalents and Table 11-4 for volume equivalents)

   d. Medications are prescribed in a specific weight per volume; for instance, a single tablet may have 100 mg of medication and the volume of that tablet is 1; a medication that comes in 80 mg per 2 mL of liquid has a volume of 2; a few liquid medications are prescribed by volume alone and are medications that come in only one strength; when the physician orders a weight of medication, the nurse determines how much medication to give based on the volume (solid or liquid) needed to include that weight

   e. Calculations: a variety of formulas are utilized in calculating medications; one is called ratio and proportion; in this calculation, the weight of the medication ordered for the client is compared to the weight and volume of the available forms of the medication; if 40 mg of furosemide (Lasix) is ordered, and the medication comes in 80 mg per 2 mL, the nurse would calculate the volume to be administered as 80/2 = 40/x or 1 mL

III. NURSE'S ROLE IN ADMINISTERING MEDICATIONS

A. Standards

1. In administering medications, the nurse must check the six "rights" of drug administration: right medication, right dose, right client, right route, right time, right documentation

2. Right medication: compare drug container label to the medication administration record (MAR) three times; note expiration date of the medication; check the drug name (many drugs have very similar names) and correctness of therapy; be knowledgeable about any medications administered, if unsure of the specific medication, review the information in an appropriate drug resource

Table 11-3	Metric System	Apothecary System
Approximate Weight Equivalents	1 mg (milligram)	1/60 grain
	60 mg	1 grain
	1000 mg = 1 gram	15 grains
	1000 grams = 1 kg	2.2 lb (pounds)

Table 11-4	Metric	Apothecary	Household
Approximate Volume Equivalents	1 mL	15 minims	15 drops (gtt)
	4–5 mL	1 fluid dram	1 teaspoon
	15 mL	4 fluid drams	1 Tbsp (tablespoon)
	30 mL	1 fluid ounce	2 Tbsp
	250 mL	8 fluid ounces	1 cup
	500 mL	16 fluid ounces	1 pint
	1000 mL	32 fluid ounces	1 quart
	4000 mL	64 fluid ounces	1 gallon

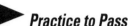

Practice to Pass

Upon entering a client's room to administer her daily dose of Betapace, a drug for ventricular arrhythmias, the client tells the nurse that she doesn't want to take the medication. What are the nursing actions and why?

3. Right dose: check the recommended dose for the drug and the appropriateness of the dose for the client, confirm calculations, and verify laboratory results or serum levels that could alter the drug dose; check heparin, insulin, and digitalis doses with another nurse; validate medication orders requiring multiple unit doses to be administered at one given time

4. Right client: have client state name and check the room and bed number and client's identification band before administering the medication

5. Right route: confirm the route of administration with the MAR and note on the medication label that the specific medication preparation can be administered by the prescribed route and that it is the correct route for the client's condition

6. Right time: confirm the time of day with the time of administration noted on the MAR and when the last dose was given; verify that the schedule for the drug is consistent with maintaining therapeutic levels; if not on military time, validate the time as either A.M. or P.M.

7. Right documentation: chart each medication completely and correctly
   a. The nurse records in the client's chart the administration details
   b. Included in the record would be the exact time of administration, name and dosage of drug, along with the route of administration
   c. Any pertinent information associated with the drug such as heart rate with digitalis or blood pressure with methergine should be recorded
   d. The nurse must sign the administration record
   e. Each agency will have specific policies regarding where and how the medication is documented
   f. If the drug was a prn medication for a specific complaint, the nurse should note follow-up assessment data indicating the success or failure of the medication effects

B. Maintaining client's rights in relation to medications
   1. Clients have the right to have medications administered safely
   2. The nurse is responsible to ensure drug administration safety by following the 6 rights
   3. Right of client to refuse medication
      a. The nurse needs to inform the client of the name of the medication, its intended action, and possible side and adverse effects so that the client can make an informed decision about whether to take the medication
      b. If the client refuses the medication, note this information on the medical record indicating the client's rationale and attempts by the nurse to correct any misinformation and allay fears

C. Nursing process

1. Assessment: psychosocial and biophysical parameters are used to assess clients' needs for the medication and response to drug therapy

   a. History: general, allergies, medication use, and diet history

      1) A general history provides baseline information essential to the safe administration of drugs

      2) The database reveals information concerning potential contraindications, drug incompatibilities, client knowledge deficits, and physical or psychological conditions that could affect the pharmacokinetics of the medication

      3) Allergies: includes client's allergic responses to drugs, food, products, or environmental allergens; obtain specific information about the type of reaction; an allergy to one prototype drug will often cause an allergic reaction with other prototype drugs within the same class

      4) Medication use: includes information on the frequency, amount, and duration of current and recent drug use including prescription drugs, over-the-counter drugs, herbal preparations, alcohol, tobacco products, illegal drugs, and drug dependencies; question the client about the effectiveness, side effects, and if the client knows the purpose for the medications

      5) Diet: obtain data about normal eating habits through a typical 24-hour dietary recall of types and amounts of all foods and beverages consumed; this assists in determining potential food and medication incompatibilities and the need to adjust the medication schedule with mealtimes or specific food items

   b. Client's perceptual/coordination problems

      1) Perception and coordination are important elements in assessing the client's reaction to the medication as well as the client's ability to self-administer medications

      2) Baseline data including the client's orientation to time, place and person, memory, attention span, equilibrium, muscle control, and movement

      3) This information assists in assessing central nervous system (CNS) responses to medications and the client's ability to self-administer his or her drugs

      4) Assess for visual, tactile, or neuromuscular disabilities that would affect client's ability to manage the necessary equipment or route of administration (e.g., using syringes, opening medication bottles, administering a suppository)

   c. Client's experience with medications

      1) Clients with previous allergic reactions to other medications are more likely to have an allergic reaction to new medications than those who have had none

      2) In addition, clients who have demonstrated idiosyncrasies to medications should also be monitored closely when new medications are added

      3) Previous experience with medication may affect the client's attitude toward a new medication

   d. Client's knowledge/understanding of medications

      1) Is the client able to understand the action, side effects, dosage, and administration schedule?

        2) Determine whether the client can afford the drugs and if the client knows what to do should he or she encounter a side effect

    e. Client's learning needs

        1) An assessment of the client's knowledge/understanding of the medications provides insight into what client teaching is necessary

        2) Assessing the educational background assists the nurse in determining the best client education approach

        3) Determine: What is the education level? Can the client read and write English, or is another language preferred? What learning style is best—written materials, oral explanation or demonstration?

2. Planning: the following goals and expected outcomes must be met:

    a. Client/family understand medication regimen

        1) The information obtained in the history assists the nurse in individualizing the client teaching plan

        2) Using the appropriate teaching methods specific to the client's learning style, physical, emotional and psychological abilities, and finances are crucial to compliance and favorable outcomes

    b. Client achieves therapeutic effect of the medication without complications or discomfort

        1) Understanding the specific purpose for which the client receives the drug is crucial to the evaluating the effectiveness of the drug (e.g., propanolol [Inderal] is prescribed for hypertension, angina, migraine headaches, and supraventricular arrhythmias)

        2) The plan of care includes appropriate assessments to evaluate effectiveness and to minimize potential side effects of drugs (e.g., one of the actions of propanolol [a beta blocker] is reduction of the heart rate, therefore taking the apical pulse before and after drug administration should be included in the nursing care plan)

    c. Client has no complications related to route of medication

        1) Understanding the pharmacokinetics of drugs ensures the proper route of administration, preparation of the drug, and appropriate assessments to monitor the client's response

        2) The route of administration alters the absorption, distribution, and excretion of drugs

        3) Validate that the route and preparation of the drug is appropriate for the medication as well as for the client's physical condition (e.g., evaluate the swallowing ability of a client admitted for a stroke prior to administering an oral medication; don't crush enteric-coated, or extended-release drugs)

    d. Client safely self-administers medications

        1) Develop teaching methods that include evaluation of the client's ability to self-administer his or her medications

        2) Cognitive, psychomotor, and affective learning are all aspects impacting successful outcomes

        3) Direct observation, tests, oral questioning, and monitoring through follow-up contacts with the client can evaluate the effectiveness of cognitive learning

        4) Psychomotor skills are best evaluated by direct observation

5) Affective learning relates to the client's values or attitudes and can significantly affect the client's follow-through with the treatment plan; evaluation of the client's attitudes or values can be inferred by listening to the client's responses to your questions and attentiveness to the client's behavior and feelings

3. Implementation

a. Receive medication order

1) A medication must have a physician or nurse practitioner order or prescription prior to administration

2) The order can be written or computerized

3) A written order is recorded in the client's chart or file

4) A telephone order is recorded by the nurse as a "telephone order" in the client's chart for signature by the prescriber, usually within 24 hours

5) Orders can be prescribed as one-time-only, PRN (as needed), or routine (according to instructions until the order is cancelled)

b. Correctly transcribe/communicate order: in noncomputerized medical records, medications are transcribed from the client's chart or file onto a MAR; it is the nurse's responsibility to ensure accuracy of the transcription and that all essential parts of the drug order are present:

1) Client's name and room number

2) Name of the drug

3) Date and time the order was written

4) Dosage

5) Route

6) Frequency

7) Signature of the person writing the order

c. Accurate dose calculation/measurement

1) The drug dosage includes the amount and also the strength when medications are available in varying strengths

2) If a fractional dose is administered, accuracy depends upon correct calculations using the metric or apothecary system and matching the dosage with the appropriate administration device (e.g., insulin requires a syringe that measures in units, liquid oral medications may require measurement in a syringe that is calculated by tenths)

3) When pouring liquid medications into a medication cup, read the solution at eye level using the bottom of the meniscus (crescent-shaped upper surface of a column of liquid)

d. Correct administration

1) Use the six rights

2) Organize the supplies (e.g., IV pump, alcohol swabs, medicine cups)

3) Compare the label of the medication with the MAR—if they are not identical, check the order in the client's chart; if there is still a discrepancy, check with the pharmacist

4) Prepare the medication using **aseptic** technique, free from germs, and according to the guidelines for the specific medication (e.g., proper diluent solution and amount)

    5) Separate **narcotics,** strong opioid analgesics that in moderate doses depress the central nervous system, from other medications requiring specific assessments (e.g., pulse or blood pressure)

    6) Administer only the medications you prepare

    7) Do not leave medications at the bedside with certain exceptions such as nitroglycerine when there is a corresponding order to do so

    8) Ensure that the client takes the medication through direct observation

    9) If a medication error is made, report it immediately according to agency policies

e. Record administration

    1) Document the name of the drug, time, dosage, route, and relevant data such as pulse with digoxin (Lanoxin) on the MAR

    2) Initial the drug and identify your initials with your signature

    3) Circle the time of withheld or refused drugs, document the reason, and report this to the healthcare provider

    4) Assess and record the client's response to the drug, particularly related to PRN medications

f. Special considerations

    1) Infants/children: children metabolize many drugs differently than adults and have immature systems for handling drugs; many drugs list recommended pediatric dosages, others can be converted to pediatric dosages based on the child's age, weight, or body surface area; oral preparations are usually prepared as elixirs (sweetened, aromatic liquids); do not mask the taste of medications in foods such as milk because the child may develop an unpleasant association with the food; be truthful to the child about painful procedures such as injections

    2) Older adults: undergo many physical changes that may result in responses that are different from the typical pharmacokinetics:

        a) Less effective absorption

        b) Less efficient distribution

        c) Retention of fat-soluble drugs and increased potential for toxicity due to increased proportion of fat to lean body mass

        d) Altered biotransformation because of liver changes

        e) Less effective excretion due to reduced renal functioning

        f) Older adults frequently have chronic diseases resulting in polypharmacy, which increases the risk for drug interactions

    3) Over-the-counter (OTC) medications

        a) Products that are available without prescription for self-treatment or are recommended by the health care provider

        b) Clients may not consider OTC drugs to be medications and not include them in their medication history; therefore, ask specifically about OTC medication use when obtaining a medication history

        c) Some drugs previously approved as prescription drugs were found to be safe and useful for clients without the need of a prescription when provided in smaller doses

        d) Some of these drugs were not rigorously screened and tested according to the current drug evaluation protocols because they were developed and marketed before the current laws were put into effect

      e) Taking these drugs could mask the signs and symptoms of underlying disease

      f) Taking these drugs with prescription medications may result in drug interactions and could interfere with drug therapy

    4) Misuse of medications

      a) Improper use of OTC and prescription drugs can lead to acute and chronic toxicity

      b) Frequently overused drugs include cough and cold medications, laxatives and antacids, which could cause harmful effects or delay the diagnosis of more serious problems

      c) Drug abuse that can lead to drug dependence and illicit drugs (street drugs) are forms of misuse

    5) Noncompliance: failure or refusal to take medications according to the instructions; can be related to many factors, such as finances, values or attitudes, cognitive and physical ability, and knowledge/understanding of the medication

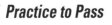

Practice to Pass

The nurse is preparing a client for discharge from the hospital. He is going home with several prescriptions. What client teaching needs to be done regarding the medications?

  4. Evaluation

    a. Monitor response: continually evaluate the client for therapeutic response, the occurrence of adverse effects, and occurrence of drug-drug or drug-food interactions

    b. Use various evaluation measures (e.g., direct observation, checklist, BP); use psychosocial and biophysical parameters to assess the client's need for and response to drug therapy (see Table 11-5)

D. Procedure for administering medications

  1. See Box 11-1

  2. Oral medications

    a. Break only scored tablets

    b. Crush only medications approved for crushing or chewing

      1) Extended-release medications are designed to be released over an extended period of time; some scored formulations can be broken without affecting the release mechanism; some mixed-release capsules can be opened and the contents sprinkled on food

      2) Abbreviations used in brand names identifying drugs as extended-release include CR (controlled release), CRT (controlled-release tablet), LA (long acting), SR (sustained release), TR (timed release), SA (sustained action), and XL or XR (extended release)

      3) Enteric-coated drugs are designed to allow the drug to pass through the stomach intact with the drug being released in the intestines

  3. Enteral tube

    a. Position the client in semi-Fowler's position

    b. Determine correct placement (it may not be possible to reliably determine placement of small-bore enteral tubes by any technique other than radiography, which is also most reliable)

      1) Nasogastric tube: aspirate stomach contents and check pH (should be 4 or less) or auscultate air insufflation; secretions should be greenish, tan to clear

      2) *Nasointestinal tubes:* aspirate stomach contents and check for pH greater than 6; duodenal secretions should be deep yellow

Table 11-5	Parameter	Evaluation Measures
Biophysical Evaluation Parameters	Cardiovascular	Blood pressure Cardiac rate and rhythm Presence or absence of chest pain Presence and strength of peripheral pulses Color, temperature, and turgor of the skin Presence or absence of edema Cardiac enzymes Electrolytes Serum concentrations of cardiac-related drugs Complete blood count
	Respiratory	Respiratory rate, rhythm, and effort Lung sounds, especially for the presence or absence of adventitious sounds Dyspnea Need for supplemental oxygen Use of accessory muscles Cyanosis Clubbing Cough and sputum production Arterial blood gases Oxygen saturation values obtained by pulse oximetry
	Renal	Presence of flank pain Adequacy of urinary output (30 mL/hr) Color and clarity of urine Specific gravity of urine Blood urea nitrogen (BUN) and creatinine levels Culture and sensitivity urine testing Serum and urine protein levels Serum electrolytes
	Central nervous system	Glasgow Coma Scale Level of cognitive functioning in comparison to baseline level of alertness and orientation Intactness of the cranial nerves Motion and sensation in the extremities Blood glucose levels Serum metabolic toxin levels Arterial blood gases Analysis of cerebrospinal fluid (CSF)
	Laboratory studies	Those mentioned under specific parameters White blood cell count (WBC)

3) Percutaneous endoscopic gastrostomy (PEG) and percutaneous endoscopic jejunostomy (PEJ) tubes do not require placement verification prior to each medication administration

c. Flush the enteral tube with approximately 30 mL of water

d. Administer medication in solution or elixir forms when available; crush tablets to a fine powder and mix in warm water to make a solution or suspension; do not mix medications—administer each medication separately; flush well between medications

e. If the client is receiving enteral feeding, ensure that the medication and the feeding are compatible; if they are not compatible, turn off the tube feeding

Box 11-1	1. Validate the medication order for consistency of drug, dose, time intervals, and route of administration.
General Medication Preparation Procedures	2. Compare the prescriber's most recent medication orders with the medication administration record (MAR).
	3. Wash your hands.
	4. Start at the top of the MAR and compare each medication with the drug label, checking for dose, time, and route of administration. Recheck information 3 times.
	5. Prepare medication as indicated.
	6. Ask client to state name and check identification band.
	7. Assist client to appropriate position for the administration route.
	8. Explain the medication to the client.
	9. Perform appropriate assessments if indicated.
	10. Using aseptic technique, administer the medication. If the medication is dispensed in the unit-dose package, open the package at the client's bedside and place in a medication cup. The packaging allows identification and keeps the medication clean.
	11. Properly dispose of medication equipment.
	12. Wash your hands.
	13. Document the name, dose, time, and route of the drug, and other assessments as indicated in the MAR.

for 30 to 60 minutes before and after the administration of the medication; if the tube is connected to suction, disconnect from suction for at least 30 minutes after administering the medication

f. Flush the enteral tube with approximately 30 mL of water following each medication

g. Maintain the client in semi-Fowler's position for at least 30 minutes following the administration of the medication

4. Skin

a. Put on gloves—prevents absorption of the medication through fingertips

b. Remove prior applications remaining on the skin unless otherwise specified

c. Remove ointments and creams from their containers and apply to the skin with tongue depressors or cotton tipped applicators in thin layers unless otherwise specified

d. Transdermal patch or premeasured paper—read package insert for application directions

1) Remove previously applied patch or paper and cleanse skin

2) Record date and time of application and your initials directly onto the transdermal patch and remove the protective covering

3) Place prescribed amount of medication directly on premeasured paper and apply immediately; secure paper with tape

4) Rotate application areas to prevent skin irritation and apply to clean, dry, intact, and hairless skin

5. Respiratory medications

   a. Nose drops

      1) Tilt the client's head back

      2) Fill the dropper with the prescribed amount of medication

      3) Place the dropper just inside the nares and instill correct number of drops

      4) Wipe excess medication with tissue

      5) Instruct the client not to sneeze or blow nose and to keep head tilted back for 5 minutes until the medication is absorbed

   b. Metered-dose inhaled medication (MDI) (see Figure 11-1)

      1) Shake the canister before each puff to mix the medication and propellant

      2) Instruct the client to hold inhaler 2 inches away from mouth

      3) Instruct the client to exhale through pursed lips

      4) Instruct the client to depress inhalation device, inhaling slowly and deeply through mouth

      5) Instruct the client to hold the breath for 10 seconds and slowly exhale through pursed lips

      6) Instruct the client to wait 2 minutes (or longer if drug literature recommends) between puffs

      7) Clean the device according to manufacturer's instructions

   c. Spacer with MDI (see Figure 11-2)

      1) Insert MDI mouthpiece into spacer

      2) Remove the mouthpiece cover from spacer

      3) Shake MDI with spacer

      4) Hold MDI and spacer with drug canister upright

      5) Instruct the client to exhale slowly through pursed lips

      6) Instruct the client to close lips around spacer mouthpiece

      7) Activate MDI canister by pushing it further into plastic adapter

      8) Instruct the client to inhale slowly and deeply through mouth

      9) Instruct the client to hold breath 10 seconds

Figure 11-1

Metered dose inhaler with device positioned away from the opened mouth.

© Jenny Thomas

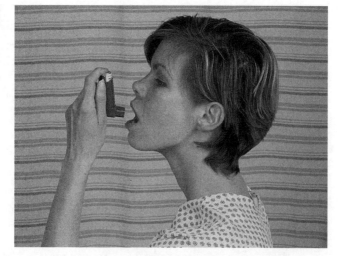

Figure 11-2

Metered-dose inhaler with extender attached to a mouthpiece placed in the mouth.

© Jenny Thomas

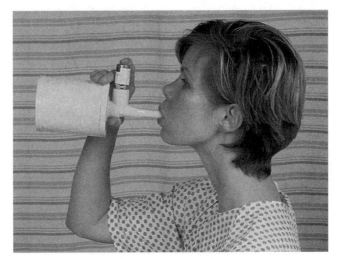

10) Instruct client to exhale and relax

11) Wipe mouthpiece after use

12) Remove rubber end of spacer, rinse with warm water and dry thoroughly

6. Optic medications

    a. Eye abbreviations include O.S.—left eye, O.D.—right eye, and O.U.—both eyes

    b. Ophthalmic drops

        1) Tilt the client's head slightly backward and ask the client to look up

        2) Give tissue to client so that the client can wipe off excess medication

        3) Hold eyedropper ½ to ¾ inch above the eyeball

        4) Expose lower **conjunctival sac** (mucosal membrane that lines the eye), by pulling down on cheek, creating a "cup"

        5) Drop prescribed number of drops into center of conjunctival sac while applying pressure to inner canthus to reduce systemic absorption of medication

        6) Instruct the client to close eyelids and move eyes

        7) Gently massage closed lid

        8) Remove excess medication with tissue

    c. Ophthalmic ointment

        1) Give tissue to client so that the client can wipe off excess medication

        2) Put on gloves

        3) Gently separate the client's eyelids with two fingers, grasping the lower lid immediately below the lashes; exert pressure downward over the bony prominence of the cheek to form a trough

        4) Instruct the client to look upward

        5) Apply eye medication along the inside edge of the entire lower eyelid, from inner canthus to outer canthus (the angles formed by the upper and lower eyelids)

        6) Instruct the client to close eyelids and move eyes to spread ointment under the lids and over the eye surface

        7) Remove excess medication with a tissue

        8) Instruct client that vision may be blurred temporarily following administration of an ointment

Figure 11-3

Instilling ear drops. Gently pull pinna up and back to instill medication in an adult or older child.

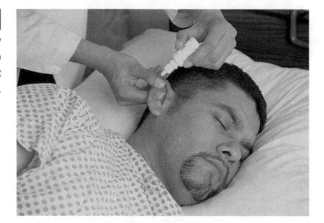

7. Otic (ear) medications
   a. Position the client on side, with ear to be treated uppermost
   b. Fill medication dropper with the prescribed amount of medication
   c. Put on gloves
   d. Straighten the ear canal
      1) Infant: pull pinna, the projected part of the upper exterior ear, gently downward and backward
      2) Adult: pull pinna gently upward and backward (see Figure 11-3)
      3) Instill medication drops, holding the medication slightly above the ear
      4) Insert cotton loosely into the ear canal, if ordered
      5) Instruct the client to remain on side for 5 to 10 minutes
8. Vagina
   a. Position the client in the dorsal recumbent or Sims' position
   b. Put on gloves
   c. Suppository: remove foil wrapper and insert the suppository into the applicator
   d. Cream: attach the tube of medication to the applicator and squeeze the tube to fill the applicator with the prescribed amount of medication; remove the tube
   e. Insert the applicator into the vaginal canal at least 2 inches, push the plunger until all of the medication is released, and remove the applicator (see Figure 11-4)

Figure 11-4

Using an applicator to instill vaginal cream.

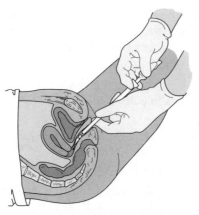

      f. Instruct the client to lie quietly for 15 minutes until the suppository or cream is absorbed

      g. Wash applicator and return it to appropriate place in the client's room

9. Rectal

      a. Place the client in Sims' (left lateral) position

      b. Wash hands and put on gloves

      c. Remove foil wrapper from the suppository

      d. Apply small amount of water-soluble lubricant to the suppository

      e. With index finger, insert the suppository flat end first (studies indicate this promotes better retention than tapered end first) beyond the internal sphincter to ensure retention

        1) Adult: insert approximately 10 cm or 4 inches (see Figure 11-5)

        2) Child or infant: insert approximately 5 cm or 2 inches

      f. Instruct the client to lie quietly for 15 minutes while medication is absorbed

10. Administering medications by **irrigation (lavage),** cleansing of a body cavity by flushing with medication (see Table 11-6)

      a. Surgical asepsis is required when there is a break in the skin (e.g., wound irrigation) or when entering a sterile body cavity (e.g., bladder)

      b. Medical asepsis is used for vaginal, rectal, or gastric irrigation; the type, strength, amount, and temperature of the irrigant are prescribed

      c. Eye

        1) Wash hands and put on gloves

        2) Supply the client with a receptacle to catch the irrigation returns (emesis basin)

        3) Gently separate the client's eyelids with two fingers, grasping the lower lid immediately below the lashes; exert pressure downward over the bony prominence of the cheek to form a trough

        4) Instruct the client to look upward

        5) Fill and hold the eye irrigator approximately 1 inch above the eye to ensure safe pressure of the irrigation solution

        6) Irrigate the eye, directing the solution on the lower conjunctival sac from the inner canthus to the outer canthus so that the irrigation returns run into the collecting basin

        7) Dry around the eye with cotton balls or tissues

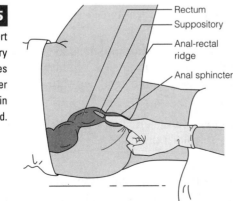

Figure 11-5

With a gloved finger, insert the rectal suppository approximately 4 inches beyond the internal sphincter in an adult and 2 inches in a child.

Rectum
Suppository
Anal-rectal ridge
Anal sphincter

Table 11-6		
Irrigation Syringes	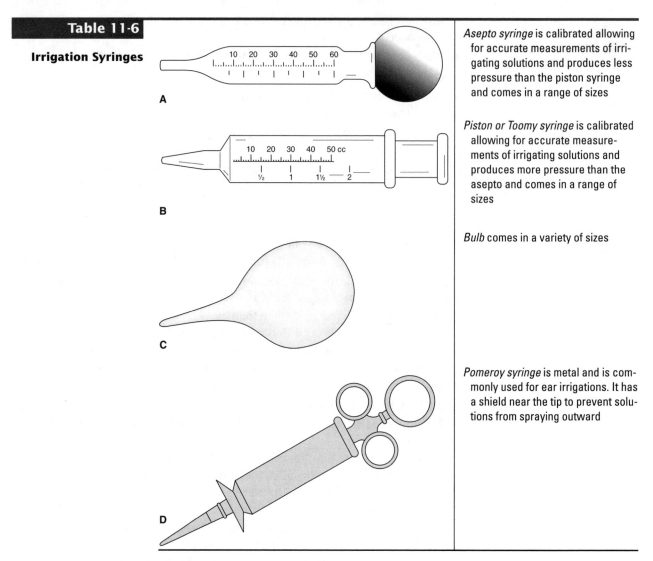	*Asepto syringe* is calibrated allowing for accurate measurements of irrigating solutions and produces less pressure than the piston syringe and comes in a range of sizes
		Piston or Toomy syringe is calibrated allowing for accurate measurements of irrigating solutions and produces more pressure than the asepto and comes in a range of sizes
		Bulb comes in a variety of sizes
		Pomeroy syringe is metal and is commonly used for ear irrigations. It has a shield near the tip to prevent solutions from spraying outward

▶ *Practice to Pass*

The nurse is to administer heparin by the subcutaneous route. What supplies will the nurse need and how will the nurse administer the medication?

    d. Ears

        1) Wash hands and put on gloves

        2) Straighten the ear canal

        3) Supply the client with a receptacle to catch the irrigation returns (emesis basin)

        4) Fill and insert the ear irrigator into the auditory canal (do not obstruct the canal with the syringe, solution must be able to escape as you are irrigating) and gently direct the solution gently upward against the top of the canal

        5) Dry the outside of the ear

        6) Position the client on the affected side and place an absorbent material under the ear to collect drainage

  11. Injections

    a. See Box 11-2 for withdrawing medications from a vial

    b. See Box 11-3 for withdrawing medications from an ampule

Box 11-2	1. Remove vial cap.
Withdrawing Medications from a Vial	2. Cleanse rubber top of the vial with alcohol.
	3. Tighten needle on syringe or use needleless syringe.
	4. Fill plunger with an amount of air equal to the amount of solution to be withdrawn.
	5. Inject air into vacant area of vial keeping the needle above the surface of medication.
	6. Invert the vial touching only the syringe barrel and plunger tip. Withdraw medication.
	7. While the syringe remains attached to the vial, expel any air bubbles from syringe by tapping the side of syringe sharply.
	8. Recheck amount of medication in syringe.
	9. Remove syringe from vial and recap needle.

   c. Maintain sterility while assembling the syringe and needle; select the appropriate size needle and syringe based on the volume and type of medication, the desired site, the client's size, and the viscosity of the medication

   d. See Table 11-7 (p. 306) for a summary of syringes, needles, and uses

   e. Using anatomical landmarks, select the site of injection appropriate for the type of injection and medication (e.g., intramuscular, intradermal, or subcutaneous); see Table 11-8 (pp. 307–309) for a summary of injection sites

   f. Wash hands and put on gloves

   g. Cleanse the area with an alcohol swab and wait for it to dry

   h. Inject the medication

   i. Discard the syringe and needle into a sharps container

   j. Specific information appropriate to injection sites

      1) Intradermal (ID): gently pull the skin taut; do not **aspirate** (draw back); inject medication slowly and observe for wheal formation and blanching at site

      2) Subcutaneous (SubQ): grasp SubQ tissue; hold syringe like a dart (between thumb and forefinger) and insert needle; release SubQ tissue; aspirate (except with heparin or insulin) and inject the medication slowly if no blood appears (if blood returns withdraw the needle, discard and prepare a new injection); with insulin administration, injection sites need to be rotated in an orderly manner to minimize tissue damage (**lipodystrophy,** atrophy or hypertrophy of the SubQ tissue), which affects absorption

      3) Intramuscular (IM): hold syringe like a dart (between thumb and forefinger); spread skin taught or grasp the skin in the pediatric and geriatric

(text continues on p. 310)

Box 11-3	1. Tap the neck of the ampule to move solution to the body of the ampule.
Withdrawing Medications from an Ampule	2. Using a pad, break ampule away from you.
	3. Use a filter needle to withdraw solution. Solution can be withdrawn from either an upright or inverted position—insert needle without touching sides of neck with the bevel down and touching the bottom of the ampule (do not add air).
	4. Return ampule to upright position.
	5. Tap barrel below bubbles to dislodge air in the syringe.
	6. Eject air with syringe in an upright position.
	7. Recheck amount of medication in syringe.
	8. Remove filter needle and replace with appropriate needle.

Table 11-7   Summary of Syringes, Needles, and Uses

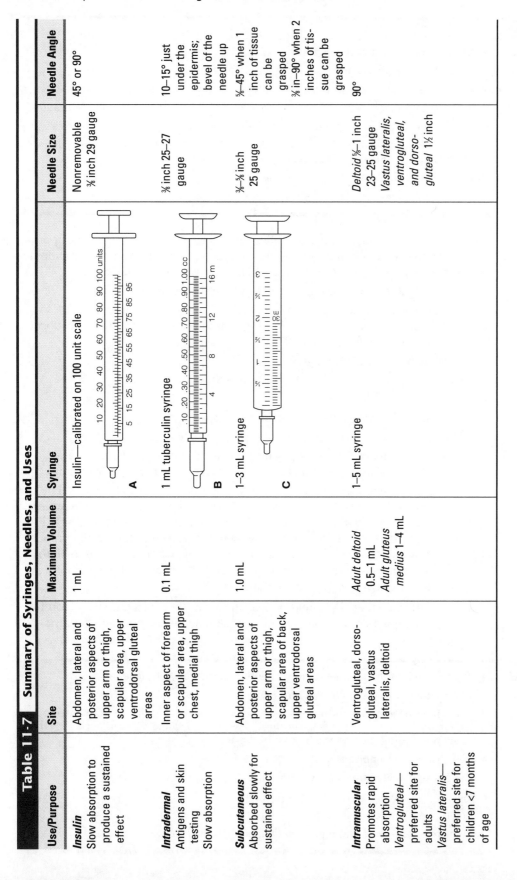

Use/Purpose	Site	Maximum Volume	Syringe	Needle Size	Needle Angle
Insulin Slow absorption to produce a sustained effect	Abdomen, lateral and posterior aspects of upper arm or thigh, scapular area, upper ventrodorsal gluteal areas	1 mL	Insulin—calibrated on 100 unit scale **A**	Nonremovable ⅜ inch 29 gauge	45° or 90°
Intradermal Antigens and skin testing Slow absorption	Inner aspect of forearm or scapular area, upper chest, medial thigh	0.1 mL	1 mL tuberculin syringe **B**	⅜ inch 25–27 gauge	10–15° just under the epidermis; bevel of the needle up
Subcutaneous Absorbed slowly for sustained effect	Abdomen, lateral and posterior aspects of upper arm or thigh, scapular area of back, upper ventrodorsal gluteal areas	1.0 mL	1–3 mL syringe **C**	⅜–⅝ inch 25 gauge	⅝–45° when 1 inch of tissue can be grasped ⅞ in–90° when 2 inches of tissue can be grasped
Intramuscular Promotes rapid absorption *Ventrogluteal*—preferred site for adults *Vastus lateralis*—preferred site for children <7 months of age	Ventrogluteal, dorso-gluteal, vastus lateralis, deltoid	*Adult deltoid* 0.5–1 mL *Adult gluteus medius* 1–4 mL	1–5 mL syringe	*Deltoid* ⅝–1 inch 23–25 gauge *Vastus lateralis, ventrogluteal, and dorso-gluteal* 1½ inch	90°

Table 11-8	*Intramuscular*
Summary of Injection Sites	*Ventrogluteal*

Ventrogluteal
- Place the client in side-lying position
- Use right hand for left anterior hip and left hand for right anterior hip
- Place palm over greater trochanter and point index finger toward the client's anterior superior iliac spine; spread out the index finger from the other three fingers to form a "V" area
- Inject at a 90° angle within the "V" area

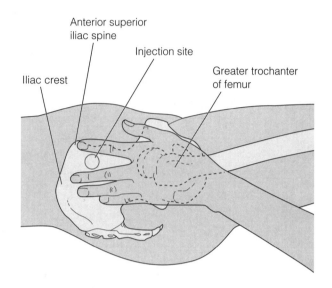

Dorsogluteal
- Place the client in the prone position with the toes pointed inward or the side-lying position with the upper knee flexed and in front of the lower leg
- Draw an imaginary line between the greater trochanter and the postero-superior spine (prominence) of iliac crest
- Inject at a 90° angle lateral and superior to the imaginary line

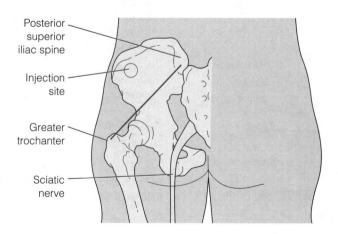

Table 11-8
Summary of Injection Sites (continued)

Vastus Lateralis
- Place the client in supine position
- Inject at a 90° angle using the anterior lateral middle third of the thigh between the greater trochanter and the lateral femoral condyle

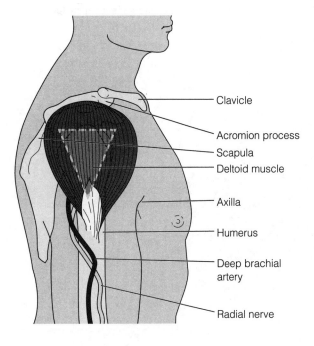

Greater trochanter of femur

Vastus lateralis (middle third)

Lateral femoral condyle

Clavicle

Acromion process

Scapula

Deltoid muscle

Axilla

Humerus

Deep brachial artery

Radial nerve

Deltoid
- Palpate the lower edge of the acromion and the midpoint of the lateral aspect of the arm. Inject at a 90° angle 2 in. below the acromion process within the triangle between the boundaries
- Alternate method—place four fingers across the deltoid muscle with the first finger on the acromion process; the site is three finger breaths below the acromion process.

Z-Track Injection
- An alternative method of intramuscular injection designed to reduce seepage of the medication into the subcutaneous tissues.
- Prior to injection, the skin is displaced; the needle is inserted at a 90° angle while the skin remains displaced; once the needle is removed, the skin is allowed to return to a neutral position, thus eliminating an intact needle tract.
- This method is used for medications that are irritating to subcutaneous tissues.

Table 11-8	
Summary of Injection Sites (continued)	

Subcutaneous

Most common sites
- Lateral posterior aspect of the upper arms
- Anterior thighs
- Lower quadrants of the abdomen (outside a 2-in. radius of the umbilicus): preferred site for heparin

Other sites
- Scapular areas
- Dorsogluteal

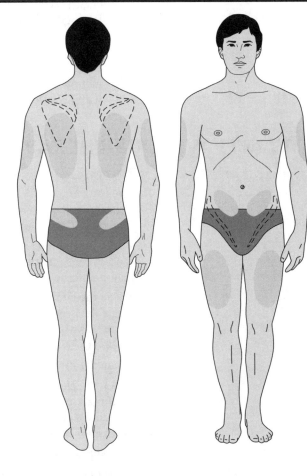

Intradermal
- Forearms
- Upper back beneath the scapula
- Upper chest

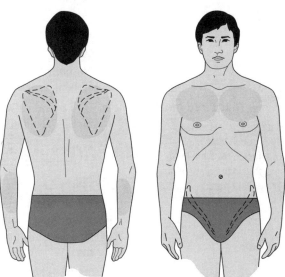

client; use a quick, darting motion to insert the needle; aspirate and inject the medication slowly unless blood returns; if blood returns, withdraw the needle, discard, and prepare a new injection); Z-track technique prevents "tracking" and is used for administering medications that are especially irritating to subcutaneous tissue (e.g., hydroxyzine)—pull the skin approximately 1 in. laterally away from the injection site, inject the medication, withdraw the needle, then release the tissue

IV. INTRAVENOUS THERAPY

A. Indications

1. The intravenous (IV) route can be used to give medications that are too irritating to be given by another route, to avoid the discomfort of frequent IM injections, or to maintain a constant therapeutic blood level of a medication

2. In life-threatening situations, it provides access for administration of medications and fluids directly into the bloodstream, ensuring prompt onset of action and the most complete absorption

3. When the client is unable to take fluids by mouth, it provides fluid and electrolyte replacement therapy for clients unable to take oral nourishment (such as with NPO status for diagnostic or surgical procedures, or problems related to swallowing or to the GI tract)

4. When the medications would be destroyed by the GI tract

5. When the client is unable to digest or absorb a diet or when the GI tract is nonfunctional because of an interruption in its continuity or impaired absorptive capacity, nutrition can be provided through the venous system, where absorption and digestion of nutrients do not depend on the GI tract

B. Types of fluids provided by the IV route

1. Hydrating solutions (see Table 11-9)

2. Blood transfusion: administration of whole blood or blood components into the venous circulation (see Box 11-4, p. 312); types of blood products include:

   a. Whole blood: replaces intravascular blood volume and all blood products; contains red blood cells, plasma, plasma proteins, fresh platelets, and other clotting factors

   b. Red blood cells: increase oxygen-carrying capacity of blood; 1 unit of red blood cells increases hematocrit approximately 2–4%

   c. Platelets: play an important role in blood coagulation, homeostasis, and blood thrombus formation

   d. Plasma: liquid part of the blood that expands blood volume and provides clotting factors

   e. Albumin: expands blood volume by providing plasma proteins; contains substances that cannot diffuse through capillary walls, resulting in increased plasma volume and increased osmotic pressure causing fluids to move into the vascular compartment; used to treat hypovolemic shock

   f. Clotting factors and cryoprecipitate provide different factors involved in blood clotting; cryoprecipitate is prepared from fresh frozen plasma and contains factor VIII, factor XIII, fibronectin, and fibrinogen; it is used to treat hypofibrinogenemia; concentrates of factor VIII and IX are also available

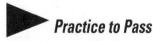

Practice to Pass

The nurse is assessing a client receiving a blood transfusion. At what intervals should the nurse monitor the vital signs?

Table 11-9	Hydrating Solutions	
Solution	**Uses**	**Nursing Implications**
Isotonic 0.9% sodium chloride (normal saline) Lactated Ringer's (LR) (Hartmann's solution) 5% dextrose in water (D$_5$W)	Has same concentration of solutes as plasma therefore remains in the vascular compartment, expanding vascular volume. Normal saline and lactated Ringer's are crystalloid solutions, increase fluid volume in both intravascular and interstitial space with minimal fluid volume expansion. Normal saline is the only solution that may be administered with blood products. D$_5$W is isotonic on initial administration but provides free water when glucose is metabolized, expanding intracellular and extracellular fluid volumes.	Assess for signs of hypervolemia. • Bounding pulse • Shortness of breath • Distended neck veins Assess for signs of hypovolemia • Urine output < 30 mL/hr • Weak, thready pulse • Subnormal temperature
Hypotonic 0.45% sodium chloride (½ normal saline) 0.225% sodium chloride (¼ normal saline)	Has lesser concentration of solutes than plasma therefore treats cellular dehydration through fluid shifting out of the vascular compartment into cells; promotes elimination by kidneys.	Do not administer to clients at risk for third-space fluid shift or accumulation (sequestration of extracellular fluid in a body space, resulting in circulatory volume loss and risk for organ failure, or increased intracranial pressure).
Hypertonic 5% dextrose in normal saline (D$_5$NS) 5% dextrose in 0.45% sodium chloride (D$_5$½NS) 5% dextrose in lactated Ringer's (D$_5$LR) 10% dextrose in water (D$_{10}$W) 20% dextrose in water (D$_{20}$W) 50% dextrose in water (D$_{50}$W)	Has higher concentration of solutes than plasma, therefore causing fluid to shift from the cells into the vascular compartment, expanding vascular volume. 10% dextrose—stand-by solution for clients receiving TPN 50% dextrose—used for hypoglycemia	Do not administer to clients with kidney or heart disease or clients who are dehydrated. Monitor for signs of hypervolemia.
Volume Expanders (colloid solutions) Albumin 5% (Albumin-5, Buminate 5%) Albumin 25% (Albumin-25, Buminate 25%) Dextran 40 (Gentran 40) Hetastarch (Hespan [HESI]) Plasma protein fraction (Plasmanate, PlasmaPlex, Plasmatein, Protenate)	Colloid solutions—contain substances that cannot diffuse through capillary walls, resulting in increased plasma volume and increased osmotic pressure causing fluids to move into the vascular compartment; used to treat hypovolemic shock.	Establish baseline vital signs, lung and heart sounds, and central venous pressure. Repeat per agency protocols. Administer with a large-gauge (18–19 gauge) needle. Monitor intake and output. Monitor for signs of hypervolemia.
Nutrient 5% dextrose (D$_5$W) 5% dextrose in 0.45% sodium chloride	Contain some form of carbohydrate (e.g., dextrose, glucose, or levulose) and water. D$_5$W provides 170 calories per liter.	Useful in preventing dehydration but does not provide sufficient calories to promote wound healing, weight gain, or normal growth in children.
Electrolyte 0.9% sodium chloride Ringer's solution (contains sodium, chloride, potassium, and calcium) Lactated Ringer's (contains sodium, chloride, potassium, calcium, and lactate) 5% dextrose in 0.45% sodium chloride	Saline and electrolytes restore vascular volume and replace electrolytes. Lactated Ringer's (LR) is also an alkalinizing solution that treats metabolic acidosis. 5% dextrose in 0.45% sodium chloride is an acidifying solution to treat metabolic alkalosis.	Monitor fluid and electrolytes. Monitor arterial blood gases. Monitor intake and output.

Box 11-4
Procedure for Blood Administration

➤ Verify client consent and obtain baseline vital signs prior to initiating transfusion (some agencies require a physician's order to administer blood with a temperature elevation greater than 100˚F).

➤ Ensure a suitable vein and appropriate gauge needle (18 or 20 gauge preferred).

➤ Set up the blood infusion equipment

➤Obtain a Y-set with a blood filter, using aseptic technique, insert the spike into a container of 0.9% normal saline and prime the tubing. Ensure that the solution covers the filter and ⅓ of the drip chamber above the filter. Back prime the other Y leg with saline. Never use a solution containing dextrose as that will cause the blood to clump.

➤Start the saline solution.

➤ Obtain the correct blood component from the blood bank checking the requisition form with the blood bag label with the lab technician. Verify client's name, identification number, blood type (A, B, AB, or O) and Rh group, the blood donor number, and the expiration date. Note any abnormal color, RBC clumping, gas bubbles, and extraneous material. Return if date is expired or any abnormalities are noted.

➤ Follow the general guidelines for medication preparation procedures in Box 11-1.

➤ With another nurse, compare the laboratory blood record: client's name and identification number (located on the client's blood identiband), number on the blood bag label, ABO group and Rh type on the blood bag label. If the information does not match exactly, notify the blood bank and do not administer the blood. Sign the appropriate form with the other nurse according to agency protocol.

➤ Immediately hang the blood—blood must be hung within 30 minutes of receiving from the blood bank:

➤Wash hands and don gloves.

➤Invert the blood bag gently several times to mix the cells with the plasma.

➤Insert remaining Y-set spike into the blood bag.

➤Open the upper clamp on the Y-set arm to the blood.

➤Close the upper clamp below the IV saline solution and open the upper clamp below the blood bag to allow the blood to run into the saline-filled drip chamber.

➤ Begin transfusion at a slow rate of about 2 mL per minute, stay with the client and check vital signs every 5–15 minutes for the first 50–100 mL of blood transfused, monitoring for reactions: bacterial, allergic, or hemolytic.

➤ After the first 15 minutes, the rate of infusion is increased. A whole unit of blood should be administered within 3–4 hours.

➤ Continue to monitor vital signs throughout blood infusion according to agency protocol.

➤ Document the procedure and client's reaction in the client's medical record.

3. Total parenteral nutrition (TPN): solutions that provide all needed calories and contain high dextrose concentrations, water, fat, proteins, electrolytes, vitamins, and trace elements

   a. Hypertonic solutions containing more than 10% dextrose require a high-flow central vein for infusion

   b. Infection control is a high priority because the glucose-rich solution promotes bacterial growth

   c. The high glucose content requires careful administration and blood glucose monitoring to prevent hypoglycemia or hyperglycemia

    d. TPN is never stopped abruptly because the sudden absence of the infusion would cause hypoglycemia

C. Equipment needed for IV therapy

  1. Catheters/needles

    a. Over-the-needle catheters: plastic catheter fits over the needle that is used to pierce the skin and vein; once in the vein, the needle is withdrawn and discarded, leaving the catheter in place; available in a variety of lengths and gauges; use the smallest length and gauge of catheter appropriate to the therapy

    b. Winged needle/butterfly: steel needles with plastic flaps (wings) attached to the shaft to facilitate the venipuncture; winged needles are commonly used for obtaining some blood samples or for short-term therapy

    c. These devices come in protected needle styles designed to reduce the risk of accidental puncture wounds and blood exposure

  2. Infusion pumps/electronic delivery devices (EDDs)

    a. Deliver fluids by exerting positive pressure on the tubing or on the fluid in order to maintain fluid flow despite increased venous resistance

    b. Regulate the rate at preset limits and have alarms that are triggered when the fluid level is low or there is air in the line

    c. Should be utilized when the volume needs to be carefully controlled

  3. Regulators/controllers/mechanical infusion devices

    a. Are devices designed to aid in the monitoring of IV flow rates; they are convenience devices and are not to be used when the flow rate must be carefully administered

    b. Because of poorer precision, they are less frequently used today

  4. Tubing: may be vented or nonvented

    a. Vented tubing is used with glass bottles while plastic bags utilize the non-vented tubing

    b. When infusions flow by gravity, the drip chamber of the tubing determines the size of the drop

    c. Drip chambers commonly are rated at 10, 12, or 15 drops per mL; pediatric sets usually are rated at 60 drops per mL

  5. Filters: devices that may be part of the infusion set or may be added to the infusion line; remove contaminants such as air, bacteria, or particulate matter; not all medications/solutions can or need to be be filtered

    a. Total parenteral nutrition requires a filter that is changed every 24 hours with the tubing change

    b. Some medications such as phenytoin (Dilantin) and pantoprazole (Protonix) require a filter change with each medication administration

    c. To prime filters, point filter downward so proximal half fills with fluid first, then invert to complete priming the filter

  6. Types of infusions

    a. Peripheral infusion: an IV device whose internal tip terminates in a peripheral vein; in adults, the internal tip lies between the fingers and the shoulder; some fluids and medications cannot be administered by peripheral line because of the characteristics of the fluids; peripheral devices are usually rotated every 3 days but this is determined by agency policy

   b. Central infusion: IV device whose internal tip lies in the central venous system, most commonly in the superior vena cava; these devices can remain in place for long periods of time; any fluid or medication that can be administered in the venous circulation can be administered by central lines; most central lines require sterile dressings to reduce the risk of contamination; agency policy and type of dressing determine the frequency of dressing changes

   c. Continuous infusion: an infusion which is uninterrupted and runs 24 hours a day

   d. Intermittent infusion: an infusion designed for clients who do not require IV fluid replacement therapy but require an IV access; a saline lock or PRN adapter is fitted to the end of the venous access device providing a connection for intermittent solution or medication administration; these devices require flushing with saline at least once every 8 hours and before and after medication administration; some central lines require the saline flush be followed by an instillation of heparin flush (10 units/mL or 100 units/mL solutions) to maintain the device; follow agency policy

D. Procedures/skills necessary to start/maintain IV therapy

  1. Peripheral infusion

    a. Start equipment includes:

     1) IV catheter

     2) IV start kit that contains a tourniquet, alcohol and betadine cleansing wipes, sterile tape, and gauze/semipermeable transparent membrane dressing materials

     3) IV fluids and appropriate tubing; filter if indicated

     4) Pump/regulator device if desired or necessary

     5) Gloves

    b. Procedure

     1) Wash hands

     2) Verify type and amount of solution with the prescriber's order, note expiration date

     3) Prepare equipment

      a) Obtain needleless adapter to connect to the venous access device if the device does not include one

      b) Remove outer wrappers from tubing, connect the tubing and filter device, and close tubing roller clamp

      c) Remove outer wrapper around IV bag, inspect bag for leaks (small amount of condensation is normal), tears, discoloration, cloudiness, or particulate matter; do not use the bag if present

      d) Hang IV bag on pole

      e) Using aseptic technique, remove port cap on IV bag and the plastic protector from IV tubing spike (end with the drip chamber) and insert the spike into the IV bag

      f) Squeeze drip chamber until it is partially full

      g) Remove protective cap on the tubing if it is not an air-vented cap, open roller clamp on the tubing to prime tubing and filter; invert and tap Y injection sites to remove air during priming, replace protective tubing cap

     4) Start IV

      a) Follow agency policy when starting and maintaining an IV device; wear gloves for protection from bloodborne pathogens

b) Prepare the client for the infusion, explain the procedure, and obtain the client's permission for the procedure

c) Identify appropriate vein for cannulation: in adults, peripheral IVs are inserted between the fingers and shoulders; depending on age, peripheral IVs in children can include the above sites as well as scalp and leg veins; avoid sites where veins are sclerotic, inflamed, or subject to decreased blood flow (as is common in adults following a stroke or mastectomy on that side)

d) Use tourniquet to distend the vessel; verify the absence of latex allergy before applying the tourniquet; in the absence of the tourniquet, a blood pressure cuff may be used; some geriatric clients may be accessed without a tourniquet; place the tourniquet 4 to 6 inches above the proposed site tightly enough to obstruct venous circulation but not arterial circulation (use light tapping, gravity, and/or topical heat application to aid vein distention)

e) Prepare the skin; typical procedure is to clean the site with alcohol followed by a povidone iodine cleansing; the site is cleaned in a circular manner that removes bacteria from the insertion site; the cleansing agent must be allowed to dry on the skin

f) Introduce the needle at a 10- to 30-degree angle with the bevel up; once blood return occurs, advance the catheter until the hub is in contact with the insertion site

g) Release the tourniquet and remove the needle from the catheter and dispose of it in a sharps container

h) Tape the catheter in a manner to reduce accidental removal; applying tape in two directions, as is common in the H or chevron styles, reduces the risk of accidental removal

i) Connect the catheter to IV tubing and apply a sterile dressing to the insertion site; a label on the side of the insertion site identifies the length and gauge of the catheter as well as the date and time of insertion and the nurse's initials

j) Apply date sticker with time and nurse's initials to the tubing

k) Initiate the prescribed flow rate: gravity flow tubing is regulated by drops per minute, and the drops delivered per mL of solution vary with different brands and types of infusion sets (drop factor) from 10 to 20 drops/mL; microdrip sets are always 60 drops/mL; to administer 1000 mL in 8 hours with a drop factor of 15 drops/mL:

$$\frac{\text{Total infusion volume} \times \text{drop factor}}{\text{Total time of infusion in minutes}} = \text{drops/minute}$$

$$\frac{1000 \text{ mL} \times 15}{8 \times 60 \text{ min (480 min)}} = 31.25 \text{ drops/min (31)}$$

5) Document date, time, solution, amount, infusion device, rate, site location, and condition of site and dressing

6) Maintain the IV infusion

a) Ensure that the correct solution is infusing

b) Check the rate of flow every hour or more as per agency policy

c) Inspect the patency of the IV tubing and needle

d) Maintain solution container 3 feet above the IV site

e) Inspect tubing for kinks or obstructions; ensure that it is not dangling below the IV site

f) Lower the solution container below IV site and observe for a blood return or gently pinch the IV tubing adjacent to the needle site causing blood to flow into the tubing (flash back), or use a sterile syringe to withdraw fluid from the port nearest the venipuncture site, causing blood to flow into the tubing

g) Splint a joint if the IV site is positional (movement of the extremity impedes flow of the solution)

h) Ensure tight connections to prevent leakage

i) Discontinue the solution and remove the IV access device if there is no blood return and you are unable to establish an acceptable drip rate

j) Inspect the insertion site for fluid infiltration (IV access device becomes dislodged from the vessel, causing fluid to flow into interstitial tissues and other complications) (see Table 11-10, pp. 318–319)

k) Instruct the client to notify the nurse if the flow rate changes or the solution stops dripping, the solution container is nearly empty, there is blood in the IV tubing or at the insertion site, or there is discomfort or swelling at the insertion site

l) At least every 8 hours document: solution, amount, infusion device, rate, site location, and condition of site and dressing

2. Central venous access devices (CVADs): access a central vein that empties into the superior vena cava

   a. Central infusion devices

     1) Percutaneous (nontunneled) catheter: a single or multiple lumen catheter inserted by the health care provider at the client's bedside

     2) Tunneled catheter: like all central lines, it terminates in the central venous system; the remainder of the catheter passes through a subcutaneous tract and exits on the chest wall or abdomen; a dacron cuff on the catheter elicits scar formation that prevents ascending tract infection; this catheter does not require a sterile dressing once the subcutaneous tract has healed

     3) Peripherally inserted central catheter (PICC): inserted in the basilic or cephalic vein just above or below the antecubital space of the right arm by a physician or specially trained IV therapy nurse and is used for longer term inpatient or outpatient therapy; although the insertion site is in the periphery, the catheter terminates in the superior vena cava

     4) Implantable venous access devices or ports: surgically implanted into a small subcutaneous pocket, usually on the upper chest using local anesthesia; the port is attached to a catheter that terminates in the central venous system; most ports are accessed with a Huber needle to preserve the life of the port septum

     5) Peripheral access system (PAS) ports are similar to a subcutaneous port except the port itself is implanted in the antecubital area

   b. The internal tips of all central lines lie within the central venous system; placement can occur in numerous settings but all placements must be verified by x-ray

c. Internal tips: the internal tip of the catheter comes in two versions

   1) Open-tipped: the end of the catheter opens directly in the bloodstream; if flushing techniques are not performed correctly, blood can back up into the catheter causing catheter occlusion; there are two open-tipped catheters; they must be flushed with saline followed by heparin flush solution to maintain patency when not in use

   a) Hickman: the adult form of the open-tipped catheter

   b) Broviac: the pediatric version, which usually means smaller lumen size

   2) Closed-tip catheter or Groshong: this catheter has a valve on its internal tip that prevents backflow of blood; Groshong catheters are routinely flushed with double volumes of saline but do not require the instillation of heparin flush solution; advantages of the Groshong catheter are:

   a) Decreased risk of air emboli or bleeding

   b) Elimination of heparin flush

   c) Elimination of catheter clamping

   d) Reduced flushing protocols between use

d. Lumens: central catheters may have a single, double, or triple lumen; each lumen corresponds to a separate catheter and has a separate exit point

   1) Multi-lumens allow for the administration of incompatible drugs

   2) Blood drawn from one lumen will not be contaminated by the drugs administered through another lumen of the catheter

   3) Each lumen is treated as a separate catheter and is flushed according to agency policy

e. Indications

   1) Long-term IV therapy

   2) Obtaining frequent blood specimens

   3) Central venous pressure (CVP) monitoring

   4) Administration of total parenteral nutrition (TPN) and medications that are irritating to veins, thus requiring a high-flow vein for rapid dilution

   5) Sclerosed peripheral veins

   6) Limited peripheral venous access

f. Nursing care involved (dressing, inspection, flushing, etc.): special precautions need to be taken with all central venous devices to ensure asepsis and catheter patency; refer again to Table 11-10 for complications

   1) Site care: subclavian, jugular, and PICC sites

   a) Require air occlusive dressings: dressings should be changed when soiled or loose

   b) Follow agency protocol for frequency of dressing changes—usually every 2 to 7 days; gauze dressings must be changed every 48 hours; semipermeable transparent membrane dressings may remain in place for up to 1 week

   c) Follow agency protocols for cleaning solutions and types of dressings; Chloraprep® (2% chlorhexidine gluconate and 70% isopropyl alcohol) is commonly used to clean the insertion site

   d) Using surgical asepsis and a mask, clean an area 2 inches in diameter around the site using a swab with Chloraprep®, use an up-and-down mo-

Table 11-10	Complications of IV Therapy
Complication	**Nursing Implications**
Infection (catheter-related) (sepsis)—common occurrence with TPN solutions that have high glucose concentration that invites bacteria. Characterized by fever, chills, erythema or drainage at insertion site, elevated white blood count, and possibly septic shock.	• Use strict aseptic technique when working with IVs • Change IV solutions at least every 24 hours • Change IV tubing and dressings per agency protocols (TPN tubing every day) • When discontinuing central lines, remove tip of catheter and apply an occlusive dressing; monitor site for 48 hours, the catheter tip may be sent to lab for culture if sepsis is suspected

Air embolism—air is introduced into the IV line during catheter insertion, tubing change, or administration of solutions and medications. Characterized by respiratory distress, chest pain, dyspnea, hypotension, and weak and rapid pulse.	• When changing tubing or reflux valves on CVADs without Groshong valves or catheters, instruct the client to perform the Valsalva's maneuver (forcefully exhale with glottis, nose, and mouth closed)
	• Ensure all catheter connections are tight
	• All connections on central lines should be luer lock not slip lock
	• During insertion of a percutaneous central venous catheter, position the client in head down position with head turned opposite direction of insertion site
	• If an air embolism is suspected:
	  • Clamp the catheter
	  • Position the client in left Trendelenburg's position
	  • Administer oxygen and contact the physician

Hypersensitivity reaction—sensitivity to the medication. Characterized by flushing, itching, and urticaria.	• Check client allergies prior to administering medications • Stop the infusion • Notify the physician • Monitor vital signs

Circulatory overload—fluids administered faster than the circulation can accommodate. Characterized by cough, dyspnea, crackles, distended neck veins, tachycardia, hypertension, S_3 heart sounds, and cardiac rhythm.	• Use IV pumps or controllers to regulate the infusion rate
	• Do not "catch up" with IV solutions
	• Carefully monitor fluid volumes with administration of multiple concurrent IV solutions or medications
	• Check the client's IV infusion rates at least hourly per agency protocols
	• Avoid selecting an IV container whose volume is greater than the volume ordered
	• Monitor the client's vital signs, intake and output, breath and heart sounds
	• For signs and symptoms of fluid volume overload:
	  • Slow or stop the infusion rate per order
	  • Place the client in high Fowler's position
	  • Administer oxygen and diuretics per order
	  • Notify the physician

Infiltration—localized swelling, coolness, pallor, and discomfort at the IV site.	• Stop the IV and remove the venous access device • Apply a warm compress to the site of the infiltration and elevate the extremity on a pillow • Restart the infusion at another site
Phlebitis—inflammation of a vein. Characterized by warmth, swelling, red streak at vein site, pain along the course of the vein, and warm to touch.	• Inspect and palpate the IV site at least every 8 hours for redness; if phlebitis is detected, discontinue the infusion and remove the venous access device • A medical order is not required to remove and replace a peripheral catheter that shows symptoms of phlebitis • Apply warm compresses to the venipuncture site • Select a large vein when administering irritating solutions/medications

Table 11-10	Complications of IV Therapy (continued)
Complication	**Nursing Implications**
	• Dilute irritating medications (e.g., promethazine [Phenergan] and administer over prescribed amount of time on an infusion pump; if client complains of pain at the insertion site, further dilute the medication and slow the flow rate
Hypoglycemia—decreased blood glucose level related to TPN being abruptly discontinued or due to excessive insulin administration; characterized by blood glucose less than 70 mg/dL, hunger, diaphoresis, weakness and anxiety	• Monitor blood glucose per agency protocols (at least every day) • Gradually decrease infusion when discontinuing TPN • Have 10% dextrose available as stand-by (medical order required for prn use)
Hyperglycemia—increased blood glucose related to TPN administration or administration of excessive dextrose solutions to diabetic clients; characterized by blood glucose greater than 200 mg/dL, excessive thirst, fatigue, restlessness, confusion, weakness, and diuresis	• Monitor blood glucose per agency protocols (at least every day) • Check medications affecting blood glucose levels (e.g., steroids) • Begin infusion at a slow rate (40 mL/hr) and gradually increase • Do not "catch up" if infusion rate falls behind

tion starting at the center and working outward; allow Chloraprep® to dry before applying air occlusive dressing over the entire insertion site

e) Assess site for redness, swelling, tenderness or drainage, and compare the length of the external portion of the catheter with its documented length to assess for displacement

f) Document date, condition of site, and dressing

2) Site care: implantable devices

a) Follow agency protocols for cleaning solutions and types of dressings; Chloraprep® is commonly used to clean the insertion site

b) Before accessing the port, using aseptic technique, clean an area 2 inches in diameter around the port using a swab with Chloraprep®, using an up-and-down motion starting at the center and working outward; allow the Chloraprep® to dry before accessing

c) Assess site for redness, swelling, tenderness or drainage

d) Access the site with an appropriate primed needle, usually a Huber needle; assess for patency by aspirating blood and then flushing according to policy

e) Apply a sterile dressing

3) Catheter care and flushing

a) Each lumen of the catheter should be flushed according to agency policy; frequency of flush varies among catheters and may be as frequent as once a shift; subcutaneous ports that are not in use may not require flushing more often than once a month

b) The flushing volume should be at least twice the internal volume of the catheter; closed-tip catheters (Groshong) should have the flushing volume doubled

c) The flushing material is usually saline; some medications are incompatible with saline and D_5W may be substituted for the saline

d) For closed-tip catheters, the saline flush is followed by a heparin flush instillation; the volume should approximate the internal volume of the catheter

        e) Syringes smaller than 10 mL should not be used for flushing as they may contribute to catheter rupture

        f) Blood draws: use distal lumen if possible; discard appropriate amount of blood prior to obtaining sample; following blood aspiration, flush the line with a double volume of saline prior to instillation of heplock solution (if appropriate); change the injection cap following a blood draw

    4) Client teaching: provide clients with the following instructions:

        a) Do not allow anyone to take a blood pressure on the arm with a PICC line or PAS port

        b) Wear a medical identification bracelet if the device will be implanted for a long time

        c) PICC and non-implanted CVADs: no activity restriction is necessary; do not immerse site in water

        d) Implanted CVADs: no restriction of activities is necessary; there are no restrictions regarding bathing or swimming when device is not accessed

E. IV medication administration

  1. Methods of administering IV medications

    a. Mixtures of medications within large volumes of IV fluids: provide and maintain a constant, well-diluted level of a medication in the blood

      1) To add the medication to an IV solution, prepare the medication from a vial or ampule and draw into a syringe

      2) To add the medication to a new IV container

        a) Clean the injection port with an alcohol swab and allow to dry for 30 seconds

        b) Remove the cap from the syringe, insert the needle or needleless device through the center of the injection port, and inject medication into solution

        c) Mix the medication and solution by gently rotating the bag

        d) Complete and attach a medication label to the IV solution, with the name and dose of the medication, date and time, and nurse's initials

        e) Proceed with setting up the IV for administration

      3) To add the medication to an existing infusion

        a) Ensure that there is enough IV solution in the container to properly dilute the medication

        b) Proceed as with adding a medication to a new IV container

    b. Injection by **bolus,** a direct injection of a medication intravenously (push), is used to obtain rapid therapeutic serum concentrations, when medications cannot be diluted, or for administration of emergency drugs

      1) With PRN adaptor: when no solutions are running

      2) Prepare the medication, draw up into a syringe, and label the syringe so that it will not be confused with the syringe containing the normal saline irrigating solution

      3) Wash hands and put on gloves

      4) Flush IV access device per agency policy

      5) Cleanse the infusion port with an alcohol swab and let it dry for 30 seconds

      6) Remove the needle from the syringe and attach the syringe with the medication to the needleless port access device

7) Administer the medication following the recommended IV push rate

8) Flush IV access device per agency policy

c. **Tandem infusion:** an intermittent method of administering medications to an existing IV (not frequently used)

1) Ensure that the existing IV solution and the intermittent infusion are compatible and the client's condition, vein, and gauge of the access device can tolerate the volume of fluid

2) The medication will be administered in a second bag of fluid, usually 50 to 100 mL, by secondary line into the Y port of a continuously running infusion; attach a needleless adapter to the tubing of the secondary set

3) Cleanse the infusion port of the continuous infusion line Y port with an alcohol swab and let it dry 30 seconds

4) Hang the secondary infusion and the existing infusion at the same level

5) Maintain the existing IV rate and regulate the piggyback rate using the roller clamp on the secondary tubing; the existing and the secondary solutions will run concurrently at their respective rates

d. **Piggyback infusion**

1) To administer an intermittent infusion without disconnecting the existing IV

   a) Set up the secondary set following the procedure for setting up an IV

   b) Hang the existing infusion set lower than the piggyback secondary set

   c) Cleanse the uppermost infusion port with an alcohol swab and let it dry for 30 seconds

   d) Connect the secondary set to the primary set using a needleless access device, above the existing IV roller clamp

   e) Maintain the existing IV roller clamp position, and regulate the piggyback rate using the roller clamp on the secondary tubing; the piggyback solution will infuse first and when complete, the existing IV will resume at the original rate

2) To administer an intermittent infusion using an infusing pump that is regulating the existing IV:

   a) When the intermittent solution is in an IV bag, set up the secondary administration set following the procedure for setting up an IV; connect the infusion tubing to the secondary access port on the pump; follow the protocols for the specific pump for administering the intermittent medication as either a continuous infusion or an infusion interrupting the existing IV

   b) When the intermittent solution is in a syringe, connect the syringe to the secondary access port on the pump; follow the protocols for the specific pump for administering the intermittent medication as either a continuous infusion or an infusion interrupting the existing IV

Practice to Pass

The nurse is administering an IV isotonic solution of 0.9% sodium chloride (normal saline). Considering the action of isotonic solutions, what are the nursing assessments specific to this type of fluid?

Case Study

A client was diagnosed with Crohn's disease. A long-term tunneled Groshong CVAD was implanted for long-term total parenteral nutrition (TPN). The nurse is preparing the client and family for discharge. A home care nurse will visit the client each day for the first week to monitor the client's progress in self-administration of her TPN. The client will receive TPN while sleeping at night and will receive no fluids through the CVAD during the daytime. In anticipating the client's discharge learning needs, prepare answers to the following questions.

1. What is total parenteral nutrition (TPN)?
2. What is a tunneled Groshong CVAD?
3. What are the care instructions for a Groshong CVAD?
4. Why is blood glucose monitoring necessary?
5. What are the specific interventions related to TPN?

For suggested responses, see pages 338–339.

POSTTEST

1 The nurse is caring for several clients with central venous access devices (CVADs). While changing the tubing on the central lines, the nurse would need to do which of the following? Select all that apply.

1. Use strict aseptic technique.
2. Use clean technique for the tubing and dressing change.
3. Assess the insertion site for signs of redness and drainage.
4. Document the length of the external portion of the catheter.
5. Remove any sutures at the insertion site if the line has been in place more than 5 days.

2 The client is receiving 5% dextrose in 0.45% sodium chloride. The physician has ordered that the client receive one unit of packed red blood cells. Prior to hanging the blood, the nurse will prime the blood tubing with which of the following solutions?

1. 5% dextrose in water
2. Lactated Ringer's
3. 0.9% sodium chloride
4. 5% dextrose in 0.45% sodium chloride

3 While assessing a client's intravenous (IV) line, the nurse notes that the area is swollen, cool, pale, and causes the client discomfort. The nurse suspects which of the following problems?

1. Infiltration
2. Phlebitis
3. Infection
4. Air embolism

4 The client is receiving 5% dextrose in 0.45% sodium chloride intravenously (IV) and reports pain at the IV site. The nurse assesses the site and notes erythema and edema. What would be the appropriate action for the nurse to take?

1. Slow the infusion rate.
2. Discontinue the IV and apply a warm compress to the IV site.
3. Apply antibiotic ointment to the IV site.
4. Gently pull back the IV access device to reposition it within the vein.

5 The nurse has an order to administer 10 grains of aspirin. The tablets that are available contain 325 mg aspirin per tablet. The nurse would administer how many tablets? Provide a numerical response rounded to a whole number.

Answer: _____

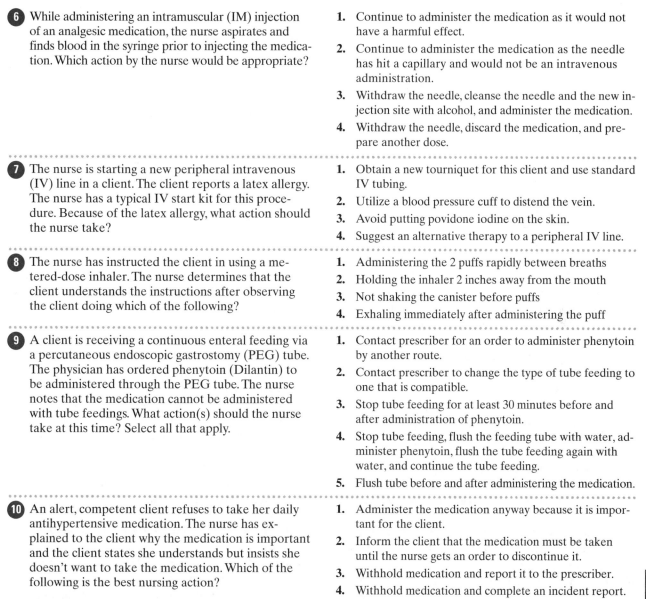

6 While administering an intramuscular (IM) injection of an analgesic medication, the nurse aspirates and finds blood in the syringe prior to injecting the medication. Which action by the nurse would be appropriate?

1. Continue to administer the medication as it would not have a harmful effect.
2. Continue to administer the medication as the needle has hit a capillary and would not be an intravenous administration.
3. Withdraw the needle, cleanse the needle and the new injection site with alcohol, and administer the medication.
4. Withdraw the needle, discard the medication, and prepare another dose.

7 The nurse is starting a new peripheral intravenous (IV) line in a client. The client reports a latex allergy. The nurse has a typical IV start kit for this procedure. Because of the latex allergy, what action should the nurse take?

1. Obtain a new tourniquet for this client and use standard IV tubing.
2. Utilize a blood pressure cuff to distend the vein.
3. Avoid putting povidone iodine on the skin.
4. Suggest an alternative therapy to a peripheral IV line.

8 The nurse has instructed the client in using a metered-dose inhaler. The nurse determines that the client understands the instructions after observing the client doing which of the following?

1. Administering the 2 puffs rapidly between breaths
2. Holding the inhaler 2 inches away from the mouth
3. Not shaking the canister before puffs
4. Exhaling immediately after administering the puff

9 A client is receiving a continuous enteral feeding via a percutaneous endoscopic gastrostomy (PEG) tube. The physician has ordered phenytoin (Dilantin) to be administered through the PEG tube. The nurse notes that the medication cannot be administered with tube feedings. What action(s) should the nurse take at this time? Select all that apply.

1. Contact prescriber for an order to administer phenytoin by another route.
2. Contact prescriber to change the type of tube feeding to one that is compatible.
3. Stop tube feeding for at least 30 minutes before and after administration of phenytoin.
4. Stop tube feeding, flush the feeding tube with water, administer phenytoin, flush the tube feeding again with water, and continue the tube feeding.
5. Flush tube before and after administering the medication.

10 An alert, competent client refuses to take her daily antihypertensive medication. The nurse has explained to the client why the medication is important and the client states she understands but insists she doesn't want to take the medication. Which of the following is the best nursing action?

1. Administer the medication anyway because it is important for the client.
2. Inform the client that the medication must be taken until the nurse gets an order to discontinue it.
3. Withhold medication and report it to the prescriber.
4. Withhold medication and complete an incident report.

➤ *See page 325–327 for Answers & Rationales.*

ANSWERS & RATIONALES

Pretest

1 **Answer: 3** Under the law, if a medication order is written incorrectly, the nurse who administers the incorrect order is responsible for the error. This includes both the right medication and the right dose (2 of the 6 "rights" of medication administration). The other responses are inaccurate conclusions about the case situation in the question.

Cognitive Level: Analysis **Client Need:** Safe, Effective Care Environment: Management of Care **Integrated Process:** Nursing Process: Evaluation **Content Area:** Fundamentals **Strategy:** The critical words in the question are *NPH insulin, IV,* and *liability.* Recall the legal role of the nurse in medication administration and use the process of elimination to make a selection about the nurse's liability. **Reference:** Kozier, B., Erb, G., Berman, A., & Snyder, S. J. (2004). *Fundamentals of nursing: Concepts, process,* *and practice* (7th ed.). Upper Saddle River, NJ: Pearson Education, p. 787.

2 **Answer: 1** The thin layer of epithelium and the vast network of capillaries under the tongue enhance sublingual absorption. This medication dissolves rapidly and is absorbed immediately. The other responses contain inaccurate information.

Cognitive Level: Application **Client Need:** Physiological Integrity: Pharmacological and Parenteral Therapies **Integrated Process:** Teaching/Learning **Content Area:** Fundamentals **Strategy:** The critical words are *sublingual* and *best response.* Recall advantages of various routes of drug administration and use the process of elimination to make a selection. **Reference:** Kozier, B., Erb, G., Berman, A., & Snyder, S. J. (2004). *Fundamentals of nursing: Concepts, process, and practice* (7th ed.). Upper Saddle River, NJ: Pearson Education, p. 793.

3 **Answer: 4** For an adult with well-developed muscle mass, the preferred medication administration injection site for medications requiring a large muscle mass is the ventrogluteal area. The vastus lateralis is the preferred IM injection site for children under 7 months of age. The other responses identify sites that are not preferred when the injection needs to go deep into a muscle.

Cognitive Level: Application **Client Need:** Physiological Integrity: Pharmacological and Parenteral Therapies **Integrated Process:** Nursing Process: Implementation **Content Area:** Fundamentals **Strategy:** The critical terms are *150-pound client* and *preferred site of injection.* Use knowledge of the advantages and disadvantages of each injection site to answer the question. **Reference:** Kozier, B., Erb, G., Berman, A., & Snyder, S. J. (2004). *Fundamentals of nursing: Concepts, process, and practice* (7th ed.). Upper Saddle River, NJ: Pearson Education, p. 826.

4 **Answer: 1** For a well-developed adult, a ⅝- to 1-inch needle is the appropriate size for an IM deltoid injection. Because this is an obese client, the longer needle (1 inch) is appropriate to ensure it reaches the muscle.

Cognitive Level: Application **Client Need:** Physiological Integrity: Pharmacological and Parenteral Therapies **Integrated Process:** Nursing Process: Planning **Content Area:** Fundamentals **Strategy:** The critical terms are *obese adult* and *deltoid.* Use basic nursing knowledge of needle sizes and their associated uses to make a selection. **Reference:** Kozier, B., Erb, G., Berman, A., & Snyder, S. J. (2004). *Fundamentals of nursing: Concepts, process, and practice* (7th ed.). Upper Saddle River, NJ: Pearson Education, p. 813.

5 **Answer: 4** Z-track technique prevents "tracking" and is used for administering medications that are especially irritating to subcutaneous tissue. With Z-track technique, the skin is pulled approximately 1 inch laterally

away from the injection site, the medication is injected, the needle is withdrawn, and the tissue is released. Using a small-gauge needle, injecting at a 45-degree angle, and applying ice to the site would not help prevent irritation to subcutaneous tissue by an irritating medication.

Cognitive Level: Application **Client Need:** Physiological Integrity: Pharmacological and Parenteral Therapies **Integrated Process:** Nursing Process: Implementation **Content Area:** Fundamentals **Strategy:** The critical words are *prevent tracking.* Recall the various injection techniques and their indications and use the process of elimination to make a selection. **Reference:** Kozier, B., Erb, G., Berman, A., & Snyder, S. J. (2004). *Fundamentals of nursing: Concepts, process, and practice* (7th ed.). Upper Saddle River, NJ: Pearson Education, p. 830.

6 **Answer: 4** Eye drops are placed in the lower conjunctival sac to prevent damage to the cornea and to facilitate coating the eye with the medication. The drops are not applied directly onto the cornea or to the sclera near either the inner or the outer canthus.

Cognitive Level: Application **Client Need:** Physiological Integrity: Pharmacological and Parenteral Therapies **Integrated Process:** Nursing Process: Implementation **Content Area:** Fundamentals **Strategy:** The core issue of the question is knowledge of the appropriate area for application of eye drops. Recall critical but basic information about proper technique to make a selection. Note that all incorrect answers involved applying the medication directly to some area of the eyeball. **Reference:** Kozier, B., Erb, G., Berman, A., & Snyder, S. J. (2004). *Fundamentals of nursing: Concepts, process, and practice* (7th ed.). Upper Saddle River, NJ: Pearson Education, p. 841.

7 **Answer: 4** Protein is responsible for a significant portion of the osmotic pressure found in the blood vessels and maintains fluid within the vessels. In burn injuries, protein is lost, allowing fluid to escape into the tissues. Albumin is used to replace the lost proteins and pull fluids from the interstitial space back into the vascular system. It does not contain clotting factors (option 1) or red blood cells (option 3) and does not have enough fluid volume to consider it as a substantial part of primary fluid resuscitation (option 2).

Cognitive Level: Application **Client Need:** Physiological Integrity: Pharmacological and Parenteral Therapies **Integrated Process:** Teaching/Learning **Content Area:** Fundamentals **Strategy:** The critical phrase is *rationale for albumin administration.* Recall first that albumin is a colloid that can be given intravenously to eliminate the options containing clotting factors and red blood cells. Choose correctly from the final 2 options, knowing that large volumes of crystalloids are used for fluid resuscitation and that albumin is a colloid. **Reference:** Kozier, B., Erb, G., Berman, A., & Snyder, S. J. (2004). *Fundamentals of nursing: Concepts, process, and practice* (7th ed.). Upper Saddle River, NJ: Pearson Education, p. 1399.

8 **Answer: 100** One way to solve the problem is to set it up as follows:

$$\frac{50 \text{ mL}}{30 \text{ min}} = \frac{x \text{ mL}}{60 \text{ min}}$$

$$30x = 3000$$

$$x = 100 \text{ mL/hour}$$

Cognitive Level: Application **Client Need:** Physiological Integrity: Pharmacological and Parenteral Therapies **Integrated Process:** Nursing Process: Implementation **Content Area:** Fundamentals **Strategy:** The core issue of the question is knowledge of how to set up and solve an IV problem. Use basic knowledge of pharmacological math procedures to answer the question. Use the "common-sense" test to check your answer by reasoning that if 50 mL should infuse in 30 minutes, then that is the equivalent speed of 100 mL infusing in an hour. **Reference:** Kozier, B., Erb, G., Berman, A., & Snyder, S. J. (2004). *Fundamentals of nursing: Concepts, process, and practice* (7th ed.). Upper Saddle River, NJ: Pearson Education, p. 1392.

9 **Answer: 4** 0.45% sodium chloride is a hypotonic solution that draws fluid from the vascular compartment into the cells; this type of solution would be used for clients with cellular dehydration. Normal saline and lactated Ringer's (options 1 and 3) are isotonic, while 5% dextrose in normal saline (option 2) is hypertonic until the body metabolizes the dextrose.

Cognitive Level: Analysis **Client Need:** Physiological Integrity: Pharmacological and Parenteral Therapies **Integrated Process:** Nursing Process: Planning **Content Area:** Fundamentals **Strategy:** The critical term is *hypotonic*. Recall commonly used hydrating solutions and their indications and use the process of elimination to make a selection. **Reference:** Kozier, B., Erb, G., Berman, A., & Snyder, S. J. (2004). *Fundamentals of nursing: Concepts, process, and practice* (7th ed.). Upper Saddle River, NJ: Pearson Education, p. 1382.

10 **Answer: 2** The client's body has adjusted to higher blood glucose levels as a result of receiving TPN with high dextrose concentrations. Abruptly stopping TPN can result in hypoglycemia. The client is not greatly at risk for hypocalcemia (option 1), sepsis (option 3), or hyperkalemia (option 4) because of the dislodgement.

Cognitive Level: Application **Client Need:** Physiological Integrity: Pharmacological and Parenteral Therapies

Integrated Process: Nursing Process: Assessment **Content Area:** Fundamentals **Strategy:** The core issue of the question is knowledge that abrupt cessation of a high-dextrose solution such as TPN places the client at risk for rebound hypoglycemia. Use nursing knowledge and the process of elimination to choose correctly. **Reference:** Kozier, B., Erb, G., Berman, A., & Snyder, S. J. (2004). *Fundamentals of nursing: Concepts, process and practice* (7th ed.). Upper Saddle River, NJ: Pearson Education, pp. 1216–1217.

Posttest

1 **Answers: 1, 3, 4** Strict aseptic technique is always required for the changing of central line tubing and/or dressings to prevent bloodborne infection. The catheter length should be documented to assess possible displacement. Removing sutures that secure the line would be inappropriate. All venous access sites should be assessed on a regular basis for signs of inflammation or infection. Clean technique would be appropriate for changing peripheral IV tubing in most cases, but not central lines.

Cognitive Level: Application **Client Need:** Physiological Integrity: Pharmacological and Parenteral Therapies **Integrated Process:** Nursing Process: Implementation **Content Area:** Fundamentals **Strategy:** The core issue of the question is knowledge of principles of safe care when working with a CVAD. Recall that the catheter is placed into a central vein to reason that strict aseptic technique is necessary and that other general assessments of intravenous lines would also be important. **Reference** Kozier, B., Erb, G., Berman, A., & Snyder, S. J. (2004). *Fundamentals of nursing: Concepts, process, and practice* (7th ed.). Upper Saddle River, NJ: Pearson Education, p. 1384.

2 **Answer: 3** 0.9% sodium chloride (normal saline) is the only solution that can be administered with blood or blood products. Other solutions may cause the blood cells to clump or cause clotting, making the other options incorrect.

Cognitive Level: Application **Client Need:** Physiological Integrity: Pharmacological and Parenteral Therapies **Integrated Process:** Nursing Process: Implementation **Content Area:** Fundamentals **Strategy:** The critical phrase is *prime the blood tubing*. Recall information about correct techniques for blood administration to answer the question. If this question was difficult, memorize that normal saline is the only solution compatible with blood products. **Reference:** Kozier, B., Erb, G., Berman, A., & Snyder, S. J. (2004). *Fundamentals of nursing: Concepts, process, and practice* (7th ed.). Upper Saddle River, NJ: Pearson Education, p. 1401.

3 Answer: 1 Infiltration is leakage of fluids into the surrounding tissues, resulting in edema around the insertion site, blanching, and coolness of skin around the site. Phlebitis and infection would result in redness, heat, and discomfort to the client at the site. Air embolism would result in sudden respiratory distress.

Cognitive Level: Analysis **Client Need:** Physiological Integrity: Pharmacological and Parenteral Therapies **Integrated Process:** Nursing Process: Analysis **Content Area:** Fundamentals **Strategy:** The core issue of the question is the ability to recognize common complications of IV therapy, such as infiltration. Use this knowledge and the process of elimination to make a selection. **Reference:** Kozier, B., Erb, G., Berman, A., & Snyder, S. J. (2004). *Fundamentals of nursing: Concepts, process, and practice* (7th ed.). Upper Saddle River, NJ: Pearson Education, p. 1394.

4 Answer: 2 Erythema and edema are consistent with phlebitis, an inflammation of the vein wall. Continuing the infusion at that site would only worsen the phlebitis. The IV should be discontinued and restarted at a new site. Applying a warm compress to an area of phlebitis dilates the vessel, improves circulation, and reduces the resistance to blood flow from within the vein reducing the pain. The other options are inaccurate statements about the method of treatment for phlebitis.

Cognitive Level: Analysis **Client Need:** Physiological Integrity: Pharmacological and Parenteral Therapies **Integrated Process:** Nursing Process: Implementation **Content Area:** Fundamentals **Strategy:** The core issue of the question is recognition that the client has developed phlebitis at the IV site and the ability to determine the appropriate actions. Review this basic information if this question was difficult. **Reference:** Kozier, B., Erb, G., Berman, A., & Snyder, S. J. (2004). *Fundamentals of nursing: Concepts, process, and practice* (7th ed.). Upper Saddle River, NJ: Pearson Education, p. 1394.

5 Answer: 2 Recall that in the apothecary system, 1 grain = 65 mg. Thus, the 10 grains can be converted to 650 mg. One way to set up the problem is as follows:

$$\frac{650 \text{ mg}}{325 \text{ mg}} = \frac{x}{1}$$

$$325x = 650$$

$$x = 2 \text{ tablets}$$

Cognitive Level: Application **Client Need:** Physiological Integrity: Pharmacological and Parenteral Therapies **Integrated Process:** Nursing Process: Implementation **Content Area:** Fundamentals **Strategy:** The core issue of the question is the ability to perform basic pharmacological math calculations. If this question was difficult, take time to review standard formulas for calculating drug dosages. **Reference:** Kozier, B., Erb, G., Berman, A., & Snyder, S. J. (2004). *Fundamentals of nursing: Concepts, process, and practice* (7th ed.). Upper Saddle River, NJ: Pearson Education, p. 800.

6 Answer: 4 If blood returns while aspirating during an IM injection, the nurse should discard and prepare a new injection. Blood indicates that the needle has entered a blood vessel, and medication injected directly into the bloodstream may be dangerous.

Cognitive Level: Application **Client Need:** Physiological Integrity: Pharmacological and Parenteral Therapies **Integrated Process:** Nursing Process: Implementation **Content Area:** Fundamentals **Strategy:** The critical phrase is *blood in the syringe.* Eliminate options 1 and 2 because they are similar and option 3 because it violates principles of aseptic technique for medication administration using needles. **Reference:** Kozier, B., Erb, G., Berman, A., & Snyder, S. J. (2004). *Fundamentals of nursing: Concepts, process, and practice* (7th ed.). Upper Saddle River, NJ: Pearson Education, p. 831.

7 Answer: 2 Tourniquets and the ports of standard IV tubing are made of latex. A blood pressure cuff can be used as an alternative method of vein distention. Povidone iodine is an unrelated item, and it is not the nurse's role to suggest alternatives to IV therapy when appropriate equipment can be obtained.

Cognitive Level: Analysis **Client Need:** Physiological Integrity: Safety and Infection Control **Integrated Process:** Nursing Process: Implementation **Content Area:** Fundamentals **Strategy:** The critical words are *latex allergy* and *typical IV start kit.* Recall what equipment contains latex and choose the option that eliminates them from contact with the client. All equipment made of rubber will cause signs and symptoms of allergy. **Reference:** Kozier, B., Erb, G., Berman, A., & Snyder, S. J. (2004). *Fundamentals of nursing: Concepts, process, and practice* (7th ed.). Upper Saddle River, NJ: Pearson Education, p. 1388.

8 Answer: 2 Clients should be instructed to hold inhaler 2 inches away from mouth, hold the breath for 10 seconds after inhalation, slowly exhale through pursed lips, and wait 2 minutes between puffs. The other options describe incorrect actions.

Cognitive Level: Application **Client Need:** Physiological Integrity: Pharmacological and Parenteral Therapies **Integrated Process:** Teaching/Learning **Content Area:** Fundamentals **Strategy:** The core issue of the question is correct administration of a dose of medication using an inhaler. Recall basic administration principles for this medication route and use the process of elimination to make a selection. **Reference:** Kozier, B., Erb, G., Berman, A., & Snyder, S. J. (2004). *Fundamentals of nursing: Concepts, process, and practice* (7th ed.). Upper Saddle River, NJ: Pearson Education, p. 850.

9 **Answer: 3, 5** When medications are administered enterally and cannot be administered with tube feedings, it is best to stop the tube feedings for at least 30 minutes prior to and after the administration of the medication. A time period of 30 minutes allows for the tube feeding to clear the GI tract and therefore not mix with the medication. The tube should be flushed before and after the dose to prevent the medication from coming in contact with the feeding. The actions listed in options 2 and 4 do not provide for safe medication administration and option 1 is unnecessary. **Cognitive Level:** Application **Client Need:** Physiological Integrity: Pharmacological and Parenteral Therapies **Integrated Process:** Nursing Process: Implementation **Content Area:** Fundamentals **Strategy:** The core issue of the question is knowledge of safe medication administration technique via a feeding tube when medication and feeding are incompatible. Choose the options that physically separate the feeding from the medication to avoid their interaction. **Reference:** Kozier, B., Erb, G., Berman, A., & Snyder, S. J. (2004). *Fundamentals of nursing: Concepts, process, and practice* (7th ed.). Upper Saddle River, NJ: Pearson Education, p. 811.

10 **Answer: 3** A client has the right to refuse a medication regardless of how important it may be to his or her health. Withholding the medication because of client refusal is not an incident and does not require an incident report, but it should be documented and reported to the prescriber. The correct choice is option 3. **Cognitive Level:** Application **Client Need:** Safe, Effective Care Environment: Management of Care **Integrated Process:** Communication and Documentation **Content Area:** Fundamentals **Strategy:** The core issue of the question is the ability to apply client rights to the procedure of medication administration. Recall the principle of client autonomy to make a selection and also realize that the prescriber should be informed of the event. **Reference:** Kozier, B., Erb, G., Berman, A., & Snyder, S. J. (2004). *Fundamentals of nursing: Concepts, process, and practice* (7th ed.). Upper Saddle River, NJ: Pearson Education, p. 82.

References

Berman, A. J., & Snyder, S. Kozier, B. & Erb, G., (2008). *Fundamentals of nursing: Concepts, process, and practice* (8th ed.). Upper Saddle River, NJ: Prentice Hall, pp. 829–901, 1455–1492.

Harkreader, H. & Hogan, M. (2007). *Fundamentals of nursing: Caring and clinical judgment* (3rd ed.). St. Louis, MO: Elsevier Science, pp. 428–495, 612–664.

LeMone, P. & Burke, K. (2008). *Medical–surgical nursing: Critical thinking in client care* (4th ed.). Upper Saddle River, NJ: Prentice Hall.

Smith, R. S., Duell, D. J., & Martin, B. C. (2005). *Clinical nursing skills: Basic to advanced skills* (6th ed.). Upper Saddle River, NJ: Prentice Hall, pp. 515–574, 993–1043.

Potter, P. & Perry, A. (2005). *Fundamentals of nursing* (6th ed.). St. Louis, MO: Mosby, pp. 821–909, 1134–1197.

Appendix

➤ Practice to Pass Suggested Answers

Chapter 1

Page 9: *Suggested Answer—*

Open: "Can you describe your pain for me?"

Closed: "On a scale of 0 to 10, with 10 being the worst pain you have ever felt, how would you rank your pain?"

Page 14: *Suggested Answer—*

- Knowledge deficit related to medication regimen; altered health maintenance related to ineffective individual coping; noncompliance related to knowledge and skill related to the regimen behavior
- Impaired skin integrity related to immobility

Page 15: *Suggested Answer—*

- PO intake will be 700 mL per 8 hours
- Urine specific gravity, weight, and laboratory studies will remain within age-appropriate parameters
- Respiratory rate will be 12 to 18 breaths per minute
- Client will remain afebrile

Page 19: *Suggested Answer—*

- Call you to assess his coccyx.
- Turn and position him so there is no weight on his coccyx.
- Cleanse reddened area gently, dry well, and do not massage it.

Page 21: *Suggested Answer—*

- When did you go to sleep?
- When did you wake up?
- Do you feel rested?

Chapter 2

Page 32: *Suggested Answer—*The interview is an important process in which the nurse attempts to extrapolate information from the client to determine healthcare needs. The nurse should first establish a rapport and attempt to make the client comfortable with the process. The nurse can use multiple skills to elicit data. The use of good communication skills and proceeding in a systematic, nonthreatening manner will facilitate the process.

Page 33: *Suggested Answer—*Clues provided by the client's complaint include:

- Client's overall health
- Client's health prior to initiating health care
- Client's perspective of health concerns
- Client's attempt to treat the disorder
- Client's perception of health needs
- Client's perception of how the healthcare team can assist the client's return to health

Page 34: *Suggested Answer—*The family history is crucial in relaying significant medical information to the healthcare team. The overall health and illnesses of a close relation will lead the healthcare team to investigate multiple areas of potential concern. All factors are significant as the healthcare team begins to build a picture of the client's current and future health status.

Page 37: *Suggested Answer—*The nurse can help alleviate the client's psychological discomfort by providing privacy, providing a gown to change into, and by ensuring that only the body part being examined is exposed at any given time. A matter-of-fact but understanding manner will also be reassuring to the client.

Page 45: *Suggested Answer—*Once the nurse detects the client has adventitious breath sounds, identification of the sounds will assist the healthcare team to choose the course of therapy. The nurse should continue to perform respiratory assessments by noting the rate, character, and depth of the respirations. Inspecting the client's mucous membranes, nail beds, and lips will indicate if the periphery of the body is being oxygenated. In addition, the nurse can percuss for diaphragmatic excursion and areas of dullness, resonance, or hyperresonance. As the assessment proceeds, the nurse questions the client about the overall state of health, duration of the symptoms, any related symptoms, cough, mucus production, chest pain,

328

palpitation, urine output, respiratory distress, and additional illnesses. The nurse can also ask the client for family history, smoking history, and exposure to asbestos.

Page 53: *Suggested Answer* —

- Brain: controls thoughts, emotions, speech
- Limbic system: emotional and behavioral responses to environmental stimuli
- Reticular formation: wake-sleep cycle
- Spinal cord: sensory and motor functions
- Peripheral nervous system: receives and transmits impulses from environment
- Autonomic nervous system: regulates internal environment
- Sympathetic nervous system: affects target organs (pupils, secretions, sweat, heart rate and rhythm, coronary arteries, bronchioles, digestion, liver, urine output, abdominal and skin blood vessels, blood clotting, metabolic rate, mental alertness)
- Parasympathetic nervous system: regulates digestion, elimination, and other activities (pupils, glandular secretions, heart rate, coronary arteries, bronchioles, peristalsis, and gastric secretions)

Chapter 3

Page 66: *Suggested Answer* — An unconscious client may hear what is being said because hearing is believed to be the last sense lost. The nurse should act as if the client can hear and should talk in a normal tone of voice. Communication should be simple and concrete.

The client should be spoken to before the nurse provides touch. Touching is a form of communication and should be done gently and smoothly. The nurse should ask closed questions that call for a simple response; for example, "If you can hear me, squeeze my hand" or "Move your head." Unavoidable environmental noises should be explained. Environmental noises should be decreased when possible to help the client focus on communication. Information regarding orientation and client care needs to be repeated frequently. Clients should be given sufficient time to respond to questions.

Page 68: *Suggested Answer* — Reduce environmental noise when possible. Decreasing environmental stimuli is likely to have a calming effect on the client. Allow the client to express his or her feelings as long as the client is not a danger to self or others. Approach the client by using his or her name. Appear accepting and not challenging. To appear nonthreatening, keep posture relaxed and have minimum eye contact. Do not react to the client's loud voice or aggressive behavior; however, listen carefully to what is said. Using simple and direct communication, explain all care measures before implementing them.

Page 70: *Suggested Answer* — Reduce environmental noise. Orient the client before initiating verbal communication. Face the client and talk in a low-pitched voice using simple sentences. Use gestures or environmental cues to augment verbal

messages. Use a word board or written messages to help convey information. Explain all procedures using pantomime as appropriate. Ensure that hearing aids are in working order.

Page 73: *Suggested Answer* — Draw a single line through the mistaken entry; write "void" or "error" above the line and initial this entry. Sign the record as per policy.

Page 74: *Suggested Answer* — Information should be complete, accurate, and relevant. Record assessment data objectively and avoid including the nurse's interpretation. Note problems as they occur, as well as nursing interventions and client options. It is not enough to document a problem without addressing it. Avoid unclear terms like "good" and "appears to be." Interventions should be documented immediately after they occur and signed by the person performing them.

Page 75: *Suggested Answer* — Important information to report would include:

- Information to identify client and medical diagnosis or major medical procedures
- Physician name including consulting services
- Significant assessment findings, including vital signs
- Diagnostic and laboratory tests scheduled, as well as results of tests done
- Information related to maintaining client safety, use of restraints, and/or sensory impairments
- Specific treatments ordered such as dressing changes, tube feedings, and intravenous therapy

Page 78: *Suggested Answer* — The nurse should consider:

- The client's developmental level
- The client's emotional state
- The client's motivation
- The client's reading ability
- What the client needs to know
- What the client already knows

Chapter 4

Page 89: *Suggested Answer* — Effective leaders adapt their style of leadership to the situation. Therefore, situational leadership is regarded as the style most compatible with a professional staff. The nurse in charge should not have to use an autocratic style to offer direction; a professional staff would be involved in making decisions and facilitating the organization in meeting its goals. A professional staff would be internally motivated, capable of making decisions, and value independence. Moreover, a style that offers no direction at all (*laissez-faire*) is incompatible with attempts to meet personal and organizational goals. Therefore, the situational leadership style would allow input from the staff and cooperation in many situations but could revert to autocratic in emergency situations.

Page 90: *Suggested Answer* — The management process provides a framework for managers and leaders to use in order to be successful in attaining organizational goals. Management functions include planning, organizing, directing, and controlling. These activities promote successful attainment of organizational goals.

Page 90: *Suggested Answer*—A new graduate does not have expert or positional power but can have referent power. As the graduate matures, the expert power can emerge. Power that is vested in the registered nurse's position generates the ability to delegate tasks and responsibilities.

Page 92: *Suggested Answer*—Delegation is the transfer of responsibility for the completion of a task. The RN should consider the nature of the task to be delegated. It should not be too complex, and it should be part of the unlicensed assistive personnel's area of responsibility. The nurse must communicate the task and responsibility to be delegated and offer guidance. The nurse retains accountability for the task and must monitor the performance of the task and its outcome.

Page 93: *Suggested Answer*—The ANA Code for Nurses is a group statement of the values held by the group. This code serves as a standard for practice and provides guidance for the professional nurse. It offers parameters for the protection of both the client and the family.

Page 95: *Suggested Answer*—Unless there is malpractice a nurse cannot be held liable for stopping to render assistance as any other reasonably prudent person would.

Page 96: *Suggested Answer*—The nurse can avoid malpractice by abiding by the ANA Code for Nurses and the state Nurse Practice Act. The nurse must be familiar with the Nurse Practice Act of the state, because it defines the practice of all nurses. In addition, the nurse will follow the policies and procedures of the agency as long as the policies are in compliance with state law. When the nurse accepts employment, the nurse must consider personal abilities versus job requirements and determine personal ability to function in a role. The nurse must communicate with supervisors when aspects of the job fall beyond the nurse's ability. The nurse should maintain a good rapport with the client—every client should be treated with kindness and respect. Also, it is crucial that the nurse participates in continuing education programs and serves as an advocate for the client and the family.

Chapter 5

Page 111: *Suggested Answer*—The client will demonstrate adaptation to current life situation, express acceptance of self, acknowledge changes in self-concept, and develop a realistic plan for adapting to life after mastectomy.

Page 113: *Suggested Answer*—Testicular cancer is the most common cancer in men aged 15 to 35. Testicular self-examination (TSE) should be done monthly on a specific day. The best place for TSE is the shower. Index and middle fingers should be under the testicle while the thumb is on top. Roll the testicle, feeling for lumps, thickenings, or hardened areas. Repeat on the other testicle. Also palpate the epididymis and

the vas deferens. After the shower, use a mirror to check for swelling or changes in skin texture. The physician should be notified of any unusual findings.

Page 121: *Suggested Answer*—Interpreters should be objective and seek to provide accurate translation of information. It is best to avoid using family members as translators because of lack of objectivity. Gender and age should be similar to that of the client in order to avoid embarrassment in sensitive issues. The interpreter should be socially and politically compatible with the client. The nurse should speak directly to the client and not the interpreter. The nurse should speak slowly and with clarity. Observe nonverbal communication from the client to validate the verbal response.

Page 122: *Suggested Answer*—Parents or guardians should be asked what religious beliefs have been taught to the preschooler. Ask the preschooler "Who is God?", "What is heaven?", "Do you pray?", "If so, can you tell me how you pray?" Ask the child about what he or she believes about religious holidays, such as Christmas, Hanukkah, or others.

Page 125: *Suggested Answer*—The nurse's response should be customized for the parent following an assessment of her grief level. Answers should be direct without detail, but sufficient to allow the parent to recognize approaching death. Symptoms of approaching death include loss of muscle tone, bowel and bladder incontinence (although urine output greatly decreases), difficulty swallowing, lack of appetite, dry mucous membranes, and low-grade fever; extremities are cyanotic, mottled, cool and clammy or may be perspiring, respirations become slow and labored often with loud lung sounds, disorientation, blurred vision, and diminished blink reflex. Ensure that the parents know that hearing is the last sense to go and encourage them to talk to their child throughout the experience.

Chapter 6

Page 135: *Suggested Answer*—General assessment data that indicate a client may be more susceptible to pathogens include:

- Poor hygiene practices.
- Inadequate nutrition.
- Being underweight or overweight.
- Having negative lifestyle habits such as cigarette smoking and lack of physical activity.

Physical assessment data that may indicate a client is susceptible to pathogens may include:

- Generalized pallor.
- Poor peripheral circulation.
- Abnormal respiratory rate with decreased lung expansion.
- Nail clubbing.
- Presence of abnormal heart sounds.
- Skin and mucous membranes not intact.
- History of chronic illness.

Page 141: *Suggested Answer—*

- The parents should be given information about proper handwashing techniques and basic infection control information.
- Information should be provided about the importance of immunizations and about accident prevention specific to the child's age.
- Parents should be instructed to seek medical treatment early in the event the child becomes ill.
- Food preparation should be discussed, including washing all fresh vegetables and fruits and ensuring meat is cooked at proper temperatures.
- Environmental controls should be discussed to prevent the spread of microorganisms. For example, toys should be washed periodically and soiled diapers handled appropriately.

Page 147: *Suggested Answer—*

- Client conditions that may cause the body temperature to be lower than normal include shock, accidental exposure to cold temperature, and postsurgical procedures. In addition, age is a factor as elderly clients experience integumentary changes and infants have immature temperature regulatory mechanisms.
- Interventions to prevent heat loss include increasing environmental temperature, providing extra blankets, keeping the client's head covered, providing warm liquids, and avoiding exposure of the skin during care.

Page 151: *Suggested Answer—*The nurse needs to consider the client's age, body type, and build. The assessment should include the client's emotional heath and evaluation of the client's stressors. Physical assessment criteria would include a body system assessment to ensure proper functioning. For instance, if the client's general color is normal, lungs are clear to auscultation, heart sounds are normal, nail beds blanch well, and urinary and bowel elimination are within normal limits, the client probably has compensated for the abnormal blood pressure measurement.

Page 151: *Suggested Answer—*The nurse could anticipate that the body temperature would be below normal. The pulse will be weak and rapid if blood loss is not too extensive. As the client loses more blood, the pulse may become very slow and difficult to palpate. The blood pressure will be slightly elevated at first as the body tries to compensate. The systolic pressure will decrease more in comparison to the diastolic, with the pulse pressure narrowing. The blood pressure will fall rapidly as the client changes position. As blood loss continues, the blood pressure continues to decline.

Chapter 7

Page 174: *Suggested Answer—*

- Provide a clutter-free environment. Depending on the degree and extensiveness of the burn, the child may try to investigate the environment. Young children are very curious and will handle anything within reach.
- Follow clean and aseptic precautions strictly (isolation, if ordered; use of sterile gloves, mask, and gown when in contact with client).
- Provide crib or bed with side rails. Sides may be padded. A toddler may need a crib that prevents him or her from crawling over the top of the rails.
- Assess child's risk for injury. The child may pull at dressings, damage blisters that form over burn area, or contaminate wounds. The child will need assistance with positioning. If needed, may use mitt or elbow restraints.

Page 180: *Suggested Answer—*

- Maintain the water seal and patency of the drainage system: tape connector sites; provide a straight line of tubing from bed to the collection system; ensure there are no kinks in tubing; do not use pins or restrain tubing.
- Assess client's vital signs and respiratory and cardiovascular status regularly.
- Maintain integrity of the drainage system: disposable system or suction bottles below level of bed; maintain suction control to create gentle bubbling.
- Strip chest tubes only with physician's orders; excessive negative pressure can damage lung tissue. If ordered, strip by pinching tube close to client chest with one hand, lubricate thumb and forefinger to compress and slide down toward the receptacle.
- Keep rubber-tipped clamps (if indicated by policy) and a sterile occlusive dressing near the client. In case connections are broken or air leaks occur, the chest tube may need to be clamped immediately or an underwater seal may need to be reestablished. If the chest tube is pulled out inadvertently, apply an occlusive dressing to the wound immediately.
- Mark drainage on the receptacle every shift and read at eye level. Report if drainage exceeds 100 mL/hr.

Page 183: *Suggested Answer—*The nurse should question the client about these common factors that interfere with sleep: heavy meals just prior to bedtime, caffeine, nicotine, or other stimulants, and environmental factors such as light, noise, and television.

Page 184: *Suggested Answer—*

- Ensure appropriate lighting, ventilation, and temperature. Keep noise level to a minimum.
- Promote rituals or routines that people are accustomed to in order to promote relaxation and encourage sleep.
- Avoid heavy meals 3 hours before bedtime, decrease fluid intake 2 hours before sleep, and avoid alcohol, caffeine, or heavily spiced foods.
- Get adequate exercise during the day to reduce stress. Pursue a nonstrenuous activity prior to sleep.
- Medications are to be used as a last resort and be taken on PRN (as necessary) basis. Clients need to be aware of the actions and desired and adverse effects of

medications used to aid sleep. Sedatives and hypnotics have different onset and duration of actions. Regular use may lead to tolerance of the drug which can lead to rebound insomnia.

Page 189: *Suggested Answer*—

- Appears tired and fatigued; listless; may be overweight or underweight; slowing of reflexes; motor restlessness; confusion, disorientation.
- Lack of appetite (anorexia); nausea, vomiting, overeating; indigestion; constipation.
- Dry, dull, sparse, brittle hair; loss of hair color; dry, flaky, or scaly skin; pale or pigmented skin; presence of petechiae or bruising; lack of subcutaneous fat; poor skin turgor; brittle, pale, ridged, or spoon-shaped nails.
- Facial edema; any swelling in the neck (enlarged lymph nodes).
- Swollen lips, red cracks at side of mouth (angular stomatitis), vertical fissures (cheilosis); dry mucous membranes in the oral cavity.
- Tongue: swollen, beefy, red or magenta-colored; coated; smooth appearance; increase or decrease in size.
- Teeth: dental caries; gums inflamed (gingivitis), spongy, bleed easily.
- Eyes: pale or red conjunctiva; dryness (xerophthalmia); soft cornea (keratomalacia); dull cornea.
- Numbness, tingling, edema of legs and feet; underdeveloped, flaccid, soft, wasting muscles.

Page 193: *Suggested Answer*—

- Drink eight 8-ounce glasses of water daily.
- Empty bladder at least every 2 to 4 hours while awake, avoiding voluntary retention.
- For women: wear cotton briefs; cleanse perineal area from front to back after voiding and defecating; void before and after sexual intercourse; avoid bubble baths, feminine hygiene sprays, and douches.
- Unless contraindicated, teach client to maintain acidity in urine by taking vitamin C or drinking at least two glasses of cranberry juice per day; avoiding excess milk products and sodium bicarbonate.
- Teach symptoms of urinary tract infection and measures to prevent it or to report promptly.

Page 196: *Suggested Answer*—

- Dietary teaching should include information on foods that cause stool odor (asparagus, beans, eggs, fish, onions, garlic); foods that increase gas; foods that thicken stool (applesauce, bananas, rice, tapioca, cheese, yogurt) and foods that loosen stool (chocolate, dried beans, fried foods, highly spiced foods, leafy green vegetables, raw fruits and vegetables).
- Skin care will need to be taught. The client will need information on protecting the exposed skin as well as changing colostomy bags. The client should be taught to assess skin and report changes.

Chapter 8

Page 208: *Suggested Answer:*—In addition to trauma or surgical interventions, any of the following serve as potential sources of pain stimuli:

- Microorganisms
- Inflammation
- Impaired blood flow
- Invasive tumor
- Radiation
- Heat
- Electricity
- Compression
- Decreased movement
- Stretching/straining
- Swelling
- Chemicals

Page 209: *Suggested Answer*—Ask the client about tolerance to pain, and assess pain location, intensity, quality, pattern, aggravating and alleviating factors, medication history, and expectations for pain relief.

Page 210: *Suggested Answer*—Acute pain usually is accompanied by fear and anxiety, while chronic pain can result in depression, despair, hopelessness, and fatigue.

Page 213: *Suggested Answer*—Common barriers include the following:

- Inadequate knowledge of pain management
- Poor assessment of pain
- Concern about regulation of controlled substances
- Fear of client addiction
- Concern about adverse effects of analgesics
- Concern about clients becoming tolerant to analgesics

Page 214: *Suggested Answer*—The client most likely is experiencing a nociceptive type of pain known as somatic.

Page 221: *Suggested Answer*—NSAIDs, tricyclic antidepressants, anticonvulsants, local anesthetics, corticosteroids, Baclofen (muscle relaxant), and capsaicin (Zostrix) can be used.

Page 224: *Suggested Answer*—The nurse should discuss with the client TENS, cutaneous stimulation, heat and cold therapy, distraction, relaxation, acupuncture, and biofeedback.

Chapter 9

Page 239: *Suggested Answer*—

- Diagnostic surgery is done to diagnose or confirm a diagnosis. In some cases, the procedure may rule out a disease process. An example of a diagnostic surgical procedure would be a breast biopsy or a craniotomy to diagnose the location of a brain tumor.
- Palliative surgery is performed to reduce or relieve symptoms of a disease. It is not performed to cure a disease. A

client with a brain tumor may have surgery to insert a ventriculoperitoneal shunt to reinstate ventricular flow and relieve (temporarily) the increased intracranial pressure.

- Ablative surgery is a surgical procedure to remove a diseased body part. An example of this would be an appendectomy or hysterectomy.
- Reconstructive surgery is performed to restore body appearance or function or to create a more normal appearance/function. An example of reconstructive surgery would be cleft lip surgery or relief of adhesions in a client with burn injuries.
- Transplant surgery replaces malfunctioning tissues (e.g., heart, kidney).
- Medication history, including current medications taken and previous medications, especially those with side effects or allergic reactions.

Page 240: *Suggested Answer*—

- Tobacco use, as it can affect the respiratory system and the client's response to anesthesia.
- Allergies, including food and medications. Contact allergies should be discussed. The nurse needs to particularly question the client about latex allergies because the client will be exposed during the surgical procedure from gloves and other equipment in use. Clients with a history of many surgeries and those with a history of spina bifida are at higher risk for latex allergies.
- Alcohol use, including type and frequency of use. The nurse should be aware of the risk of withdrawal.
- Previous surgical experiences including anesthesia. The nurse can discuss the previous experiences, which may influence how the client perceives this surgery. In addition, types of anesthesia used previously with any complications that occurred would be important to note.
- Psychosocial factors such as culture, support systems, and anxieties. Culture can influence a client's beliefs and values. For instance, if the culture values large families, a woman having a hysterectomy can have emotional distress. The adequacy of support systems will affect the client's needs for emotional support during periods of stress. Anxieties and fears (such as those related to body image) can make the stress of surgery greater for the client.

Page 241: *Suggested Answer*—

- Integumentary: rashes may indicate an infection. Poor skin turgor may indicate dehydration.
- Lungs: crackles and rhonchi heard on auscultation could indicate a respiratory infection.
- Cardiovascular: murmurs could indicate a heart defect that may interfere with the effectiveness of circulation. Clients with heart defects may be at greater risk for the development of subacute bacterial endocarditis. Prophylactic antibiotics are used to prevent this infection.
- Gastrointestinal: obesity can interfere with the body's ability to heal. The cardiovascular system can be affected

by obesity and makes the client more prone to postoperative complications.
- Genitourinary/reproductive system: urinary frequency can indicate a urinary tract infection.
- Neurologic: difficulty with memory may interfere with the client's ability to understand the procedure and postoperative teaching.

Page 242: *Suggested Answer*—

- The client's consent is voluntary. The client is not being forced or coerced to sign the consent form.
- The client's mental status allows him or her to understand the procedure to be done and make a rational decision.
- The client has the authority to consent. This means the client is by law allowed to make decisions for his/her own care. The client would be of legal age in the state where the procedure is being performed.
- The client has received the information necessary to make an informed decision.

Page 247: *Suggested Answer*—To prevent hypothermia in the surgical client, the OR nurse should cover the client's head, use warm blankets and warm IV fluids, and minimize body surface area exposures.

Page 250: *Suggested Answer*—Client goal: the lungs remain clear to auscultation.

Nursing interventions:

- Turn and reposition the client every 2 hours while awake.
- Encourage the client to use an incentive spirometer every 2 hours while awake.
- Auscultate the lungs every 4 hours.

Chapter 10

Page 265: *Suggested Answer*—The nurse should assess the wound for healing. The wound edges should be well approximated; sutures may or may not be present at this stage. Dehiscence and evisceration are less likely to occur at this stage; the time for these complications is usually 4 to 5 days postoperative. At this stage, the wound should be in the proliferative phase, which extends from day 3 to 21 after injury. The fibroblasts that surround the wound have begun to synthesize collagen. A raised "healing ridge" may be noted. The presence of granulation tissue (translucent red tissue) will be noted.

The nurse will also observe for drainage from the wound. Purulent exudate, thick pus with varying colors including yellow and green, would be present if the wound was infected. The nurse would note the color of the drainage as that may provide information on the causative organism. Clear discharge (serous) may be noted during the early stages of healing.

Page 268: *Suggested Answer*—In this stage of a pressure ulcer, there is no broken skin. The wound care would be to keep the area clean and dry. To keep pressure off the area, turn and position the client frequently. Encourage the client to remain in side-lying positions whenever possible. When moving the client up in bed, try to prevent dragging the client as this creates shearing pressure that can promote skin breakdown. Skin prep is a spray that could be used to toughen the skin. Specialty mattresses can be added to the bed that reduce pressure by means of distributing body weight more evenly or by alternating pressure on different portions of the skin. The client should avoid using doughnuts and rings that interfere with circulation to the area. Good nutrition is important; include high amounts of protein and vitamin C in food choices.

Page 270: *Suggested Answer*—Factors that add to sensory overload are pain, anxiety, and lack of sleep. The nurse would want to avoid excessive light and noise. Provide clocks and calendars in the client's line of vision. Allow for uninterrupted rest periods. Eliminate noxious odors.

Page 272: *Suggested Answer*—The nurse should face the client and speak directly facing him. The nurse should not have anything in the mouth while speaking. The voice should be kept at a moderate volume, the nurse should not shout, as that distorts the words. The nurse should avoid making excessive mouth and face movements. Use nonverbal cues whenever possible. Eliminate background noise if possible.

Page 278: *Suggested Answer*—Have the client squeeze a rubber ball several times a day. Have the client flex and extend the arms. Move from a supine to a sitting position by flexing elbows and pushing hands against the bed. Lift the body off the bed by pushing down with the palms of the hands and extending the elbow.

Chapter 11

Page 288: *Suggested Answer*—In the United States and Canada, the federal government regulates the production, prescription, distribution, and administration of drugs. Each state legislates a Nurse Practice Act for RNs and LVN/LPNs. Nurse Practice Acts define the nurses' boundaries and responsibilities regarding medications. Law also governs nursing practice involving use and management of controlled substances. It is the responsibility of local healthcare facilities to establish and implement policies and procedures that con-

form to their state's regulations. When the laws or regulations of a community, state, or institution differ from the federal laws, the stricter law generally prevails.

Page 289: *Suggested Answer*—The client is most probably experiencing an idiosyncratic effect: unexpected and unpredictable individual response to a drug manifested as an under-response, over-response, or completely different response. The nurse should withhold further doses of the medication and notify the physician.

Page 291: *Suggested Answer*—1 kilogram = 2.2 pounds. 160 pounds = 72.73 kilograms. 0.5 micrograms $\times$ 72.73 = 36.365 micrograms/kg/min.

Page 292: *Suggested Answer*—The nurse should discuss the medication with the client to ensure that the client is basing her decisions upon accurate information about the medication and how it relates to her condition, and that she is mentally competent to make an informed decision. Despite the client's medical condition warranting the need for the medication, the client has the right to refuse to take a medication and the nurse should honor the client's wishes and report this to the physician.

Page 297: *Suggested Answer*—The client should be instructed about the action and use of the drug as it pertains to his condition; adverse effects and what to do should he experience any of these effects; route; dose; frequency; and how long he should take the medication. If he received a dose of the medication in the healthcare agency, the nurse should advise him when the next dose is due.

Page 304: *Suggested Answer*—You will need a syringe appropriate for the volume of medication (generally a tuberculin syringe), #25 gauge, 3/8- to 5/8-inch needle, clean gloves, and an alcohol swab. Administer the medication in the lower abdomen fat pad at least two fingerbreadths from the umbilicus and above the iliac crest. Gently pinch an inch of subcutaneous tissue, inject at a 90-degree angle, administer the medication slowly without aspirating.

Page 310: *Suggested Answer*—The nurse should take initial vital signs before starting the transfusion. The nurse should stay with the client, taking vital signs every 5 to 15 minutes for the first 50 mL of the transfusion.

➤ Case Study Suggested Answers

Chapter 1

1. Critical assessment data includes:
   - Thorough pain assessment (using a pain scale, location of pain, characteristics of pain, onset of pain, associated signs and symptoms, aggravating factors, relieving factors, treatments tried and their effects)
   - Physical examination of abdomen and gastrointestinal system
   - Vital signs to obtain objective data related to signs and symptoms of pain
2. Nursing diagnoses could include: Pain incisional (location) related to . . . and Nausea related to . . .
3. Client outcomes could include:
   - Client will state pain at or below 3 on a 0-to-10 scale within 30 minutes after administration of pain medication and repositioning.
   - Client will deny nausea 30 minutes after administration of antiemetic medication.
   - Client will not vomit throughout shift.
4. Independent and interdependent interventions include:
   - Independent: reposition for comfort; teach coughing and deep-breathing techniques, relaxation techniques, and splinting of abdomen when changing positions
   - Interdependent: Obtain physician's order for pain and antiemetic medication; administer as ordered
5. Criteria used for evaluation:
   - Objective data: vital signs, numerical pain scale (or Wong-Baker Faces pain scale if client has language or developmental barriers), presence or absence of nausea and/or vomiting
   - Subjective data related to pain, nausea

Chapter 2

1. The nurse must first establish a rapport with the client; the appearance of warmth and understanding provides her with some comfort. Additionally the nurse must demonstrate a professional attitude and demeanor.
2. The health history is crucial in helping to determine the origin and critical nature of the client's symptoms. The nurse must be prepared before beginning the health history. A complete knowledge of the mechanics of the health history as well as methods to promote communication are essential as the client and nurse work together to investigate the health problem. The history as well as the physical must be done in a methodical, systematic manner.
3. As the nurse commences with the history and physical, some of the symptoms and physical manifestations can be linked with the chief complaint. An in-depth knowledge of anatomy and physiology will assist the nurse to link the symptoms to possible etiologies of the client's difficulties.

4. When a client has external pressures and stress, symptoms can exacerbate because of the stimulation of the sympathetic nervous system.
5. The nurse must return M. L. to bed and raise the head of the bed. Vital signs must be taken and compared to normal values and M. L.'s normal values. The nurse begins to assess her while asking pointed questions about her "spell." The nurse utilizes inspection, palpation, auscultation and percussion to determine normal and abnormal findings.

Chapter 3

1. Learning objectives that focus on client behavior need to be identified. The nurse needs to establish the content for each objective and identify the method of instruction based on the clients' learning ability. The teaching plan should include skills taught, strategies to be used, time framework, and content.

   The following is a list of items to include in the plan for this client.

   Learning Objectives
   - Client will verbalize basic anatomy of urinary system before discharge.
   - Client will verbalize reason for catheterization in own terms before discharge.
   - Client will describe measures to prevent urinary tract infection before discharge.
   - Client will identify signs and symptoms that require medical care before discharge.
   - Client will demonstrate self-catheterization technique before discharge.

   Content
   - Explanation of anatomy as relates to client's medical condition
   - Signs and symptoms of infection and urinary retention
   - Client behaviors to decrease incidence of urinary tract infection
   - Equipment required
   - Preparation for procedure guidelines

   Methods
   - Audiovisuals: diagrams of system, video on procedure
   - Discussion
   - Demonstration
   - Return demonstration

   The parts of the teaching process that should be documented in the client's chart include diagnosed learning needs, learning objectives, topics taught and client outcomes, need for additional teaching, and resources provided.
2. The nurse needs to evaluate the client's willingness to learn as well as what the client views as important. The nurse needs to evaluate the client's knowledge about the problem and how the problem affects his life. The nurse

needs to evaluate the client's sensory abilities and physical state, which may affect the learning process. Finally, the nurse should assess the client's preferred learning style.

3. The nurse should begin with open-ended questions that are associated with the impact his health problem has on his life, for example, "How has your bladder problem affected the things you enjoy doing?" The nurse should validate the client's option. The nurse could also begin by restating what the daughter has told the nurse, for example, "Your daughter has told me that recently you have not attended church or gone to the high school to help the students, and that you also have talked more about death." Then allow the client sufficient time to respond.

4. Possible nursing diagnoses include:
   - Deficient knowledge: self-urinary catheterization
   - Death anxiety related to increased discussion with daughter
   - Potential for enhanced spiritual well-being related to past history of church attendance daily
   - Hopelessness (alteration in health has altered client's church attendance and mentoring of high-school students)

5. Criteria to evaluate the nursing diagnosis of Knowledge deficit would be client's verbalization of the health problem and cause, client's ability to perform the procedure correctly, client's verbalization of signs and symptoms to report to doctor, and client's verbalization of the need to maintain adequate fluid intake.

   Criteria to evaluate Death anxiety could be verbalization of feelings, preparation for end of life, identification of unresolved issues, and planning funeral.

   Criteria to evaluate Potential for enhanced spirituality could be verbalizing importance of church in his own life, identifying an alternative to church attendance to enhance spirituality, or identifying plans to attend church again.

   Criteria to evaluate Hopelessness could be the client's verbalization how learning this new procedure will improve his quality of life so that he can resume normal activities.

Chapter 4

1. The registered nurse does not have a legal obligation to stop at the scene of the accident unless the state has a duty-to-rescue statute.

2. Good Samaritan laws differ from state to state. It is important the RN understands the state law.

3. The situation must be considered an emergency if there will be loss of life or limb without immediate assistance. The Good Samaritan law does not cover providing care in a non-emergent situation.

4. If someone willfully injures the victim, the Good Samaritan law will not protect him or her from liability.

5. The nurse can leave the scene when someone with appropriate skills such as a paramedic or EMT arrives at the scene. Until then, the nurse is bound to stay and continue assistance.

Chapter 5

1. Determine if she is serious about suicide. If so, suicide precautions are in order. If not, a spiritual assessment is the priority. Determine what religious practices are important to the client. Ask what her faith means to her. Does her faith bring her strength? Look around the home for religious artifacts. Observe for support people in the client's life and whether they visit, call, or write her notes.

2. Spiritual distress related to concerns about disease state

3. The client will renew relationships to strengthen her; find meaning in her spiritual being; and express positive feelings regarding the future

4. Help the client gather strength from her faith by supporting her religious practices.

   Encourage the client to have increased contact with the support people in her life.

   Allocate more time per visit to listen closely to the client.

   Ask the client if you may call her priest for a home visit. If she agrees, make the call and encourage him to make a visit with the client a priority.

5. Observe and inquire whether relationships have helped to strengthen the client; discuss with the client the utilization and effectiveness of her spiritual practices; inquire whether the client's perception of the future has been modified.

Chapter 6

1. The tests likely to be ordered for this client include culture and sensitivity of the wound exudate, erythrocyte sedimentation rate, white blood count with differential, and fasting blood glucose. The fasting blood glucose will be ordered to determine if the client's blood glucose level is within normal limits because a high level promotes pathogen growth.

2. The body defense mechanism activated was the inflammatory response. In response to injury, dilatation of the blood vessels caused increased permeability of fluids and an influx of leukocytes to the site. This allowed phagocytosis to occur resulting in destruction of the pathogen. The inflammatory response accounts for some of the symptoms the client is experiencing.

3. Possible diagnoses include:
   - Risk for injury: criteria to support this diagnosis are presence of a wound on the bottom of foot interfering with normal gait, and client statement of pain.
   - Impaired tissue integrity: the criterion to support this diagnosis is a wound at bottom of foot.
   - Impaired mobility: criteria to support this diagnosis are wound on bottom of foot, swollen foot, and statement of pain.

4. Expected outcomes include:
   - Pain: the criterion to support this diagnosis is the client's statement of pain.

- Expected outcome for Risk for injury: client will be free of injury.
- Expected outcome for Impaired tissue integrity: client's foot will show signs of healing by discharge as indicated by decreased redness and decreasing size of wound.
- Expected outcome for Pain: client will verbalize decreased pain each hospitalized day.
- Expected outcome for Impaired mobility: client will demonstrate walking with assistance of cane until foot is healed.

5. Implementation of standard precautions and medical asepsis including handwashing, use of gloves when in contact with body fluids, proper disposal of soiled dressings and linens, and following procedures for disinfecting room. In addition, ensure that the client does not use a communal shower or bathtub. Sterile (surgical aseptic) technique should be used with any dressing changes ordered for client.

Chapter 7

1. Assessments about client's ability to meet basic needs:
   - Self-care abilities for hygiene and toileting
   - Risk factors related to safety: poor eyesight; use of equipment such as a cane; use of medications that cause postural hypotension and changes in mental status; environmental factors such as presence of clutter, ability to use call bell, use of side rails
   - Factors affecting sleep: illnesses, emotional stress, drugs and other substances, exercise, usual sleep patterns
   - Factors affecting air exchange: lifestyle factors (exercise, smoking, anxiety)
   - Self-care abilities for nutrition, urinary and bowel elimination
   - Factors affecting nutrition: ability to chew, special or therapeutic diets, drugs
   - Factors affecting urinary and bowel elimination: fluid intake, activity, psychological factors, personal habits, and problems
2. Measures to ensure safety:
   - Give clear instructions to client regarding use of call bell, necessity of side rails
   - Provide a nightlight
   - Make frequent checks on client
   - Have a clutter-free environment
   - Follow protocol for safe medication administration
   - Use preventive measures for fire safety
   - Do proper maintenance of equipment
   - Keep needed objects within client's reach
3. Interventions to promote sleep:
   - Alleviate pain: relaxation techniques, back massage, medication
   - Assist in performing bedtime rituals
   - Encourage toileting prior to bedtime
   - Avoid strenuous exercise or anxiety producing conversations immediately prior to bedtime
   - Make environment conducive for sleep
   - Avoid heavy meal 3 hours before bedtime
   - Decrease fluid intake 2 hours before sleep
   - Avoid alcohol, caffeine, or heavily spiced foods
4. Measures to assist with adequate air exchange:
   - Assess client's respiratory and cardiovascular status
   - Assist client to a Fowler's position to promote adequate chest expansion
   - If client has dyspnea, instruct client to do slow, rhythmic breathing and assist with relaxation
   - If pain interferes with breathing, use pain distraction methods
5. Promote healthy urinary elimination:
   - Instruct about sufficient (2 liters) fluid intake
   - Teach Kegel exercises; contract perineal muscles and hold for a count of 3 to 5 seconds and relax; do 10 contractions 5 times daily
   - Empty bladder at least every 2 to 4 hours while awake, avoiding voluntary retention; for bladder training if client is incontinent, instruct to void according to a timetable rather than urge to void
   - Unless contraindicated, teach client to maintain acidity in urine by drinking at least two glasses of cranberry juice per day or taking vitamin C; avoiding excess milk products and sodium bicarbonate

Chapter 8

1. Common physiologic responses for acute pain includes nausea and vomiting, tachycardia, rapid, shallow respirations, hypertension, sweating, pallor, and dilated pupils.
2. Due to the type of trauma (a fractured hip), this client may benefit from medications having anti-inflammatory effects such as NSAIDs and corticosteroids. In addition, a muscle relaxant such as Baclofen may be helpful.
3. The initial priority is client teaching about the purpose and correct use of the device, and to provide information regarding any questions the client or family members have. The control button must always be in reach for client use. The nurse should provide regular pain assessments, including vital signs, and check the pump settings to assure accuracy of the physician's orders. Side effects such as pruritis, sedation, and respiratory compromise need to be monitored and documented according to agency policies.
4. Application of cold, repositioning, massage, and a variety of distraction techniques may be helpful.
5. Based on the information provided, the following nursing diagnoses could be anticipated:
   - Ineffective coping (individual), related to persistent pain that may add stress affecting the client's ability to cope
   - Deficient knowledge related to lack of information or misinformation regarding pain treatment strategies
   - Impaired physical mobility related to movement limited by pain
   - Disturbed sleep pattern related to persistent pain
   - Anxiety related to loss of control
   - Fear related to pain

- Activity intolerance related to pain and/or depression
- Self-care deficit (total or partial) related to pain

Chapter 9

1. This client is not allowed by law to make decisions about her own care. However, because of her age and mental capacity, the nurse would want to ensure that the client is included with the parents when information is shared related to her condition and proposed treatments. The nurse would encourage communication between the girl and her parents that allow both sides to express their feelings and concerns.
2. The nurse would want to ask the usual questions about her medical/surgical history including medications, previous illnesses, chronic illnesses, and alcohol and drug use including tobacco. The nurse would want to ask the client about her concerns and fears related to the surgery. This discussion should be done in private to allow the client to express thoughts she may be unwilling to share with her parents. In addition to the usual lab tests, a pregnancy test might be indicated if there is evidence the client is sexually active. The client will be allowed to select the support person that stays with her as allowed by hospital policies.
3. Two preoperative diagnoses would include:
   - Deficient knowledge related to the postoperative experience.
   - Anxiety related to the uncertainty of the diagnosis and surgical outcome.
4. Postoperative care to be taught would include the need for coughing and deep breathing in the postoperative period. The use of an incentive spirometer would be taught, as well as abdominal splinting. The client will also receive initial instructions about the expected wound appearance. Pain control methods will be discussed, and she will be assured that her needs will be met.
5. The nurse will discuss what occurs as the anesthesia is being administered, as well as what she will see and hear during the induction and as she is coming out of anesthesia.

Chapter 10

1. The compression bandage should be applied from the bottom aspect of the foot going upward towards the calf in even spiral turns. In order to properly apply a compression bandage to an extremity you must go from distal to proximal (in the flow of venous return).
2. Teach the three-point gait. The client must be able to bear the entire weight on the unaffected (uninjured) leg. The two crutches and the unaffected leg are used to walk and bear weight alternately.
3. To obtain a proper fit, the client should lay in a supine position. The nurse should measure from the anterior fold of the axilla to the heel and add 2.5 cm. Alternately, have the client stand erect holding the crutch in position. The arm rest should fall 3 finger widths below the axilla.
4. The client had a closed wound. There was no break in the skin. Inflammation can take up to ten days to resolve.
5. Teach the client to wear non-skid shoes and to make sure crutches have rubber tips to help prevent falls. Using good lighting and keeping the environment free of clutter are other general measures to prevent falls.

Chapter 11

1. Total parenteral nutrition (TPN) are solutions that provide all needed calories and contain high-dextrose concentrations, water, fat, proteins, electrolytes, vitamins, and trace elements. Hypertonic solutions containing greater than 10% dextrose require a high-flow central vein for infusion. Infection control is a high priority because the glucose-rich solution invites bacteria. The high-glucose content requires careful administration and blood glucose monitoring to prevent hypoglycemia or hyperglycemia.
2. A tunneled Groshong CVAD is a catheter that provides long-term access to a central vein for the purpose of medication administration, blood draws, or hyperalimentation administration. The tip is inserted into a central vein and advanced to the superior vena cava. The remainder of the catheter passes through a subcutaneous track and exits on the chest wall or abdomen. It contains a three-way pressure-sensitive valve that remains closed at normal vena caval pressure. When closed, it restricts air from entering the venous system or a backflow of blood from the catheter. Advantages of the Groshong valve and catheter include:
   - Decreased risk of air emboli or bleeding
   - Elimination of heparin flush
   - Elimination of catheter clamping
   - Reduced flushing protocols between use
3. Caring for the Groshong catheter involves:
   - Maintenance flush—according to agency policy, usually 10 to 20 mL saline vigorously weekly
   - Medication flush—5 to 10 mL saline before and vigorously after medication administration
   - Blood draws—double the normal flushing volume of saline with 10 mL saline after blood sampling
     - Waste—5 mL blood for routine sampling
     - Waste—10 mL blood for PT or PTT
     - TPN—flush with 20 mL saline before blood sampling
   - TPN flush—20 mL saline vigorously upon discontinuing TPN
   - Always use a 10 mL or larger size syringe
   - All lumens must have a luer-locked cap or needleless adaptor with reflux valves
   - Lumens *do not* require clamping when not in use
   - Does not require heparin
4. TPN has a high dextrose concentration thus increasing blood glucose levels. It is therefore important to test blood

glucose per agency protocols (at least once each day) to ensure that the values remain within normal limits (70–110). Should the client's blood glucose levels consistently be elevated, frequently insulin will be added to the TPN solution to maintain a normal serum glucose level.

5. Interventions include:

- If the dextrose solution is greater than 10 percent, a high flow central
- vessel is required for administration
- Blood glucose monitoring per agency protocols (at least once each day)

- Requires a filter
- Tubing and filter changes every 24 hours
- Air occlusive dressings
- Sterile technique for dressing changes at a frequency per agency
- protocol (usually every 3–7 days)
- Change solution every 24 hours
- Gradually increase and decrease the rate when instantiating and discontinuing the treatment

Index

Page numbers followed by b indicate box; those followed by f indicate figure; those followed by t indicate table.